Obesity and Cardiovascular Disease: Mechanistic Insights and Nutritional Management Strategies

Obesity and Cardiovascular Disease: Mechanistic Insights and Nutritional Management Strategies

Guest Editors

Ehud Grossman
Dror Dicker
Nagila Raquel Teixeira Damasceno
Anabelle Retondario

MDPI

Basel • Beijing • Wuhan • Barcelona • Belgrade • Novi Sad • Cluj • Manchester

Guest Editors
Ehud Grossman
Adelson School of Medicine
Ariel University
Ariel
Israel

Dror Dicker
Gray Faculty of Medical and Health Sciences
Tel Aviv University
Tel Aviv
Israel

Nagila Raquel Teixeira Damasceno
Department of Nutrition
University of São Paulo
São Paulo
Brazil

Anabelle Retondario
Departamento de Nutrição
Federal University of Paraná (UFPR)
Curitiba
Brazil

Editorial Office
MDPI AG
Grosspeteranlage 5
4052 Basel, Switzerland

This is a reprint of the Special Issue, published open access by the journal *Nutrients* (ISSN 2072-6643), freely accessible at: https://www.mdpi.com/journal/nutrients/special_issues/XTN58117TB.

For citation purposes, cite each article independently as indicated on the article page online and as indicated below:

Lastname, A.A.; Lastname, B.B. Article Title. *Journal Name* **Year**, *Volume Number*, Page Range.

ISBN 978-3-7258-7154-4 (Hbk)
ISBN 978-3-7258-7155-1 (PDF)
https://doi.org/10.3390/books978-3-7258-7155-1

Contents

About the Editors

Ehud Grossman

Ehud Grossman received his medical education at the Sackler Medical School of Tel-Aviv University, earning an M.D. degree magna cum laude in 1975. He completed his training in Internal Medicine and Hypertension at the Chaim Sheba Medical Center. Between 1987 and 1990, he completed a research fellowship in the USA. Here, he spent one year at the Ochsner Clinic in New Orleans, studying hemodynamic changes in hypertension, and two years at the Hypertension section of the National Institute of Health, studying the relationship between the sympathetic nervous system and hypertension.

Between 1997 and 2018, he was the head of Internal Medicine Department and the hypertension unit, and from 2018 to 2023, he was the Chairman of Medicine at the Chaim Sheba Medical Center. Since 2023, he has been the President of Ariel University.

At Tel Aviv University, Ehud Grossman became a Professor of Medicine on 2000 and the incumbent of the Hella Gertner Cathedra for research of high blood pressure on 2005.

Ehud Grossman was the Vice-Chairman of the Scientific Council and the Chairman of the Specialization Committee of the Scientific Council of the Israeli Medical Association.

Between 2003 and 2005, Ehud Grossman was the president of the Israeli Society of Hypertension, and between 2014 and 2022, he was the Dean of the Faculty of Medicine at Tel-Aviv University.

Ehud Grossman has written more than 400 publications in peer-reviewed journals and 20 book chapters on hypertension and internal medicine.

Ehud Grossman conducts multiple clinical studies and basic research in hypertension.

Dror Dicker

Dror Dicker received his medical education at the Technion Institute Haifa, earning an M.D. degree magna cum laude in 1990. He completed his training in Internal Medicine in Hasharon Hospital Rabin Medical Center.

In 1995, he opened the Multidisciplinary Clinic for CVD Risk Factors & Obesity Management, at which he is still working, focusing on promoting obesity management. Since 1999, Dror Dicker has been the head of the Internal Medicine D and Obesity Clinic. Between 2010 and 2015, Dror Dicker served as the President of the Israeli Association for Internal Medicine, and between 2021 and 2023, he served as the President of the European Federation of Internal Medicine (EFIM). He is currently the President of the Israeli Association for the Study of Obesity and the Co-Chair of the Collaborating Centers for Obesity Management (COM'S), part of the European Association for the Study of Obesity (EASO). Dicker's goal is to contribute, promote and advance the quality of internal medicine and obesity, striving to improve conditions, expertise, and work environments and to attract new young doctors to work in internal and obesity medicine, thus achieving the best possible patient health. As the President of the Israeli Association for the Study of Obesity and Co-Chair of the COM'S, he strives to promote educational activities, aiming to broaden knowledge of internal and obesity medicine. Dror Dicker has published more than 150 papers in peer-reviewed journals and book chapters, as well as several international guidelines regarding obesity medicine and CVD risk factors. Recently, he co-authored the new framework of obesity definition published by the EASO.

Nagila Raquel Teixeira Damasceno

Nagila Raquel Teixeira Damasceno is an Associate Professor at the Department of Nutrition, Faculty of Public Health, University of São Paulo (FSP-USP). She leads the research group on Biological Oxidations and Lipid Metabolism Applied to Chronic Non-Communicable Diseases (OxLIPID) and coordinates the Laboratory of Biochemistry of Nutrition Applied to Chronic Diseases.

Her research focuses on Nutrition and Chronic Diseases, including CVD, obesity, cancer, epilepsy, and neurodegenerative diseases, with emphasis on lipid, oxidative, and inflammatory aspects modulated by fatty acids and other nutritional components. She supervises students in the Postgraduate Programs in Nutrition and Public Health (FSP-USP) and Cardiology (FM-USP).

She served as the Director of the Nutrition and Dietetics Division at the University Hospital (HU-USP, 2010–2024) and has previously been a member of the Deliberative Council of the National Institute of Complex Fluids (INCT-FCx, 2018–2025) and the Research Center for Complex Fluids (NAP-FCx, 2018–2022). She currently serves on the Council of the Department of Nutrition (FSP-USP, 2024–2026) and the Board of Directors of the Department of Nutrition at SOCESP (2014–2026).

She coordinated the Brazil–Sweden International Cooperation Program (CAPES-STINT, 2014–2018) and collaborates on a Brazil–Germany project (FAPESP-FAPESC-Greifswald, since 2018). Her national and international collaborators include UECE, UFC, UFF, FURB, Harvard University, the University of Barcelona, the University of Umeå, and the University of Greifswald.

She is actively involved in university extension, with over 50 interviews and 20+ projects in the last decade. In partnership with SOCESP, Centro Universitário São Camilo, and INCT-FCx, she coordinates the PEDUCA platform, an EAD initiative training school teachers on Food and Nutrition Education for cardiovascular disease prevention. Her research group has received over 20 awards in the past two decades.

Anabelle Retondario

Anabelle Retondario is an Adjunct Professor in the Department of Nutrition at the Federal University of Paraná (UFPR), Brazil. She is a member of the Research Group on Dietary Exposure (Gupea) and the Food Quality and Nutrition Research Group.

Her research focuses on the living conditions and health of vulnerable populations. She coordinates the research project *"Life and Health of Homeless People"*, which aims to understand the lifestyle and health habits of people experiencing homelessness, including chronic non-communicable diseases, as well as their perceptions of services provided by public facilities and social organizations.

In addition to her research activities, she coordinates two outreach projects focused on socially vulnerable groups: the *"On-Street Extension"* project, which works with people experiencing homelessness, and the *"Origin Food"* project, which supports migrant populations within the university.

Her research interests include nutrition and public health, cardiovascular and other non-communicable diseases, child and adolescent nutrition and behavior, school feeding programs, and nutritional requirements.

nutrients

torial

besity and Cardiovascular Disease: Mechanistic Insights and utritional Management Strategies

ıd Grossman

Adelson School of Medicine, Ariel University, Ariel 4077625, Israel; ehud.grossman@ariel.ac.il; Tel.: +972-39066153

Obesity and overweight represent a growing global epidemic. As of 2021, an estimated 1.0 billion men and 1.1 billion women over the age of 25 were affected by overweight and obesity. Projections suggest that by 2050, more than half of the world's adult population—approximately 3.8 billion individuals—will be classified as overweight or obese [1]. A recent study further reported that between 1990 and 2021, the combined prevalence of overweight and obesity in children and adolescents doubled, while the prevalence of obesity alone tripled [2].

Globally, the rise in obesity is driven by a convergence of factors, including sedentary behavior, energy-dense diets, and broader socioeconomic influences. Obesity is associated with reduced life expectancy and increased risk for numerous comorbidities, including type 2 diabetes, hypertension, dyslipidemia, non-alcoholic fatty liver disease (NAFLD), cardiovascular diseases (e.g., myocardial infarction, heart failure, atrial fibrillation, stroke), obstructive sleep apnea, osteoarthritis, and certain cancers [3]. While BMI is widely used to define obesity, it is now well recognized that central (abdominal) adiposity is a more accurate predictor of cardiometabolic risk. Anthropometric measures such as waist circumference, waist-to-hip ratio, and waist-to-height ratio offer better estimates of visceral fat burden [3,4].

Adipose tissue functions not merely as an energy storage depot but as a metabolically active endocrine organ. It secretes various adipokines—such as leptin, adiponectin, and resistin—that influence inflammation, insulin sensitivity, and vascular homeostasis [3]. Dysregulation of these signals can lead to endothelial dysfunction and a chronic pro-inflammatory state, which are key contributors to atherosclerosis.

In individuals with obesity, adipose tissue is marked by hypertrophic adipocytes, ectopic fat deposition, dysregulated adipocytokine profiles, and the induction of chronic low-grade inflammation and fibrosis. These processes contribute to insulin resistance and the eventual development of type 2 diabetes [3].

Obesity is a well-established risk factor for hypertension [5]. Several mechanisms may mediate this link, including increased sympathetic nervous system activity, activation of the renin–angiotensin–aldosterone system, insulin resistance with sodium retention, and elevated leptin levels [3,6]. Weight loss has been shown to improve blood pressure control through the reversal of these mechanisms [7,8]. However, its benefits depend on sustained weight reduction; even modest weight regain can negate the improvements [9]. Shlomai et al. showed that minor, unintentional weight gain can lead to elevated blood pressure [10].

Obesity is also associated with ectopic fat accumulation in various organs. Hepatic steatosis is a well-documented consequence, and NAFLD is closely linked to BMI and waist circumference [11]. Emerging data indicate that fat accumulation in the kidneys may also occur. Importantly, renal fat accumulation may induce inflammation and fibrosis, serving

 https://doi.org/10.3390/nu17142281

as a potential early marker for chronic kidney disease (CKD) development in patients with obesity. Renal steatosis has also been associated with diabetes, CKD progression, and hypertension, and its early identification may have important clinical implications for risk stratification and prevention [12].

Management of obesity-associated cardiovascular disease involves both aggressive control of cardiometabolic risk factors and implementation of weight reduction strategies. Risk factor management focuses on blood pressure, glucose, and lipid control, along with smoking cessation [3].

Lifestyle modification, including a calorie-restricted carbohydrate-reduced diet and regular physical activity, is recommended for all individuals with obesity. These interventions can be effective in achieving weight loss. For patients unable to maintain such changes or who do not respond adequately, pharmacological therapy may be appropriate [3].

Recent advances have shown that GLP-1 receptor agonists (e.g., semaglutide, orforglipron) and dual GLP-1/GIP receptor agonists (e.g., tirzepatide) not only lower glucose levels but also result in significant weight loss, improved metabolic parameters, and reduced cardiovascular events [13–15]. SGLT2 inhibitors may also support modest weight loss and confer cardiovascular protection [3,16].

In cases of severe obesity, or when pharmacologic treatments are poorly tolerated or ineffective, bariatric surgery should be considered. These procedures are associated with substantial and sustained weight loss, metabolic improvement, and reduction in cardiovascular morbidity [3,17,18].

This Issue offers a comprehensive overview of the multifaceted relationship between obesity and cardiovascular disease. It addresses diagnostic approaches, nutritional and environmental etiologies, the renal consequences of obesity, and the impact of behavioral and weight changes on cardiometabolic risk.

Funding: This research received no external funding.

Conflicts of Interest: The authors declare no conflicts of interest.

List of Contributions:

1. Xia, Z.; Li, Y.; Yin, J.; Gong, Z.; Sun, J.; Shen, S.; Yang, Y.; Liu, T.; Wang, L.; Huo, J. Integrating Metabolomics and Gut Microbiota to Identify Key Biomarkers and Regulatory Pathways Underlying Metabolic Heterogeneity in Childhood Obesity. *Nutrients* **2025**, *17*, 1876. https://doi.org/10.3390/nu17111876.
2. Akritidis, J.; Mérida, D.M.; Torrijo-Belanche, C.; Moreno-Franco, B.; Gimeno-Ruiz, S.; Rey-García, J.; Morales-Suarez-Varela, M.; Guallar-Castillón, P. Phthalate Metabolites and Their Relationship with Abdominal and General Obesity: Evidence from the Aragon Workers' Health Study (AWHS). *Nutrients* **2025**, *17*, 1869. https://doi.org/10.3390/nu17111869.
3. Fontalba-Navas, A.; Echeverria, R.; Larrea-Killinger, C.; Gracia-Arnaiz, M.; Soar, C.; Arrebola, J.P. Association Between the Healthy Eating Index and the Body Mass Index of Older Adults: An Analysis of Food Frequency and Preferences. *Nutrients* **2025**, *17*, 1717. https://doi.org/10.3390/nu17101717.
4. Zeiler, E.; Gabriel, S.; Ncube, M.; Thompson, N.; Newmire, D.; Scharf, E.L.; Goldhamer, A.C.; Myers, T.R. Prolonged Water-Only Fasting Followed by a Whole-Plant-Food Diet Is a Potential Long-Term Management Strategy for Hypertension and Obesity. *Nutrients* **2024**, *16*, 3959. https://doi.org/10.3390/nu16223959.
5. Gordito Soler, M.; López-González, Á.A.; Vallejos, D.; Martínez-Almoyna Rifá, E.; Vicente-Herrero, M.T.; Ramírez-Manent, J.I. Usefulness of Body Fat and Visceral Fat Determined by Bioimpedanciometry versus Body Mass Index and Waist Circumference in Predicting Elevated Values of Different Risk Scales for Non-Alcoholic Fatty Liver Disease. *Nutrients* **2024**, *16*, 2160. https://doi.org/10.3390/nu16132160.

6. Raphael, H.; Klang, E.; Konen, E.; Inbar, Y.; Leibowitz, A.; Frenkel-Nir, Y.; Apter, S.; Grossman, E. Obesity Is Associated with Fatty Liver and Fat Changes in the Kidneys in Humans as Assessed by MRI. *Nutrients* **2024**, *16*, 1387. https://doi.org/10.3390/nu16091387.
7. Weinstein, S.; Maor, E.; Kaplan, A.; Hod, T.; Leibowitz, A.; Grossman, E.; Shlomai, G. Non-Interventional Weight Changes Are Associated with Alterations in Lipid Profiles and in the Triglyceride-to-HDL Cholesterol Ratio. *Nutrients* **2024**, *16*, 486. https://doi.org/10.3390/nu16040486.
8. Cheung, K.; Chan, V.; Chan, S.; Wong, M.M.H.; Chung, G.K.-K.; Cheng, W.-Y.; Lo, K.; Zeng, F. Effect of Intermittent Fasting on Cardiometabolic Health in the Chinese Population: A Meta-Analysis of Randomized Controlled Trials. *Nutrients* **2024**, *16*, 357. https://doi.org/10.3390/nu16030357.

ferences

GBD 2021 Adult BMI Collaborators. Global, Regional, and national prevalence of adult overweight and obesity, 1990–2021, with forecasts to 2050: A forecasting study for the Global Burden of Disease Study 2021. *Lancet* **2025**, *405*, 813–838. [CrossRef] [PubMed]

GBD 2021 Adult BMI Collaborators. Global, regional, and national prevalence of child and adolescent overweight and obesity, 1990–2021, with forecasts to 2050: A forecasting study for the Global Burden of Disease Study 2021. *Lancet* **2025**, *405*, 785–812. [CrossRef] [PubMed]

Bluher, M. An overview of obesity-related complications: The epidemiological evidence linking body weight and other markers of obesity to adverse health outcomes. *Diabetes Obes. Metab.* **2025**, *27* (Suppl. 2), 3–19. [CrossRef]

De Lorenzo, A.; Gratteri, S.; Gualtieri, P.; Cammarano, A.; Bertucci, P.; Di Renzo, L. Why primary obesity is a disease? *J. Transl. Med.* **2019**, *17*, 169. [CrossRef]

Guo, T.; Zhou, Y.; Yang, G.; Sheng, L.; Chai, X. Association between cardiometabolic index and hypertension among US adults from NHANES 1999–2020. *Sci. Rep.* **2025**, *15*, 4007. [CrossRef] [PubMed]

Grossman, E.; Eshkol, A.; Rosenthal, T. Diet and weight loss: Their effect on norepinephrine renin and aldosterone levels. *Int. J. Obes.* **1985**, *9*, 107–114. [PubMed]

Zevallos, A.; Sanches, E.E.; Parmar, C.; Ribeiro, R.; Pouwels, S. Remission of hypertension after laparoscopic sleeve gastrectomy versus Roux-en-Y-gastric bypass: A systematic review of randomized control trials. *Surg. Obes. Relat. Dis.* **2025**, *21*, 271–278. [CrossRef] [PubMed]

Sowers, J.R.; Nyby, M.; Stern, N.; Beck, F.; Baron, S.; Catania, R.; Vlachis, N. Blood pressure and hormone changes associated with weight reduction in the obese. *Hypertension* **1982**, *4*, 686–691. [CrossRef] [PubMed]

Sjostrom, C.D.; Peltonen, M.; Wedel, H.; Sjostrom, L. Differentiated long-term effects of intentional weight loss on diabetes and hypertension. *Hypertension* **2000**, *36*, 20–25. [CrossRef] [PubMed]

Shlomai, G.; Ovdat, T.; Klempfner, R.; Leibowitz, A.; Grossman, E. Non-interventional weight changes affect systolic blood pressure in normotensive individuals. *J. Clin. Hypertens.* **2021**, *23*, 990–998. [CrossRef] [PubMed]

Zhang, W.; Zou, M.; Liang, J.; Zhang, D.; Zhou, M.; Feng, H.; Tang, C.; Xiao, J.; Zhou, Q.; Yang, W.; et al. Association of cardiovascular health with MAFLD and mortality in overweight and obese adults and mediation by inflammation and insulin resistance. *Sci. Rep.* **2025**, *15*, 18791. [CrossRef] [PubMed]

Raphael, H.K.; Konen, E.; Leibowitz, A.; Frenkel-Nir, Y.; Apter, S.; Grossman, E. Renal Fat Accumulation Assessed by MRI or CT and Its Association with Clinical and Metabolic Disorders: A Systematic Imaging Review. *J. Clin. Med.* **2025**, *14*, 4305. [CrossRef]

McGuire, D.K.; Marx, N.; Mulvagh, S.L.; Deanfield, J.E.; Inzucchi, S.E.; Pop-Busui, R.; Mann, J.F.E.; Emerson, S.S.; Poulter, N.R.; Engelmann, M.D.M.; et al. Oral Semaglutide and Cardiovascular Outcomes in High-Risk Type 2 Diabetes. *N. Engl. J. Med.* **2025**, *392*, 2001–2012. [CrossRef]

Aronne, L.J.; Horn, D.B.; le Roux, C.W.; Ho, W.; Falcon, B.L.; Gomez Valderas, E.; Das, S.; Lee, C.J.; Glass, L.C.; Senyucel, C.; et al. Tirzepatide as Compared with Semaglutide for the Treatment of Obesity. *N. Engl. J. Med.* **2025**, *393*, 26–36. [CrossRef]

Wharton, S.; Rosenstock, J.; Konige, M.; Lin, Y.; Duffin, K.; Wilson, J.; Banerjee, H.; Pirro, V.; Kazda, C.; Mather, K. Treatment with orforglipron, an oral glucagon like peptide-1 receptor agonist, is associated with improvements of CV risk biomarkers in participants with type 2 diabetes or obesity without diabetes. *Cardiovasc. Diabetol.* **2025**, *24*, 240. [CrossRef] [PubMed]

Ferdinand, K.C.; Izzo, J.L.; Lee, J.; Meng, L.; George, J.; Salsali, A.; Seman, L. Antihyperglycemic and Blood Pressure Effects of Empagliflozin in Black Patients With Type 2 Diabetes Mellitus and Hypertension. *Circulation* **2019**, *139*, 2098–2109. [CrossRef] [PubMed]

17. Aminian, A.; Al-Kurd, A.; Wilson, R.; Bena, J.; Fayazzadeh, H.; Singh, T.; Albaugh, V.L.; Shariff, F.U.; Rodriguez, N.A.; Jin et al. Association of Bariatric Surgery With Major Adverse Liver and Cardiovascular Outcomes in Patients With Biopsy-Pro Nonalcoholic Steatohepatitis. *JAMA* **2021**, *326*, 2031–2042. [CrossRef] [PubMed]
18. Carlsson, L.M.S.; Sjoholm, K.; Jacobson, P.; Andersson-Assarsson, J.C.; Svensson, P.A.; Taube, M.; Carlsson, B.; Peltonen, Life Expectancy after Bariatric Surgery in the Swedish Obese Subjects Study. *N. Engl. J. Med.* **2020**, *383*, 1535–1543. [CrossR [PubMed]

nutrients

MDPI

icle

teractive and Joint Effects of Obesity and Insulin Resistance on ypertension in Adolescents and the Mediating Role of Insulin esistance—Five Provinces, China

yuan Zhu [1], Zebang Zhang [1], Yumei Feng [1], Qiqi Wu [1], Runquan Zhang [1], Tao Liu [1], Dan Liu [2], Xiongfei Chen [3] Xiaomei Dong [1,*]

[1] Department of Public Health and Preventive Medicine, School of Medicine, Jinan University, Guangzhou 510632, China; jnuzhu007@stu2023.jnu.edu.cn (H.Z.); zhangzb117@163.com (Z.Z.); 15573415243@163.com (Y.F.); hestiawu1121@163.com (Q.W.); zhangrunquan3@163.com (R.Z.); gztt_2002@163.com (T.L.)

[2] Department of Epidemiology, School of Public Health, Southern Medical University, Guangzhou 510515, China; liudan0717@smu.edu.cn

[3] Department of Primary Public Health, Guangzhou Center for Disease Control and Prevention, Guangzhou 510440, China; chenxf_1975@163.com

* Correspondence: tdongxm@jnu.edu.cn

Abstract: Background: The global prevalence of pediatric hypertension is on the rise. Adolescence is a period of high prevalence of childhood hypertension. Obesity and insulin resistance (IR) are important risk factors in the development of hypertension, but their interaction and combined effects on adolescent hypertension remain unclear. **Methods:** This cross-sectional study utilized data from the China National Nutrition and Health Surveillance of Children and Lactating Mothers (2016–2017). A total of 7031 adolescents aged 12–17 years from five provinces were included. The triglyceride-glucose index (TyG) was used as an indicator of IR. Multivariable logistic regression and generalized linear mixed-effect models were used to assess the interaction and joint effects of IR and obesity (measured by body mass index [BMI] and waist circumference [WC]) on hypertension. Relative excess risk due to interaction (RERI), proportion attributable to interaction (AP), and synergy index (SI) were calculated to evaluate additive interactive effects. Mediation analysis explored the potential mediating role of the TyG in the association between obesity and hypertension. **Results:** IR and obesity were positively associated with adolescent hypertension ($p < 0.001$). Interaction analyses revealed a robust synergistic interaction between obesity and IR on hypertension, with the AP being approximately 40% ($p < 0.001$). TyG significantly mediated the association between obesity and adolescent hypertension (6.30% for high BMI and 8.54% for high WC, both $p < 0.001$). **Conclusions:** This study suggests that obesity and IR could synergistically contribute to the prevalence of hypertension in adolescents. For the primary prevention and management of hypertension in adolescents, strategies targeting both factors should be considered.

Keywords: adolescent; China Nutrition and Health Surveillance; hypertension; insulin resistance; obesity; TyG

1. Introduction

Pediatric hypertension is a growing public health concern, with its prevalence increasing in recent decades worldwide [1,2]. A systematic review covering 22,431,861 children reported that in 2020, the overall prevalence of hypertension among Chinese individuals aged 6–18 years was 3.11%, equivalent to 6.80 million affected children [3]. Research shows that the age-specific prevalence rises rapidly from the onset of puberty and peaks at 14–15 years of age [2]. Notably, elevated blood pressure (BP) in childhood can not only induce early cardiovascular damage but also increase the risk of cardiovascular diseases (CVD) and mortality in adulthood [1,4], which highlights the importance of normal BP during childhood and adolescence [4]. Although the BP of minors increases with age, it may rise more during puberty, possibly due to hormonal changes and rapid growth spurts [5,6]. This might also explain why the prevalence of hypertension in children peaks at the end of puberty [2]. Adolescence thus becomes a special period in which individuals are more susceptible to hypertension. Given the long-term health impacts of untreated and unmanaged pediatric hypertension, the importance of early prevention and intervention cannot be overstated.

Obesity is a widely recognized risk factor for hypertension [1,2], particularly abdominal obesity [7]. Body mass index (BMI) and waist circumference (WC) are commonly used to assess the condition of obesity. Obesity can cause fat accumulation in body tissues, which is associated with insulin resistance (IR), a condition characterized by reduced sensitivity and responsiveness to insulin [8]. IR leads to dysfunction in insulin regulation of glucose metabolism [9] and is thought to play a crucial role in the progression and development of hypertension [10,11]. The gold standard for measuring IR, the hyperinsulinemic-euglycemic clamp (HEC) test, is invasive and costly, whereas the triglyceride-glucose index (TyG) is a reliable and cost-effective indicator of IR [10,11] and has been proven to be a useful surrogate marker for IR in adolescents [12]. Obesity and IR are increasingly prevalent metabolic conditions among adolescents, largely driven by modern lifestyle factors such as high intake of sugar and fat and insufficient physical activity [13]. Both conditions could increase the risk of hypertension, and there may be a mechanistic interrelationship between fat accumulation and IR [14].

This study aims to examine the interactive and joint effects of obesity and IR (assessed by TyG) on adolescent hypertension, and to evaluate whether TyG mediates the association between obesity and hypertension among adolescents. To date, no studies have systematically explored the interaction and combined effect of obesity and IR on hypertension from an epidemiological perspective among individuals in adolescence. Considering the potential links and overlaps between obesity and IR, further evaluation into the effects of combined obesity and IR on adolescent hypertension is warranted. The findings may help enhance the understanding of the underlying mechanisms of adolescent hypertension, facilitate risk stratification, and inform targeted interventions for adolescent BP control, reducing their risk of developing CVD in adulthood.

2. Methods

2.1. Data Sources and Study Population

The data analyzed in the present study came from a nationwide survey, the China Nutrition and Health Surveillance of Children and Lactating Mothers in 2016–2017, which was led by the Chinese National Health Commission (NHC) and conducted by the Chinese Center for Disease Control and Prevention (China CDC), using a multi-stage stratified random sampling. Detailed multi-stage sampling procedures and sample selection processes are available in a published article [15]. In short, for children and adolescents aged 6–17 years, participants were selected from monitoring sites across 31 provincial-level administrative divisions in mainland China, with 280 students recruited at each site. Students with serious physical and mental illnesses did not participate in the program. Subsequently, participants completed face-to-face questionnaires, anthropometric measurements, and provided blood and urine samples for laboratory tests. Eventually, the data collected were nationally and provincially representative.

However, the database of this surveillance is not publicly available. We endeavored to seek sectoral cooperation of the relevant authorities to obtain the data and ended up with data for five provinces (Shandong, Jiangsu, Guangdong, Guizhou, and Inner Mongolia). These provinces are located in various regions of China: Northeast, East, South, Southwest, and North. The broad geographic distribution of participants ensured sufficient variability in the study population. Finally, we extracted 7031 adolescents aged 12–17 years from our dataset for our study. However, 1328 participants were excluded due to missing data, as detailed in Figure 1. The specific missingness of data and the details of participants included and not included are shown in Supplementary Materials: Figure S1 and Table S1.

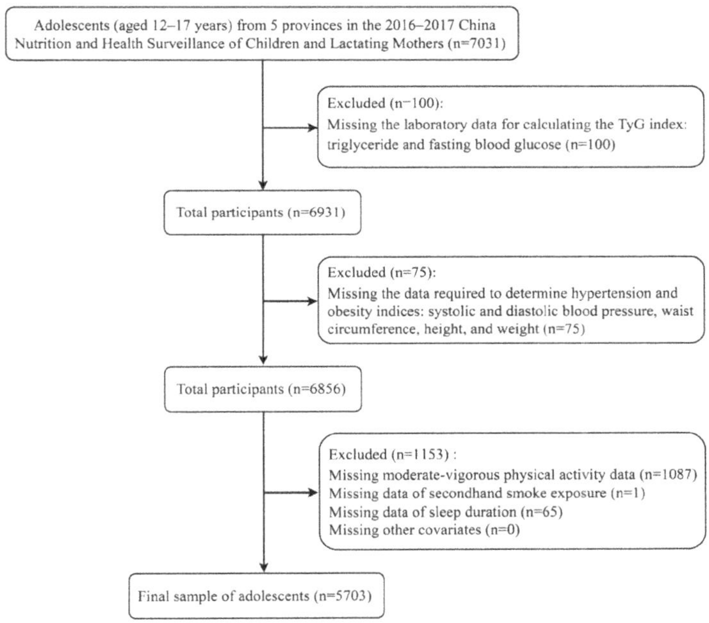

Figure 1. Exclusion flowchart of study participants in our surveillance dataset.

2.2. Ethical Considerations

This study received ethical approval from the Ethics Committee of the Chinese Center for Disease Control and Prevention (Protocol Code: 201614). Children and adolescents were included in the program only after their guardians and/or the participants themselves had signed an informed consent form. The study was conducted in accordance with the Declaration of Helsinki.

2.3. Assessment of BMI, WC, and TyG

Participants at each survey site were measured using anthropometric equipment selected by the national project team [15] and Chinese health industry standard measurement methods [16]. Height measurements were performed using a TZG-type stadiometer (accuracy up to 0.1 cm) with participants in a standing position having removed their shoes. Body weight was measured to the nearest 0.01 kg using an electronic scale (TANITA HD-390,Tokyo, Japan), with participants wearing only a single layer of clothing and no shoes or outerwear. All equipment was calibrated prior to the physical examination, and measurements were conducted in the morning when participants were in a fasting state. Body mass index (BMI, kg/m^2) was calculated as weight in kilograms divided by the square of height in meters. Definitions of overweight and obesity in adolescents in this study were based on the standard thresholds of the health industry in China [17]. We classified participants who were overweight or obese as having a high BMI, and otherwise as having a low BMI.

Waist circumference (WC) was measured in the fasting state with participants standing upright. A non-elastic tape was placed horizontally at the midpoint between the lower margin of the costal arch and iliac crest along the mid-axillary line, lightly applied to the skin, and readings were taken at the end of a normal expiration. Two measurements were taken, and both were recorded only if the difference was less than 2 cm; otherwise, the measurement was repeated. In the present study, the average of the two readings was used as the participants' WC. Abdominal obesity was defined as a WC at or above the 90th percentile for age and sex, determined according to the cut-off points specified in the national health industry criteria of China for children and adolescents [18,19]. We referred to abdominal obesity as high WC, and non-abdominal obesity as low WC.

In order to test their laboratory indicators, including triglyceride (TG) and fasting blood glucose (FG), 6 mL of fasting blood and 8–10 mL of random urine were collected from participants. TG levels were measured via enzymatic colorimetry using the Roche Cobas C701 automated analyzer, and FG was assessed using the glucokinase method with a Roche P800 biochemical analyzer (Roche, Basel, Switzerland). TyG was calculated as $\ln[\text{TG (mg/dL)} \times \text{FG (mg/dL)}/2]$ [11], and the median (8.18) was used as the cut-off point in this study, classifying the TyG into 'low' and 'high' categories. Notably, 8.18 is thought to be the TyG cut-off for diagnosing IR in adolescents [12].

2.4. Assessment of Hypertension

BP was measured in the morning using an electronic sphygmomanometer (OMRON HBP-1300, Tokyo, Japan), accurate to 1 mmHg. Participants were instructed to avoid exercise, eating, or drinking (except water) for at least one hour before the measurement. Unless contraindicated, BP measurements were performed on the left arm. A total of three measurements were taken at 1 min intervals. The average of the two closest values among the three BP measurements was used in this study. Hypertension in adolescents was defined as systolic BP and/or diastolic BP $\geq$ 95th percentile for sex, age, and height, based on the reference of screening for Chinese children and adolescents [20].

2.5. Assessment of Covariates

Data on sociodemographic information, including date of birth (month/day/year), sex (male or female), father's and mother's education levels ($\leq$primary education, secondary education, or $\geq$bachelor's degree), and residence (rural or urban), were collected through a structured questionnaire by interviewing participants face to face. The age used as a covariate was derived from the interval between the date of birth and the date of data collection, rounded down to the nearest whole year. To avoid collinearity, father's and mother's education levels were combined into a single variable—parental education level—classified as low (both parents $\leq$ primary education, or one $\leq$ primary and the other received secondary education), medium (both secondary, or one $\leq$ primary and the other $\geq$ bachelor's degree), and high (both $\geq$ bachelor's, or one secondary and the other $\geq$ bachelor's).

Investigators also collected health-related information such as frequency of moderate-vigorous physical activity (MVPA), bedtime and wake-up time, secondhand smoke, alcohol intake, and family history of hypertension using the questionnaire. The frequency of MVPA (continuous) was obtained by asking participants about the number of days they typically engaged in MVPA per week. Participants' sleep duration was calculated as the interval between their bedtime and wake-up time. By the minimum sleep duration recommendations for children and adolescents (≥8 h/day for high school students, ≥9 h/day for middle school students, and ≥10 h/day for primary school pupils) issued by the Ministry of Education of the People's Republic of China [21], participants meeting these criteria were considered to have adequate sleep; otherwise, they were considered insufficient. Family history of hypertension was considered present if at least one of the following relatives had been diagnosed with hypertension: father, mother, paternal grandparents, or maternal grandparents.

We also considered the impact of dietary patterns on outcome variable, so we used dietary data in the database obtained from a Food Frequency Questionnaire (FFQ), which surveyed participants on their frequency of consumption of various foods over the past month, to calculate an unhealthy dietary score for each adolescent, representing a potential confounder from different diets. The scoring criteria were based on the Chinese Dietary Guidelines [22], and the detailed scoring process is accessible in our previously published article [23].

Other covariates were laboratory-tested, including serum uric acid, serum total protein, total cholesterol (TC), urine sodium, and serum creatinine. We calculated estimated glomerular filtration rate (eGFR) as a covariate based on values of serum creatinine to consider a confounder of kidney disease, which can independently contribute to hypertension. A formula recommended by the Chinese guideline for early screening of pediatric chronic kidney disease was used: eGFR = K × height (cm) × 88.4/serum creatinine (μmol/L) (children age 2–12 years: K= 0.55; adolescents age > 12 years: K = 0.77 for boys and 0.55 for girls) [24]. In post-modeling diagnostics, the variance inflation factors of covariates in all models of the present study were less than 5, indicating that there was no major collinearity affecting our regression estimates.

2.6. Statistical Analysis

All statistical analyses were performed using R software version 4.2.3 (R Foundation, Vienna, Austria). A two-tailed $p < 0.05$ was considered statistically significant. Quantitative data were presented as means and standard deviations (SDs), while qualitative data were described as numbers and percentages. Pearson's chi-square test, Student's t test, or Wilcoxon rank sum test were used to compare the differences in variables between groups where appropriate.

Multivariable logistic regression models were used to estimate the odds ratios (ORs) and 95% confidence intervals (CIs) of hypertension associated with TyG, BMI, and WC. In Model 1, age and sex were adjusted. Model 2, the fully adjusted model, was adjusted for sex, age, MVPA, unhealthy dietary score, sleep adequacy, secondhand smoke, alcohol intake, family history of hypertension, parental education level, residence, serum uric acid, serum total protein, eGFR, TC, and urine sodium. Furthermore, we performed restricted cubic spline (RCS) regression to explore potential non-linear relationships, with the knots set to 3 for smooth curve fitting.

The 'interactionR' package (version 0.1.7) in R software was used for the calculations of additive interaction and to assess the joint effects of IR and obesity on hypertension in the main analysis. Relative excess risk due to interaction (RERI), proportion attributable to interaction (AP), and synergy index (SI) were used to evaluate additive interactive effects. Multiplicative interactions were assessed through likelihood ratio tests, comparing models with and without the interaction term.

We proceeded to conduct mediation analysis to explore whether IR mediates the link between obesity and adolescent hypertension. The analysis was performed using the 'mediation' package (version 4.5.0), incorporating linear and logistic regression models to assess the direct and indirect associations. In the process, a nonparametric bootstrap approach was applied, with continuous TyG as a mediator, allowing us to quantify the proportion of the total effect of obesity on hypertension mediated by TyG.

To investigate the potential heterogeneity of interactive and joint effects in individuals with different characteristics, subgroup analyses stratified by age, sex, MVPA, and sleep adequacy were conducted, and the p values for interaction of stratification variables with the interaction terms of 'TyG × high obesity indices' were simultaneously calculated. Based on the subgroup results, interaction analysis was re-performed in age groups of 12–14 years and 15–17 years, separately.

Furthermore, several sensitivity analyses were conducted to validate the robustness of the main analysis of interaction in this study. First, a generalized linear mixed-effect model (GLMM) with a logit link function was fitted, with the province included as a random intercept to account for geographical clustering and unmeasured contextual factors (e.g., climatic conditions, pollution levels) that may contribute to between-province differences in hypertension risk. Second, the original entire dataset was used (n = 7031). The missing values were renamed 'unknown' for qualitative variables alcohol intake, secondhand smoke, MVPA, and sleep adequacy, which were covariates with missing values exceeding 15% (Supplementary Materials: Figure S1). For the variables with less than 3.5% missing values, their missing values were assumed to be randomly missing, and therefore, multiple imputation based on chained equations using baseline characteristics was used for imputation. We created an imputed dataset using the 'mice' package (version 3.16.0) to re-examine previous main findings. Finally, E-values were calculated to estimate the potential impact of unmeasured confounders in the association of TyG and obesity indices with adolescent hypertension.

3. Results

3.1. Characteristics of Adolescents and the Prevalence of Hypertension

Table 1 presents the characteristics of the participants. A total of 5703 adolescents were finally included in the main analysis, of which 47.07% were boys and 52.93% were girls. The mean age was 14.2 years (SD = 1.7 years). Participants with hypertension exhibited significantly higher levels of BMI, WC, serum uric acid, serum total protein, TG, FG, and TyG, compared with those without hypertension, while the frequency of MVPA was higher in the non-hypertension group (all $p < 0.05$). In addition, compared with the non-hypertension group, the hypertension group had a greater proportion of high BMI (37.06% for hypertension vs. 15.82% for non-hypertension, $p < 0.001$) and high WC (30.39% for hypertension vs. 13.08% for non-hypertension, $p < 0.001$). Further, alcohol consumption, family history of hypertension, and province differed significantly between the two groups (all $p < 0.01$).

The overall prevalence of adolescent hypertension in five provinces was 19.4%, with regional variations: Guangdong, 11.1%; Jiangsu, 25.1%; Shandong, 23.4%; Guizhou, 20.3%; and Inner Mongolia, 18.4%. Figure 2 illustrates the prevalence of hypertension across groups of different combinations of TyG and obesity indices, and the prevalence reaches approximately 40% when high TyG is combined with high BMI or high WC.

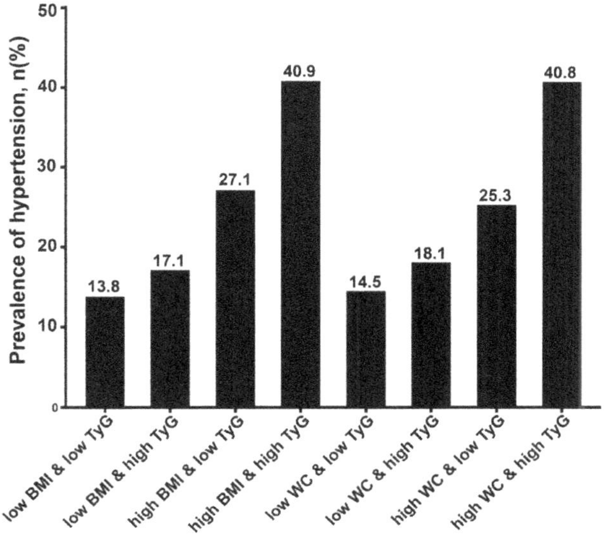

Figure 2. Prevalence of adolescent hypertension across groups of different combinations of obesity and TyG (n = 5703). The cut-off value for defining low/high TyG is its median (8.18), while the cutoffs for low/high obesity indices refer to the sex- and age-specific thresholds set by the Chinese national health industry standards for children and adolescents. TyG, triglyceride-glucose index; BMI, body mass index; WC, waist circumference.

Table 1. The characteristics of the adolescents from five provinces (n = 5703).

ariables	Hypertension		Total (n = 5703)	*p*-Value
	No (n = 4594)	Yes (n = 1109)		
ge, year	14.2 (1.7)	13.9 (1.7)	14.2 (1.7)	<0.001
ex, male	2326 (50.63%)	522 (47.07%)	2848 (49.94%)	0.033
MI, kg/m^2	19.8 (3.3)	22.0 (4.8)	20.3 (3.7)	<0.001
igh BMI (overweight/obesity) *	727 (15.82%)	411 (37.06%)	1138 (19.95%)	<0.001
aist circumference, cm	68.0 (9.0)	72.3 (12.2)	68.8 (9.8)	<0.001
igh WC (abdominal obesity) *	601 (13.08%)	337 (30.39%)	938 (16.45%)	<0.001
VPA, days/week †	4.0 (2.0, 5.0)	3.0 (2.0, 5.0)	4.0 (2.0, 5.0)	0.006
nhealthy dietary score	5.9 (1.0)	5.9 (1.0)	5.9 (1.0)	0.156
dequate sleep	1386 (30.17%)	363 (32.73%)	1749 (30.67%)	0.097
econdhand smoke				0.462
almost none	3388 (73.75%)	832 (75.02%)	4220 (74.00%)	
1–3 days/week	626 (13.63%)	135 (12.17%)	761 (13.34%)	
4–6 days/week	175 (3.81%)	37 (3.34%)	212 (3.72%)	
everyday	405 (8.82%)	105 (9.47%)	510 (8.94%)	
lcohol intake				0.002
never	3577 (77.86%)	917 (82.69%)	4494 (78.80%)	
30 days ago	712 (15.50%)	131 (11.81%)	843 (14.78%)	
within 30 days	305 (6.64%)	61 (5.50%)	366 (6.42%)	
arental education level				0.143
low	1718 (37.40%)	411 (37.06%)	2129 (37.33%)	
medium	2453 (53.40%)	617 (55.64%)	3070 (53.83%)	
high	354 (7.71%)	64 (5.77%)	418 (7.33%)	
unknown	69 (1.50%)	17 (1.53%)	86 (1.51%)	

Table 1. *Cont.*

Variables	Hypertension		Total (n = 5703)	*p*-Value
	No (n = 4594)	Yes (n = 1109)		
Family history of hypertension	1599 (34.81%)	381 (34.36%)	1980 (34.72%)	0.008
Rural residence	2042 (44.45%)	459 (41.39%)	2501 (43.85%)	0.065
Province				<0.001
Guangdong	1256 (27.34%)	157 (14.16%)	1413 (24.78%)	
Jiangsu	875 (19.05%)	293 (26.42%)	1168 (20.48%)	
Shandong	1090 (23.73%)	332 (29.94%)	1422 (24.93%)	
Guizhou	598 (13.02%)	152 (13.71%)	750 (13.15%)	
Inner Mongolia	775 (16.87%)	175 (15.78%)	950 (16.66%)	
Urine sodium, mmol/L	144.6 (69.6)	147.2 (71.4)	145.2 (70.0)	0.434
Serum uric acid, μmol/L	363.2 (90.8)	371.3 (96.3)	364.8 (92.0)	0.035
Serum total protein, g/L	76.4 (5.0)	77.7 (5.2)	76.6 (5.1)	<0.001
eGFR, mL/(min·1.73 m^2)	147.3 (28.6)	147.6 (28.1)	147.4 (28.5)	0.552
TC, mg/dL	149.6 (28.6)	150.8 (30.0)	149.9 (28.9)	0.299
TG, mg/dL	80.8 (33.8)	90.2 (42.0)	82.7 (35.7)	<0.001
FG, mg/dL	93.3 (10.4)	94.8 (11.9)	93.6 (10.7)	<0.001
TyG	8.2 (0.4)	8.3 (0.4)	8.2 (0.4)	<0.001

* The cut-off values for low/high obesity indices refer to the sex- and age-specific thresholds set by the Chinese national health industry standards for children and adolescents. † MVPA was present as median (interquartile range), other variables were presented as mean (standard deviation) or count (percentage). Abbreviation: BMI, body mass index; WC, waist circumference; MVPA, moderate-vigorous physical activity; eGFR, estimated glomerular filtration rate; TC, total cholesterol; TG, triglyceride; FG, fasting blood glucose; TyG, triglyceride-glucose index.

3.2. Relationships of TyG, BMI, and WC with Adolescent Hypertension

TyG, BMI, and WC, whether continuous or categorical, were consistently associated with adolescent hypertension prevalence in Model 1 and Model 2 (all $p < 0.001$), as shown in Table 2. After full adjustment (Model 2), the ORs were 1.52 (95%CI: 1.33, 1.75, $p < 0.001$) in high TyG, 3.07 (95%CI: 2.63, 3.58, $p < 0.001$) in high BMI, and 2.71 (95%CI: 2.31, 3.19, $p < 0.001$) in high WC. RCS models (Figure 3) revealed a linear relationship between TyG and hypertension (p for non-linear > 0.05), while a non-linear relationship was observed between obesity indices and hypertension (p for non-linear < 0.05). Supplementary Materials: Figure S2 shows non-linear relationships of BMI and WC with TyG (p for non-linear < 0.001).

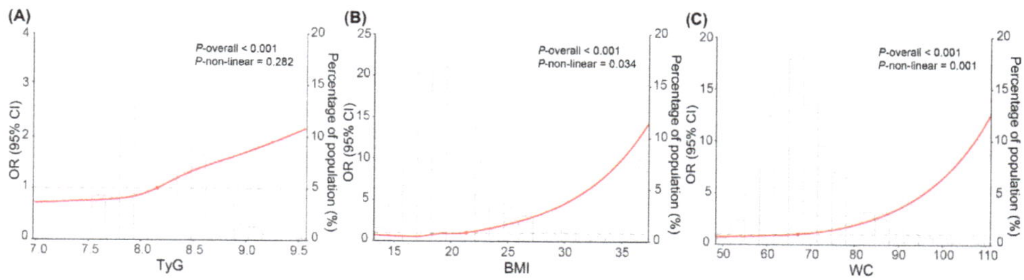

Figure 3. Non-linear relationship of TyG, BMI, and WC with adolescent hypertension, as modeled by restricted cubic spline regression (n = 5703). (**A**) TyG and hypertension; (**B**) BMI and hypertension; (**C**) WC and hypertension. Models were adjusted for sex, age, moderate-vigorous physical activity, unhealthy dietary score, sleep adequacy, secondhand smoke, alcohol intake, family history of hypertension, parental education level, residence, serum uric acid, serum total protein, estimated glomerular filtration rate, total cholesterol, and urine sodium. TyG, triglyceride-glucose index; BMI, body mass index; WC, waist circumference. Shadow shapes indicate 95%CIs.

Table 2. Independent association of TyG and obesity indices with hypertension (n = 5703).

Variables *	Model 1		Model 2	
	OR (95%CI)	*p*-Value	OR (95%CI)	*p*-Value
ontinuous TyG	1.95 (1.66, 2.31)	<0.001	1.86 (1.56, 2.22)	<0.001
w TyG	Reference		Reference	
gh TyG	1.59 (1.40, 1.82)	<0.001	1.52 (1.33, 1.75)	<0.001
ontinuous BMI (kg/m^2)	1.17 (1.15, 1.19)	<0.001	1.16 (1.14, 1.19)	<0.001
w BMI	Reference		Reference	
gh BMI	3.22 (2.78, 3.74)	<0.001	3.07 (2.63, 3.58)	<0.001
ontinuous WC (cm)	1.05 (1.04, 1.06)	<0.001	1.05 (1.04, 1.06)	<0.001
w WC	Reference		Reference	
gh WC	2.94 (2.52, 3.43)	<0.001	2.71 (2.31, 3.19)	<0.001

Model 1 was adjusted for age and sex. Model 2 was adjusted for sex, age, moderate-vigorous physical activity, unhealthy dietary score, sleep adequacy, secondhand smoke, alcohol intake, family history of hypertension, parental education level, residence, serum uric acid, serum total protein, estimated glomerular filtration rate, total cholesterol, and urine sodium. * The cut-off value for defining low/high TyG is its median (8.18), while the cutoffs for low/high obesity indices refer to the sex- and age-specific thresholds set by the Chinese national health industry standards for children and adolescents. Abbreviations: OR, odds ratio; CI, confidence interval; TyG, triglyceride-glucose index; BMI, body mass index; WC, waist circumference.

3.3. *Interactive, Joint, and Mediating Effects*

Table 3 presents the calculation results of interaction and joint effects. The results suggested that a synergistic interaction exists between IR and obesity on adolescent hypertension. Specifically, significant multiplicative interactions were observed ($p < 0.05$), and SI > 1 further indicated synergistic interactions; RERI > 0 suggested that the joint effect of high TyG and high obesity indices surpassed the sum of their independent effect; and the AP quantified the proportion of excess risk attributable to the combined exposure. In the multivariable logistic regression, the ORs for hypertension were 4.11-fold (95%CI: 3.37, 5.01) and 3.69-fold (95%CI: 3.01, 4.53) higher in the high BMI & high TyG group and the high WC & high TyG group than their corresponding low combined groups. The APs showed that nearly 40% of the hypertension risk associated with concurrent high obesity indices and high TyG in adolescents could be attributed to their interaction.

Table 3. Interacting and joint effects of obesity and insulin resistance on adolescent hypertension (n = 5703).

Variables *			OR (95%CI)	*p* for Interaction †	Additive Interaction Measures		
MI	TyG	WC			RERI (95%CI)	AP (95%CI)	SI (95%CI)
w	low		Reference	0.015	1.60 (0.77, 2.43)	0.39 (0.23, 0.55)	2.06 (1.35, 3.15)
w	high		1.21 (1.03, 1.43)				
gh	low		2.30 (1.78, 2.96)				
gh	high		4.11 (3.37, 5.01)				
	low	low	Reference	0.007	1.60 (0.79, 2.41)	0.43 (0.26, 0.60)	2.46 (1.42, 4.26)
	high	low	1.23 (1.05, 1.44)				
	low	high	1.86 (1.39, 2.50)				
	high	high	3.69 (3.01, 4.53)				

Models were adjusted for sex, age, moderate-vigorous physical activity, unhealthy dietary score, sleep adequacy, secondhand smoke, alcohol intake, family history of hypertension, parental education level, residence, serum uric acid, serum total protein, estimated glomerular filtration rate, total cholesterol, and urine sodium. * The cut-off value for defining low/high TyG is its median (8.18), while the cutoffs for low/high obesity indices refer to the sex- and age-specific thresholds set by the Chinese national health industry standards for children and adolescents. † The significance of the multiplicative interaction was evaluated through a likelihood ratio test, comparing models with and without the interaction term. Abbreviations: OR, odds ratio; CI, confidence interval; RERI, relative excess risk due to interaction; AP, proportion attributable to interaction; SI, synergy index; TyG, triglyceride-glucose index; BMI, body mass index; WC, waist circumference.

Mediation analysis (Figure 4) demonstrated that TyG significantly mediated the total effect of obesity on adolescent hypertension ($p < 0.001$). The proportions mediated were 6.30% for high BMI and 8.54% for high WC.

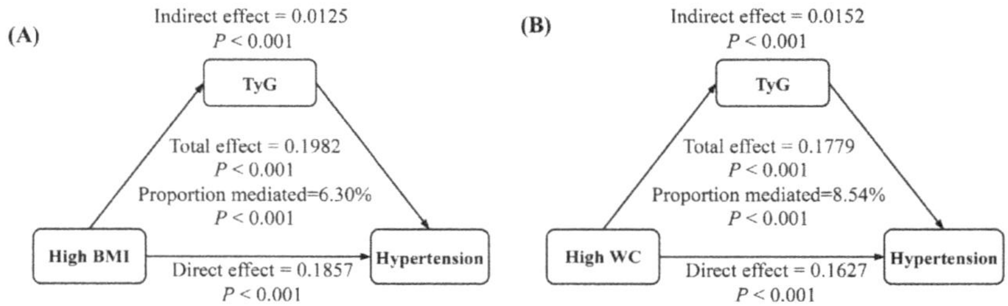

Figure 4. Mediation effects of TyG on the association between obesity and adolescent hypertension (n = 5703). (**A**) Mediation effect of TyG on the high-BMI–hypertension association; (**B**) Mediation effect of TyG on the high-WC–hypertension association. Models were adjusted for sex, age, moderate-vigorous physical activity, unhealthy dietary score, sleep adequacy, secondhand smoke, alcohol intake, family history of hypertension, parental education level, residence, serum uric acid, serum total protein, estimated glomerular filtration rate, total cholesterol, and urine sodium. The cut-off values for low/high obesity indices refer to the sex- and age-specific thresholds set by the Chinese national health industry standards for children and adolescents. TyG, triglyceride-glucose index; BMI, body mass index; WC, waist circumference.

3.4. Subgroup and Sensitivity Analyses

Table 4 shows that no significant interactions were observed between the stratification variables and the joint effect of TyG and obesity indices on hypertension (p for interaction > 0.05), except for age, suggesting that the combined impact of IR and obesity on hypertension varies between individuals aged 12–14 years and 15–17 years. Specifically, adolescents aged 15–17 with high TyG and high obesity indices had greater odds of hypertension than adolescents aged 12–14 (high BMI & high TyG: OR = 3.54 for 12–14 years vs. OR = 5.50 for 15–17 years; high WC & high TyG: OR = 3.17 for 12–14 years vs. OR = 4.85 for 15–17 years). The results of the re-analysis of the interaction in these two age groups show that AP was greater in the adolescents aged 15–17 years than in those aged 12–14 years (Table 5).

Table 4. Joint effects of obesity and insulin resistance on adolescent hypertension stratified by age, sex, physical activity, and sleep adequacy.

Subgroup (Cases/Total)	Variables *	BMI		WC	
		OR (95%CI) †	*p* for Interaction ‡	OR (95%CI) †	*p* for Interaction ‡
Age, year			0.019		0.045
12–14 (709/3259)	low BMI/WC & low TyG	Reference		Reference	
	low BMI/WC & high TyG	1.26 (1.02, 1.56)		1.27 (1.04, 1.55)	
	high BMI/WC & low TyG	2.09 (1.50, 2.92)		1.63 (1.10, 2.41)	
	high BMI/WC & high TyG	3.54 (2.75, 4.57)		3.17 (2.44, 4.13)	
15–17 (400/2444)	low BMI/WC & low TyG	Reference		Reference	
	low BMI/WC & high TyG	1.05 (0.79, 1.39)		1.10 (0.84, 1.43)	
	high BMI/WC & low TyG	2.66 (1.78, 3.97)		2.24 (1.45, 3.47)	
	high BMI/WC & high TyG	5.50 (3.98, 7.60)		4.85 (3.49, 6.75)	

Table 4. *Cont.*

Subgroup (Cases/Total)	Variables *	BMI		WC	
		OR (95%CI) †	*p* for Interaction ‡	OR (95%CI) †	*p* for Interaction ‡
x			0.806		0.237
ale (522/2848)	low BMI/WC & low TyG	Reference		Reference	
	low BMI/WC & high TyG	1.06 (0.82, 1.38)		1.05 (0.83, 1.34)	
	high BMI/WC & low TyG	2.30 (1.64, 3.24)		1.91 (1.27, 2.89)	
	high BMI/WC & high TyG	3.87 (2.94, 5.10)		3.87 (2.91, 5.14)	
nale 37/2855)	low BMI/WC & low TyG	Reference		Reference	
	low BMI/WC & high TyG	1.34 (1.07, 1.67)		1.39 (1.12, 1.72)	
	high BMI/WC & low TyG	2.37 (1.60, 3.53)		1.91 (1.26, 2.89)	
	high BMI/WC & high TyG	4.26 (3.17, 5.71)		3.40 (2.51, 4.59)	
VPA, ys/week			0.338		0.360
3 (594/2841)	low BMI/WC & low TyG	Reference		Reference	
	low BMI/WC & high TyG	1.40 (1.11, 1.76)		1.41 (1.13, 1.76)	
	high BMI/WC & low TyG	2.49 (1.76, 3.53)		2.11 (1.43, 3.12)	
	high BMI/WC & high TyG	4.05 (3.06, 5.36)		3.70 (2.77, 4.96)	
7 (515/2862)	low BMI/WC & low TyG	Reference		Reference	
	low BMI/WC & high TyG	1.03 (0.80, 1.31)		1.04 (0.82, 1.31)	
	high BMI/WC & low TyG	2.09 (1.43, 3.07)		1.62 (1.04, 2.54)	
	high BMI/WC & high TyG	4.05 (3.04, 5.39)		3.61 (2.70, 4.83)	
lequate sleep			0.065		0.239
(746/3954)	low BMI/WC & low TyG	Reference		Reference	
	low BMI/WC & high TyG	1.19 (0.97, 1.46)		1.23 (1.01, 1.50)	
	high BMI/WC & low TyG	2.34 (1.72, 3.20)		1.94 (1.36, 2.75)	
	high BMI/WC & high TyG	4.83 (3.80, 6.15)		4.29 (3.35, 5.50)	
s (363/1749)	low BMI/WC & low TyG	Reference		Reference	
	low BMI/WC & high TyG	1.24 (0.93, 1.66)		1.21 (0.92, 1.60)	
	high BMI/WC & low TyG	2.26 (1.43, 3.57)		1.72 (1.01, 2.94)	
	high BMI/WC & high TyG	2.90 (2.03, 4.14)		2.60 (1.86, 3.87)	

* The cut-off value for defining low/high TyG is its median (8.18), while the cutoffs for low/high obesity indices refer to the sex- and age-specific thresholds set by the Chinese national health industry standards for children and adolescents. † Models were adjusted for, if not stratified, sex, age, moderate-vigorous physical activity, unhealthy dietary score, sleep adequacy, secondhand smoke, alcohol intake, family history of hypertension, parental education, residence, serum uric acid, serum total protein, estimated glomerular filtration rate, total cholesterol, and urine sodium. ‡ *p* for interaction was derived from logistic regression models by comparing models including and not including the stratification variable in the interaction terms (TyG with BMI or WC) to test for heterogeneity of the studied interactive effects across subgroups. Abbreviations: OR, odds ratio; CI, confidence interval; TyG, triglyceride-glucose index; BMI, body mass index; WC, waist circumference; MVPA, moderate-vigorous physical activity.

Table 5. Interactive effects of obesity and insulin resistance on hypertension in adolescents aged 12–14 years and 15–17 years.

nteractive Items *	Measures †	12–14 Years Old (n = 3259)		15–17 Years Old (n = 2444)	
		Coefficients (95%CI)	*p*-Value	Coefficients (95%CI)	*p*-Value
	Additive effects				
MI and TyG	RERI	1.18 (0.25, 2.12)	0.007	2.79 (1.03, 4.55)	0.001
	AP	0.33 (0.11, 0.56)	0.002	0.51 (0.29, 0.73)	<0.001
	SI	1.87 (1.07, 3.29)	0.014	2.63 (1.35, 5.14)	0.002

Table 5. *Cont.*

Interactive Items *	Measures †	12–14 Years Old (n = 3259)		15–17 Years Old (n = 2444)	
		Coefficients (95%CI)	*p*-Value	Coefficients (95%CI)	*p*-Value
WC and TyG	Additive effects				
	RERI	1.28 (0.36, 2.19)	0.003	2.51 (0.87, 4.16)	0.002
	AP	0.40 (0.17, 0.64)	<0.001	0.52 (0.28, 0.75)	<0.001
	SI	2.42 (1.10, 5.33)	0.014	2.88 (1.30, 6.39)	0.005

* Additive interaction measures were calculated based on the reference group with low TyG & low BMI or low WC. The cut-off value for defining low/high TyG is its median (8.18), while the cutoffs for low/high obesity indices refer to the sex- and age-specific thresholds set by the Chinese national health industry standards for children and adolescents. † Models were adjusted for sex, moderate-vigorous physical activity, unhealthy dietary score, sleep adequacy, secondhand smoke, alcohol intake, family history of hypertension, parental education level, residence, serum uric acid, serum total protein, estimated glomerular filtration rate, total cholesterol, and urine sodium. Abbreviations: CI, confidence interval; RERI, relative excess risk due to interaction; AP, proportion attributable to interaction; SI, synergy index; TyG, triglyceride-glucose index; BMI, body mass index; WC, waist circumference.

Sensitivity analysis revealed that the results using the GLMM modeling approach or using the imputed dataset were consistent with our main analysis, indicating our findings were robust and not affected by province and missing data (Supplementary Materials: Tables S2–S4). The E-value supported the robustness of the association of TyG and obesity indices with adolescent hypertension (Supplementary Materials: Table S5).

4. Discussion

Based on a provincially representative surveillance database including five provinces, this study provides a comprehensive perspective regarding the interaction and combined effect of IR and obesity on adolescent hypertension, and the mediating role of IR in the pathway of obesity leading to hypertension in adolescents. The results demonstrated that individuals with both obesity and higher TyG levels had the highest odds of hypertension. Statistically, a synergistic interaction existed between IR and obesity on adolescent hypertension. Moreover, IR mediated the association of obesity with hypertension (Figure 4).

The primary suggestive evidence for pediatric hypertension is currently considered to be excessive weight, salted food intake, and family history of hypertension [3,25]. As a modifiable condition, obesity is a well-recognized risk factor for high blood pressure in both children and adults [26,27]. An umbrella review combined accumulated observational (associative) and genetics-driven (causal) research to gather mutually complementary insights and elucidate the perplexing epidemiological relationship between obesity and cardiovascular disease (including hypertension) [28]. The review found that these two types of studies were concordant, with Mendelian randomization studies supporting adiposity (including general obesity measured by BMI and central obesity measured by WC) as a causal factor for hypertension development. However, not all children with obesity develop hypertension, as some remain normotensive despite excess adiposity [25]. This suggests the need to consider additional metabolic factors when evaluating hypertension risk. As a promising non-insulin-based IR index, a study in 2010 laid the cornerstone for accepting it as a reliable surrogate indicator for evaluating IR [29]. It was reported that TyG showed excellent correlation with the HEC test in diagnosing IR, with an area under the curve (AUC) of 0.858 [29]. Based on simple and low-cost biochemical parameters, TyG is particularly suitable for large-scale epidemiological investigations and resource-limited settings. A substantial body of epidemiological research has demonstrated the link between elevated TyG and the risk of hypertension, including cross-sectional studies and longitudinal cohort studies [8,30–32]. Notably, a 2019 study in Mexico was the first to report this association in pediatric populations [30]. Our results on the correlation of TyG with hypertension align with previous literature.

In the development of diseases, especially chronic conditions, the pathogenic factor rarely acts in isolation. Instead, they typically result from a complex interplay of multiple contributing causes. At present, it is thought that obesity-driven fat accumulation leads to hypertension primarily through chronic vascular inflammation, physical compression of the kidney, and overactivation of the sympathetic nervous system (SNS) and the renin–angiotensin–aldosterone system [33,34]. IR contributes to elevating BP through several proposed mechanisms, including SNS activation and increased renal sodium reabsorption [11]. IR can also impair vascular function and structure, promoting the onset and progression of hypertension [33]. Importantly, the accumulation of fat (including visceral fat) can decrease the sensitivity of tissues and cells to insulin, and conversely, IR impairs lipid metabolism, leading to lipid accumulation [33,35]. These intricate pathophysiological networks may underlie the mechanism of the synergistic effects observed between IR and obesity on adolescent hypertension and provide a theoretical foundation for the mediating effects found in our study (Table 3, Figure 4). Although IR may exhibit a physiological increase during puberty, our data emphasize the significance of maintaining relatively low levels of TyG in adolescents. Since obesity can lead to IR, excessive adiposity may transform a physiological increase in IR into a pathological condition. Therefore, weight management is essential for pubertal adolescents.

In the present study, adolescents with a concurrent high obesity index and high TyG had at least a 13.8% higher prevalence of hypertension than those with either factor alone (Figure 2). As expected, our results showed that there were significant biological interactions between the two factors on the prevalence of adolescent hypertension, which epidemiologically confirms the interrelationship between obesity and IR. Our findings are consistent with some studies in adults: IR has a synergistic effect on the obesity–hypertension association among Black and white adults [36]. We also found that the synergistic interaction observed might be influenced by the individuals' puberty stage, as age subgroups interact with this synergistic effect (p for interaction < 0.05) (Table 4). Further analysis showed that the synergistic interaction between obesity and IR was stronger in mid-to-late adolescence (15–17 years) compared with adolescents aged 12–14 years (Table 5). This suggests that adolescents in the age group of 15–17 years who are both obese and have IR may be at a higher risk of developing hypertension.

Given previous research that hypertension prevalence in China is higher in the north than in the south—possibly due to climatic conditions, pollution, or socio-economic factors [37]—we built a GLMM with 'province' as a random effect, confirming the robustness of the observed interactions. Actually, we have further tested the effect of province on the interaction term in the main analysis but found no significant heterogeneity (p for interaction > 0.05). These results suggest that provinces have no effect on our observation, and given the provincial representativeness of our dataset, this evidence thus supports the generalizability of our results to the national adolescent population.

Between 1990 and 2021, the global prevalence of obesity in children and adolescents tripled [38]. The epidemic of obesity is accompanied by an increasing number of pediatric patients with chronic diseases, including hypertension. However, obesity and IR are both modifiable factors. Healthy lifestyles are helpful to keep IR at an appropriate level, including good sleep, a healthy diet (e.g., more intake of fruits and vegetables, less consumption of added sugars and trans-fats), limiting alcohol, avoiding smoking, and lowering stress through proper means [39]. Furthermore, regular exercise is particularly encouraged because weight loss interventions can significantly lower the risk of hypertension and, importantly, also improve IR, as our findings show [33,39].

Of note, the prevalence of hypertension observed in this study (19.4%) was higher than that reported in most previous studies among children and adolescents [2,3]. However, using the entire national database from this nutrition surveillance, it was found that the prevalence among children and adolescents nationwide in China was 24.9% [40], which is similar to our results. Several factors may account for the relatively high prevalence of hypertension in this surveillance. First, BP was measured using an electronic sphygmomanometer, and prior research has shown that readings obtained with electronic devices tend to be higher than those from mercury sphygmomanometers [41]. In addition, though BP was measured three times at one-minute intervals, it was on a single occasion, which may lead to an overestimation of hypertension prevalence [3,42]. Finally, as mentioned earlier, the growing epidemic of childhood obesity in recent years may have led to dramatic changes in BP levels.

The results in the present study indicated that adolescents with both obesity and IR require particular attention, as obesity and IR might strengthen each other's association with adolescent hypertension. The combined use of the obesity index and a simple marker of IR could help identify high-risk individuals for hypertension and is beneficial for the prevention and management of hypertension. Future large-scale longitudinal cohort studies will help provide higher-level evidence.

Limitations

This study has several limitations. First, IR was evaluated by TyG instead of the HEC test, and obesity was estimated by BMI and WC rather than electronic instruments. Studies in the future using more precise measurements could provide more accurate results. Second, considering that our study population consists only of Chinese adolescents and the relationship between IR and BP varies by race [43], it is unclear whether the results of this study can be extended to other ethnicities.

Third, some biases cannot be overlooked. The surveillance data used in this study were collected under strict quality control procedures. A 10% non-response rate was considered during the survey design process. Participants were selected using a standardized sampling method across all survey sites, with strict adherence to randomization principles at each stage of the survey process. Consequently, selection bias was relatively small. All investigators received standardized training before the investigation, and those who did not meet preset criteria underwent additional training to ensure data quality. In addition, certain information regarding participants was collected based on validated structured questionnaires. However, several questionnaire-based covariates may be prone to recall bias, such as secondhand smoke exposure and alcohol use. Single-occasion BP measurement may also lead to misclassification bias. Further, though E-values were calculated to support the robustness of the association of TyG and obesity with adolescent hypertension, residual confounding from unmeasured or unknown factors cannot be excluded, as obesity and IR are intricately related and share many other risk factors.

Fourth, although obesity is a well-established risk factor for hypertension, and IR is thought to be involved in the development of hypertension, the cross-sectional design of this study precludes establishing temporal relationships and thus limits causal inference. Meanwhile, despite some support from the proposed physiological mechanisms, the mediation analysis in this study should be regarded as exploratory due to the constraints of the temporal relationship. Future longitudinal cohort studies are warranted to address this limitation. Finally, it should be noted that it remains unclear whether hypertension in adolescents is a concomitant condition to obesity or obesity is considered as a trigger, or if other interactions between these factors exist. The results of this study should be interpreted with caution.

5. Conclusions

This study reveals that IR warrants attention when adolescents are obese, as the two conditions synergistically increase the odds of adolescent hypertension. Our findings indicate that incorporating both obesity and IR into early risk stratification models may help identify adolescents at high risk before the onset of hypertension. Also, strategies simultaneously targeting both obesity and IR should be emphasized for the primary prevention of adolescent hypertension.

Supplementary Materials: The following supporting information can be downloaded at: https://www.mdpi.com/article/10.3390/nu17172783/s1, Figure S1. Missing variables in our original dataset of 7031 adolescents aged 12–17 years old. Figure S2. Non-linear relationship of body mass index and waist circumference with triglyceride-glucose index (n = 5703). Table S1. Baseline characteristics between adolescents included and not included. Table S2. Interacting and joint effects of obesity and insulin resistance on adolescent hypertension based on generalized linear mixed-effect models. Table S3. The characteristics of the adolescents from five provinces after multiple imputation. Table S4. Interacting and joint effects of obesity and insulin resistance on adolescent hypertension in samples after multiple imputation. Table S5. E-values of high TyG, high BMI, and high WC with adolescent hypertension.

Author Contributions: Conceptualization, H.Z.; methodology, H.Z. and Z.Z.; software, H.Z., Z.Z. and Y.F.; formal analysis, H.Z.; data curation, Q.W., R.Z., T.L. and D.L.; writing—original draft preparation, H.Z.; writing—review and editing, X.D. and H.Z.; project administration, T.L., D.L. and X.C. All authors have read and agreed to the published version of the manuscript.

Funding: This research received no external funding.

Institutional Review Board Statement: Received ethical approval from the Ethics Committee of the Chinese Center for Disease Control and Prevention (Protocol Code: 201614; approval date: 3 June 2016).

Informed Consent Statement: All subjects participating in the study gave informed consent.

Data Availability Statement: The datasets used and/or analyzed during the current study are not publicly available due to ethical and privacy reasons, but are available from the corresponding author upon reasonable request.

Acknowledgments: We are grateful for the collaboration of the data-providing departments, particularly the Centers for Disease Control and Prevention (CDCs) in the five provinces, as well as the contributions of investigators and the cooperation of participants.

Conflicts of Interest: The authors declare no conflicts of interest.

Abbreviations

TyG, triglyceride-glucose index; BMI, body mass index; WC, waist circumference; BP, blood pressure; MVPA, moderate-vigorous physical activity; eGFR, estimated glomerular filtration rate; TC, total cholesterol; TG, triglyceride; FG, fasting blood glucose; OR, odds ratio; CI, confidence interval; RERI, relative excess risk due to interaction; AP, proportion attributable to interaction; SI, synergy index; AUC, area under the curve.

ferences

Robinson, C.H.; Chanchlani, R. High Blood Pressure in Children and Adolescents: Current Perspectives and Strategies to Improve Future Kidney and Cardiovascular Health. *Kidney Int. Rep.* **2022**, *7*, 954–970. [CrossRef]

Song, P.; Zhang, Y.; Yu, J.; Zha, M.; Zhu, Y.; Rahimi, K.; Rudan, I. Global Prevalence of Hypertension in Children: A Systematic Review and Meta-Analysis. *JAMA Pediatr.* **2019**, *173*, 1154. [CrossRef]

Zhou, J.; Wu, J.; Jiang, D.; Cai, S.; Zhang, C.; Ying, J.; Cao, J.; Song, Y.; Song, P. National, Regional and Provincial Prevalence of Childhood Hypertension in China in 2020: A Systematic Review and Modelling Study. *Lancet Child Adolesc. Health* **2024**, *8*, 872–881. [CrossRef]

4. Yang, L.; Magnussen, C.G.; Yang, L.; Bovet, P.; Xi, B. Elevated Blood Pressure in Childhood or Adolescence and Cardiovasc Outcomes in Adulthood: A Systematic Review. *Hypertension* **2020**, *75*, 948–955. [CrossRef]
5. Shankar, R.R.; Eckert, G.J.; Saha, C.; Tu, W.; Pratt, J.H. The Change in Blood Pressure during Pubertal Growth. *J. Clin. Endocr Metab.* **2005**, *90*, 163–167. [CrossRef]
6. Ewald, D.R.; Haldeman, L.A. Risk Factors in Adolescent Hypertension. *Glob. Pediatr. Health* **2016**, *3*, 1–26. [CrossRef]
7. Din-Dzietham, R.; Liu, Y.; Bielo, M.-V.; Shamsa, F. High Blood Pressure Trends in Children and Adolescents in National Surv 1963 to 2002. *Circulation* **2007**, *116*, 1488–1496. [CrossRef]
8. Tsai, K.-Z.; Chu, C.-C.; Huang, W.-C.; Sui, X.; Lavie, C.J.; Lin, G.-M. Prediction of Various Insulin Resistance Indices for the Ris Hypertension among Military Young Adults: The CHIEF Cohort Study, 2014–2020. *Cardiovasc. Diabetol.* **2024**, *23*, 141. [Cross
9. Zhao, X.; An, X.; Yang, C.; Sun, W.; Ji, H.; Lian, F. The Crucial Role and Mechanism of Insulin Resistance in Metabolic Dise *Front. Endocrinol.* **2023**, *14*, 1149239. [CrossRef]
10. Wang, K.; He, G.; Zhang, Y.; Yin, J.; Yan, Y.; Zhang, Y.; Wang, K. Association of Triglyceride-Glucose Index and Its Interaction v Obesity on Hypertension Risk in Chinese: A Population-Based Study. *J. Hum. Hypertens.* **2021**, *35*, 232–239. [CrossRef]
11. Chen, Y.; Hu, P.; He, Y.; Qin, H.; Hu, L.; Yang, R. Association of TyG Index and Central Obesity with Hypertension in Middle-A and Elderly Chinese Adults: A Prospective Cohort Study. *Sci. Rep.* **2024**, *14*, 2235. [CrossRef] [PubMed]
12. Kang, B.; Yang, Y.; Lee, E.Y.; Yang, H.K.; Kim, H.-S.; Lim, S.-Y.; Lee, J.-H.; Lee, S.-S.; Suh, B.-K.; Yoon, K.-H. Triglycerides/Gluc Index Is a Useful Surrogate Marker of Insulin Resistance among Adolescents. *Int. J. Obes.* **2017**, *41*, 789–792. [CrossRef] [PubM
13. Calcaterra, V.; Verduci, E.; Vandoni, M.; Rossi, V.; Fiore, G.; Massini, G.; Berardo, C.; Gatti, A.; Baldassarre, P.; Bianchi, A.; e The Effect of Healthy Lifestyle Strategies on the Management of Insulin Resistance in Children and Adolescents with Obesit Narrative Review. *Nutrients* **2022**, *14*, 4692. [CrossRef]
14. Yazıcı, D.; Sezer, H. Insulin Resistance, Obesity and Lipotoxicity. *Adv. Exp. Med. Biol.* **2017**, *960*, 277–304. [CrossRef] [PubMe
15. Yu, D.; Zhao, L.; Zhang, J.; Yang, Z.; Yang, L.; Huang, J.; Fang, H.; Guo, Q.; Xu, X.; Ju, L.; et al. China Nutrition and He Surveys (1982−2017). *China CDC Wkly.* **2021**, *3*, 193. [CrossRef]
16. Anthropometric Measurements Method in Health Surveillance. WS/T 424—2013. Available online: https://www.nhc.gov wjw/yingyang/201308/1f27caef0b22493e93a1da8aec2cd63a/files/1739783545878_39188.pdf (accessed on 25 March 2025).
17. Screening for Overweight and Obesity Among School-Age Children and Adolescents. WS/T 586—2018. Available onl http://www.nhc.gov.cn/ewebeditor/uploadfile/2018/03/20180330094031236.pdf (accessed on 25 March 2025).
18. Cheng, X.; Guo, Q.; Ju, L.; Gong, W.; Wei, X.; Xu, X.; Zhao, L.; Fang, H. Association between Sedentary Behavior, Screen Time Metabolic Syndrome among Chinese Children and Adolescents. *BMC Public Health* **2024**, *24*, 1715. [CrossRef]
19. High Waist Circumference Screening Threshold Among Children and Adolescents Aged 7−18 Years. WS/T 611—2018. Avail online: http://www.nhc.gov.cn/ewebeditor/uploadfile/2018/07/20180704145130574.pdf (accessed on 25 March 2025).
20. Reference of Screening for Elevated Blood Pressure Among Children and Adolescents Aged 7−18 Years. WS/T 610—2 Available online: http://www.nhc.gov.cn/ewebeditor/uploadfile/2018/07/20180705095101600.pdf (accessed on 25 March 2(
21. The State Council of the People's Republic of China. China Sets Minimum Sleeping Hours for Children, Teens. Avail online: https://english.www.gov.cn/statecouncil/ministries/202104/03/content_WS6067ac56c6d0719374afc027.html?u source=chatgpt.com (accessed on 25 March 2025).
22. The Chinese Nutrition Society. The Chinese Dietary Guidelines. Available online: http://dg.cnsoc.org/imgnewslist_0602_2. (accessed on 26 April 2025).
23. Zhu, H.; Wu, Q.; Zhang, R.; Zhang, Z.; Feng, Y.; Liu, T.; Liu, D.; Chen, X.; Dong, X. Protective Association of Weekend Catch-up S with Metabolic Syndrome in Chinese Children and Adolescents with Sleep Insufficiency. *Sleep Med.* **2025**, *133*, 106654. [CrossRef]
24. Subspecialty Group of Nephrology, the Society of Pediatrics, Chinese Medical Association; Editorial Board, Chinese Journa Pediatrics. Clinical practice guideline for early screening of pediatric chronic kidney disease in China (version 2021). *Chi Pediatr.* **2022**, *60*, 858–868. [CrossRef]
25. Astudillo, Y.; Kibrom, S.; Pereira, T.; Solomon, S.; Krishnan, S.; Samsonov, D. Association between Anxiety and Elevated Bl Pressure in Adolescent Patients: A Single-Center Cross-Sectional Study. *J. Hypertens.* **2024**, *42*, 644. [CrossRef]
26. Rutigliano, I.; De Filippo, G.; Pastore, L.; Messina, G.; Agostoni, C.; Campanozzi, A. Obesity-Related Hypertension in Pediat the Impact of American Academy of Pediatrics Guidelines. *Nutrients* **2021**, *13*, 2586. [CrossRef]
27. Roush, G.C. Obesity-Induced Hypertension: Heavy on the Accelerator. *J. Am. Heart Assoc. Cardiovasc. Cerebrovasc. Dis.* **2** *8*, e012334. [CrossRef]
28. Kim, M.S.; Kim, W.J.; Khera, A.V.; Kim, J.Y.; Yon, D.K.; Lee, S.W.; Shin, J.I.; Won, H.-H. Association between Adiposity Cardiovascular Outcomes: An Umbrella Review and Meta-Analysis of Observational and Mendelian Randomization Stuc *Eur. Heart J.* **2021**, *42*, 3388–3403. [CrossRef]
29. Guerrero-Romero, F.; Simental-Mendía, L.E.; González-Ortiz, M.; Martínez-Abundis, E.; Ramos-Zavala, M.G.; Hernández-Gonz S.O.; Jacques-Camarena, O.; Rodríguez-Morán, M. The Product of Triglycerides and Glucose, a Simple Measure of Insulin Sensiti Comparison with the Euglycemic-Hyperinsulinemic Clamp. *J. Clin. Endocrinol. Metab.* **2010**, *95*, 3347–3351. [CrossRef]

Simental-Mendía, L.E.; Hernández-Ronquillo, G.; Gamboa-Gómez, C.I.; Gómez-Díaz, R.; Rodríguez-Morán, M.; Guerrero-Romero, F. The Triglycerides and Glucose Index Is Associated with Elevated Blood Pressure in Apparently Healthy Children and Adolescents. *Eur. J. Pediatr.* **2019**, *178*, 1069–1074. [CrossRef]

Xu, J.; Xu, W.; Chen, G.; Hu, Q.; Jiang, J. Association of TyG Index with Prehypertension or Hypertension: A Retrospective Study in Japanese Normoglycemia Subjects. *Front. Endocrinol.* **2023**, *14*, 1288693. [CrossRef]

Xin, F.; He, S.; Zhou, Y.; Jia, X.; Zhao, Y.; Zhao, H. The Triglyceride Glucose Index Trajectory Is Associated with Hypertension: A Retrospective Longitudinal Cohort Study. *Cardiovasc. Diabetol.* **2023**, *22*, 347. [CrossRef]

Parvanova, A.; Reseghetti, E.; Abbate, M.; Ruggenenti, P. Mechanisms and Treatment of Obesity-Related Hypertension—Part 1: Mechanisms. *Clin. Kidney J.* **2023**, *17*, sfad282. [CrossRef]

Dorresteijn, J.A.N.; Visseren, F.L.J.; Spiering, W. Mechanisms Linking Obesity to Hypertension. *Obes. Rev. Off. J. Int. Assoc. Study Obes.* **2012**, *13*, 17–26. [CrossRef]

Lin, M.; Chen, X.; Wu, M.; Xiao, J.; Li, S.; Tang, H.; Tan, X.; Chen, Y. Interactive Effects of Abdominal Obesity and Insulin Resistance on Cardiometabolic Risk. *Rev. Espanola Cardiol. Engl. Ed.* **2025**, *in press*. [CrossRef]

Zhang, T.; Zhang, H.; Li, S.; Li, Y.; Liu, Y.; Fernandez, C.; Harville, E.; Bazzano, L.; He, J.; Chen, W. Impact of Adiposity on Incident Hypertension Is Modified by Insulin Resistance in Adults: Longitudinal Observation from the Bogalusa Heart Study. *Hypertension* **2016**, *67*, 56–62. [CrossRef]

Li, Y.; Wang, L.; Feng, X.; Zhang, M.; Huang, Z.; Deng, Q.; Zhou, M.; Astell-Burt, T.; Wang, L. Geographical Variations in Hypertension Prevalence, Awareness, Treatment and Control in China: Findings from a Nationwide and Provincially Representative Survey. *J. Hypertens.* **2018**, *36*, 178–187. [CrossRef] [PubMed]

Kerr, J.A.; Patton, G.C.; Cini, K.I.; Abate, Y.H.; Abbas, N.; Magied, A.H.A.A.A.; ElHafeez, S.A.; Abd-Elsalam, S.; Abdollahi, A.; Abdoun, M.; et al. Global, Regional, and National Prevalence of Child and Adolescent Overweight and Obesity, 1990–2021, with Forecasts to 2050: A Forecasting Study for the Global Burden of Disease Study 2021. *Lancet* **2025**, *405*, 785–812. [CrossRef] [PubMed]

Li, M.; Chi, X.; Wang, Y.; Setrerrahmane, S.; Xie, W.; Xu, H. Trends in Insulin Resistance: Insights into Mechanisms and Therapeutic Strategy. *Signal Transduct. Target. Ther.* **2022**, *7*, 216. [CrossRef] [PubMed]

Yang, Y.; Li, Y.; Yuan, H.; Tang, Z.; Chen, M.; Cai, S.; Piao, W.; Nan, J.; Li, F.; Yu, D.; et al. Hypertension-Related Status and Influencing Factors among Chinese Children and Adolescents Aged 6~17 Years: Data from China Nutrition and Health Surveillance (2015–2017). *Nutrients* **2024**, *16*, 2685. [CrossRef]

Cao, Q.; Li, D.; Yu, W.; Guo, Q.; Zhao, L.; Yu, D.; Wang, Y. Consistency between the electronic and mercury sphygmomanometer in children and adolescents on blood pressure measuring. *Wei Sheng Yan Jiu* **2016**, *45*, 758–765.

Dong, J.; Dong, H.; Yan, Y.; Cheng, H.; Zhao, X.; Mi, J. Prevalence of Hypertension and Hypertension Phenotypes after Three Visits in Chinese Urban Children. *J. Hypertens.* **2022**, *40*, 1270–1277. [CrossRef]

Saad, M.F.; Lillioja, S.; Nyomba, B.L.; Castillo, C.; Ferraro, R.; De Gregorio, M.; Ravussin, E.; Knowler, W.C.; Bennett, P.H.; Howard, B.V. Racial Differences in the Relation between Blood Pressure and Insulin Resistance. *N. Engl. J. Med.* **1991**, *324*, 733–739. [CrossRef]

nutrients

MDPI

Article

Integrating Metabolomics and Gut Microbiota to Identify Key Biomarkers and Regulatory Pathways Underlying Metabolic Heterogeneity in Childhood Obesity

Zhiwei Xia [1,2], Yan Li [1], Jiyong Yin [1], Zhaolong Gong [1], Jing Sun [1], Shi Shen [1], Yi Yang [3], Tingting Liu [1], Liyuan Wang [1] and Junsheng Huo [1,*]

1 NHC Key Laboratory of Public Nutrition and Health, National Institute of Nutrition and Health, Chinese Center for Disease Control and Prevention, Beijing 100050, China; yinjy@ninh.chinacdc.cn (J.Y.); wangly@ninh.chinacdc.cn (L.W.)

2 Department of School Health, Beijing Center for Disease Control and Prevention, Beijing 100013, China

3 Key Laboratory of Diagnostic and Traceability Technologies for Food Poisoning, Beijing Center for Disease Control and Prevention, Beijing 100013, China

* Correspondence: huojs@ninh.chinacdc.cn

Abstract: Background/Objectives: Individuals with childhood obesity exhibit significant metabolic heterogeneity, necessitating precise biomarkers for risk stratification and assessment. This multi-omics investigation characterizes metabolic and microbial signatures underlying divergent metabolic phenotypes in the context of pediatric obesity. Methods: We analyzed 285 Chinese children (5–7 years) stratified into five groups: wasting (WAS, $n = 55$), metabolically healthy/unhealthy and normal weight (MHWH, $n = 54$; MUWH, $n = 67$), and metabolically healthy/unhealthy obesity (MHO, $n = 36$; MUO, $n = 73$). Untargeted metabolomics (Orbitrap ID-X Tribrid™) and 16S rRNA sequencing were integrated with multivariate analyses (OPLS-DA with VIP > 1, FDR < 0.05; Maaslin 2 with TSS normalization and BH correction, FDR < 0.10). Results: Analysis identified 225 differential metabolites and 12 bacterial genera. The proportion of steroids and their derivatives among differential metabolites in the MUO/MHO group was significantly lower than that in the OVOB/NOR and OVOB/WAS groups (2.12% vs. 7.9–14.1%). MUO displayed elevated C17 sphinganine and LysoPC (O-18:0) levels but reduced PI (16:0/14:1) levels. In contrast, OVOB showed upregulated glycerol phospholipids (LPCs and PSs) and downregulated PE species (e.g., PE(16:0/16:0)) as well as gut microbiota dysbiosis characterized by a higher Firmicutes/Bacteroidetes (F/B) ratio (2.07 vs. 1.24 in controls, $p = 0.009$) and reduced α diversity (Ace index, Chao1 index, and Shannon index values were lower in the OVOB group, Shannon index: 2.96 vs. 3.45, $p = 0.03$). SCFA-producing genera were negatively correlated with the OVOB group, while positively associated with PE(16:0/16:0). Internal validation showed differential metabolites had potential predictive efficacy for MUO/MHO (AUC = 0.967) and OVOB/NOR (AUC = 0.888). Conclusions: We identified distinct lipid disruptions characterizing obesity subtypes, including steroid/terpene deficits and sphingolipid/ether lipid dysregulation in the MUO/MHO groups as well as phospholipid imbalance (↑LPC/PS↓PE) in the OVOB/NOR groups. The gut microbiota exhibited a profile characterized by low diversity, an increased F/B ratio, and a reduced abundance of SCFA-producing genera. These findings suggest potential biomarkers for childhood obesity stratification, though further validation is warranted.

Keywords: childhood obesity; multi-omics; metabolic heterogeneity; gut microbiota; metabolomics

 https://doi.org/10.3390/nu17111

1. Introduction

1.1. Global Burden and Clinical Significance of Childhood Obesity

Obesity has emerged as a major public health crisis, significantly increasing the risk of chronic diseases such as cardiovascular disorders, type 2 diabetes, and metabolic syndrome, thereby imposing substantial economic and societal burdens [1,2]. In particular, childhood obesity is alarmingly prevalent, with global rates quadrupling since 1990, affecting approximately 159 million children and adolescents in 2022 [1]. In China, the obesity rate among school-aged children surged from 0.1% in 1985 to 7.9% in 2020 [3,4], with projections exceeding 15% by 2030 [5]. Beyond its role as an independent risk factor for cardiometabolic diseases, obesity exhibits marked metabolic heterogeneity, which critically influences clinical outcomes [6]. For instance, children with metabolically unhealthy obesity (MUO) face a 3- to 5-fold higher risk of cardiovascular events compared to those with metabolically healthy obesity (MHO) [7]. However, conventional metrics such as body mass index (BMI) and popular biomarkers (e.g., blood lipids and insulin resistance indices) lack the sensitivity to distinguish these phenotypes [8]. These methods exhibit certain limitations in early monitoring and warning, risk assessment, and providing insights into specific molecular and biochemical changes during the development of obesity [9]. Consequently, these limitations hinder classified management as well as precise prevention and control of obesity [10].

1.2. Metabolic Heterogeneity in Pediatric Obesity: Challenges in Phenotyping

MHO refers to individuals who reach the obesity criteria but do not exhibit adverse metabolic effects, including IR, impaired glucose tolerance, dyslipidemia, and hypertension [7,11]. The transition from "metabolically healthy" to "unhealthy" states in pediatric obesity is driven by multifaceted interactions among genetic predisposition, epigenetic modifications, and environmental exposures [12]. Although adult obesity studies have identified branched-chain amino acids (BCAAs), aromatic amino acids (AAAs), and acylcarnitines as key obesity risk factors [13,14], these findings cannot be directly extrapolated to children due to developmental dynamics. One study reported that further metabolic pathway analysis of fatty acid biosynthesis, phenylalanine metabolism, and leucine and valine degradation can help to distinguish differences between childhood MHO and MUO individuals [15]. A study on the lipid profile characteristics of Danish children and adolescents showed that 142 lipid types showed significant differences in obese children; in particular, sphingolipids (such as ceramide) and PE (phosphatidylethanolamine) were significantly increased, whereas lysophospholipids (such as LysoPE and LysoPC) were significantly decreased in the obesity group [16]. However, these results were not observed in all populations of children due to different races, regions, ages, and lifestyle influences such as diet and exercise [17]. In addition, the diagnostic criteria of MHO and MUO in obese children are controversial, and simple indicators such as blood pressure, lipid, blood glucose, and waist circumference cannot accurately distinguish their metabolic differences and subsequent complications [11]. Such limitations highlight the necessity of pediatric-specific multi-omics investigations to elucidate metabolic pathways unique to childhood obesity.

1.3. Gut Microbiota in Obesity: Current Evidence and Controversies

The gut microbiota constantly interacts with the host and plays an important role in maintaining the host's energy metabolism balance and immunity [18]. Over the past 5 years, numerous cross-sectional studies have shown that the gut microbiota of obese children is characterized by an increase in the relative abundance of Firmicutes, a decrease in the abundance of Bacteroidetes, an increase in the abundance of opportunistic pathogens, and a decrease in the abundance of probiotics [19,20]. However, studies and observations that dispute the above results have also been reported. For example, Chen compared the fecal flora of 28 obese children and 23 healthy children and did not observe a significant difference in the ratio of Firmicutes to Bacteroides (F/B) between the two groups [21]. Existing studies have not reached a consensus on the characteristics of the intestinal flora unique to obese children. Challenges remain, including population heterogeneity, an excessive focus on the differences in dominant bacteria genera, and a lack of dedicated databases. For example, *Akkerman mucophilic* has been identified as part of the next generation of probiotics that are highly beneficial to human metabolic health, despite its low proportion in the overall flora [22].

1.4. Objective of This Study

Childhood obesity combined with metabolic heterogeneous phenotypes shows different characteristics of gut microbiota composition and serum metabolomic profiles [7,23]. Studies have shown that the gut microbiota and its metabolites can interact with the enteric nervous system and the central nervous system in a bidirectional manner through two pathways: enteroendocrine and neurosecretion [18,24,25]. This bidirectional pattern is called the gut–brain axis [26]. The metabolic active products of the gut microbiota, such as short-chain fatty acids (SCFAs), bile acids, and acidic metabolites, as well as vitamin K, vitamin B12, biotin, and folic acid, affect hypothalamic inflammation, satiety signals, energy expenditure, and food intake through the gut–brain axis, thereby establishing a connection with the occurrence and development of obesity [18,27]. Meanwhile, lifestyle behaviors related to obesity, such as diet and exercise, can directly act on the gut microbiota. One study reported that a high-fat or high-carbohydrate diet induces an inflammatory response at the base of the hypothalamus through the gut–brain axis, causing central resistance to leptin (an appetite-regulating hormone) [28].

Therefore, this study conducted an untargeted metabolomic and 16S rRNA sequencing analysis of 285 Chinese children aged 5–7 years to uncover multiple omics features and potential biomarkers of childhood obesity and its associated metabolic phenotypes. This study also sought to explore possible biological pathways leading to obesity and abnormal metabolic phenotypes. We conducted a correlation analysis between differential metabolites and differential bacterial genera to explore possible metabolic or regulatory networks. In addition, this study not only focuses on the overall characteristics of obese children but also further subdivides metabolic phenotypes (such as MHO and MUO) to identify the metabolic and microbial differences between different phenotypes. This study identifies the significant differences between MUO and MHO in terms of metabolic pathways (lipid metabolism and sphingoid metabolism) and key metabolites (LysoPC and PE), highlighting the correlations between key differentiator genera and serum metabolites. We hypothesize that different obese children exhibit different characteristics of the gut microbiota and serum metabolites (for example, a reduction in the taxonomic groups that produce SCFA and dysregulation of lipid metabolites), and the interaction between bacterial genera and metabolites could be observed.

2. Materials and Methods

2.1. Study Design and Participants

This cross-sectional study utilized data from "Nutrition and Health Influencing Factors Cohort Survey and Intervention" (Project No. 102393220020070000016). Participants were recruited from a population of 1078 children aged 5–7 years in 2023. Anthropometric measurements (height and weight), dietary behaviors, and biological samples (blood and feces) were collected using standardized questionnaires.

Nutritional status was classified according to the 2007 WHO growth standards using age- and sex-specific BMI Z-scores (BMIZ) as follows: wasting (WAS), BMIZ < −2 SD (n = 55); overweight/obesity (OVOB), BMIZ > +1 SD (n = 109); and normal weight (NOR), BMIZ between −2 SD and +1 SD (n = 121, matched according to gender and age). Exclusion criteria included the following: (1) incomplete blood samples or unqualified specimens (hemolysis and chylous blood); (2) antibiotic/probiotic use within three months prior to enrollment; (3) diarrhea, constipation, and fever or diseases such as pediatric diarrhea and pediatric constipation diagnosed by a doctor within the past two weeks; and (4) severe clinically diagnosed metabolic diseases or neuroendocrine diseases (e.g., diabetes and congenital hypothyroidism). Metabolic phenotypes were further stratified based on consensus definitions [29], including triglycerides (TG) $\leq$ 1.7 mmol/L, high-density lipoprotein cholesterol (HDL-C) $\geq$ 1.03 mmol/L, fasting blood glucose (FBG) < 5.6 mmol/L, and systolic and diastolic blood pressure (SBP: systolic blood pressure; DBP: diastolic blood pressure) $\leq$ 90th percentile. When all criteria were met, the individual was considered to have a normal metabolic phenotype. Individuals with one unsatisfactory item were further classified as having an abnormal metabolic phenotype. The final groups included metabolically healthy and weight healthy (MHWH, n = 54); metabolically unhealthy and weight healthy (MUWH, n = 67); metabolically healthy obesity (MHO, n = 36); and metabolically unhealthy obesity (MUO, n = 73). Fecal samples were collected from a subset (n = 42) matched by age, sex, and BMIZ (OVOB (n = 13), WAS (n = 8), and NOR (n = 21)).

All procedures were approved by the Ethics Committee of the National Institute of Nutrition and Health, Chinese Center for Disease Control and Prevention (Approval No. 2018-017), with written informed consent obtained from legal guardians. The research flow design chart is shown in Figure 1.

2.2. *Questionnaire Survey*

A self-designed questionnaire was used to collect demographic characteristics (age, sex, parental occupation/education level, primary caregiver status, and annual household income), perinatal factors (birth weight, birth length, breastfeeding duration, formula feeding, and micronutrient supplementation), semi-quantitative food frequency questionnaire (FFQ), health status survey (antibiotic/probiotic use in the past three months; diseases and related symptoms, such as diarrhea, constipation, and fever in the past two weeks), and parents' attitude toward nutrition knowledge. The questionnaire was completed by the child and the guardian. The on-site quality control officer checked the logic and completeness, and the errors or missing items were corrected immediately.

2.3. *Anthropometry*

Certified technicians performed measurements in compliance with WS/T 424-2013 national standards [30]. A height measuring instrument (accuracy 0.1 cm) and electronic weight scale (accuracy 0.05 kg), which were verified by the quality inspection department, were used to measure height and weight. Measurements were performed in a quiet, spacious, level, and solid environment according to the requirements of pediatric hygiene. Blood pressure was measured in accordance with the American Heart Association pediatric guidelines (Flynn et al., 2017 [31]). After a 10 min rest in a seated position, three consecutive readings were obtained from the right arm using a validated oscillometric device (OMRON HEM-7121, OMRON Healthcare Co., Ltd.,Kyoto, Japan) with appropriate cuff sizes (covering 80–100% of the arm circumference). The average of the last two measurements was recorded for analysis.

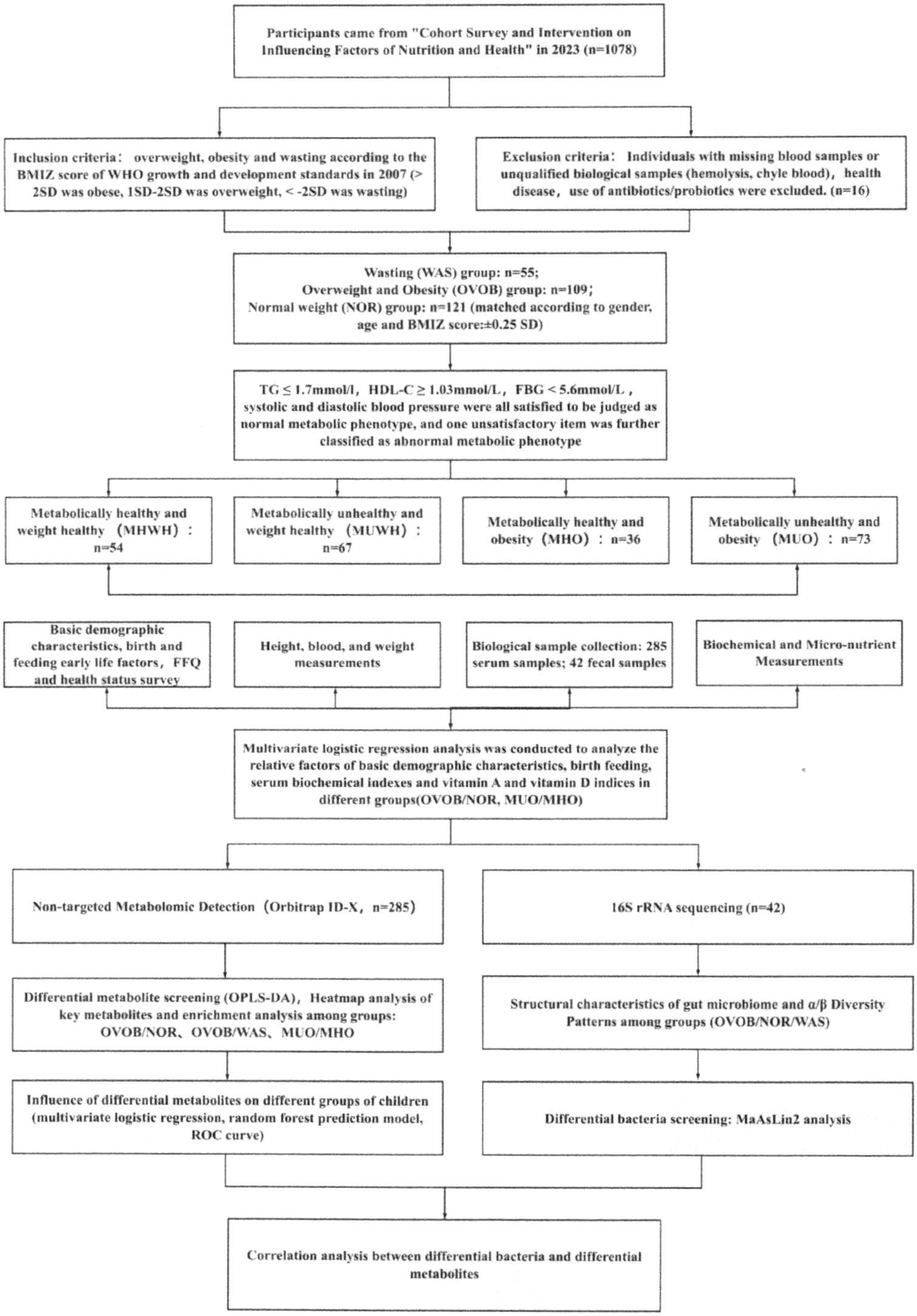

Figure 1. Research flow design chart.

2.4. Biological Sample Collection

Sample collection and processing: (1) Blood sample: A 3 mL sample of venous blood from the survey subjects was collected using vacuum blood collection tubes, and the blood was inverted 5 times immediately after blood collection. After leaving at room temperature for 20–30 min, the sample was centrifuged at 3000 RPM for 15 min to separate the serum. The serum was transferred to a serum freezing tube for temporary storage at −20 °C and then transported to −80 °C for long-term storage. (2) Fecal samples: A sterile fecal collection tube with spoon and fecal protection solution were used to collect the subjects' first stool in the morning. A spoonful of central inner stool (about 2 g) free of water and urine contamination was obtained using the plastic spoon. After adding the fecal protection solution, it was temporarily stored at −20 °C and transported to −80 °C for storage. All samples were tested for serum metabolomics and fecal 16S rRNA in the same batch.

2.5. Biochemical and Micronutrient Measurements

Serum biochemical parameters, including total cholesterol (TC), TG, HDL-C, low-density lipoprotein cholesterol (LDL-C), FBG, alanine aminotransferase (ALT), aspartate aminotransferase (AST), high-sensitivity C-reactive protein (CRP-H), adenosine diphosphate (ADP), and minerals (calcium, Ca; iron, Fe; and zinc, Zn), were analyzed using a Hitachi 7020 Automatic Biochemical Analyzer (Hitachi High-Technologies Corporation, Tokyo, Japan) with commercial assay kits (Leadman Biochemistry Co., Ltd., Beijing, China). Two-level quality controls (Leadman Biochemistry Co., Ltd., Beijing, China) were analyzed daily.

According to the "WS/T 553-2017" [32] and "WS/T 677-2020" [33] methods, serum vitamin A and 25(OH)D2/D3 levels were determined using high-performance liquid chromatography mass spectrometry (HPLC-MS/MS: Waters Corporation, Milford, MA, USA). Quantitative determination was performed using the isotope internal standard method.

2.6. Nontargeted Metabolomic Detection

2.6.1. Reagents and Instrumentation

Mass spectrum-grade solvents (methanol and acetonitrile) and formic acid were procured from Fisher Scientific (Hampton, NH, USA). Ultra-pure water (18.2 MΩ·cm) was generated using a Milli-Q® Integral system (MilliporeSigma, Burlington, MA, USA). Sample preparation involved a refrigerated centrifuge (Eppendorf 5430 R, Hamburg, Germany), ultrasonic processor (KQ5200E, Kunshan Ultrasonic Instruments Co., Ltd., Kunshan, China), and a Thermo Scientific™ Orbitrap ID-X Tribrid™ mass spectrometer equipped with a heated electrospray ionization (HESI) source (Thermo Fisher Scientific, San Jose, CA, USA).

2.6.2. Sample Preparation

Serum aliquots (100 μL) were subjected to a methanol-based extraction protocol: (1) rapid thawing at 4 °C; (2) protein precipitation with 900 μL ice-cold methanol (1:9 *v/v*) with 1 min of vortex mixing; (3) ultrasonication in an ice bath (20 min); (4) centrifugation (13,000× *g*, 4 °C, 10 min); and (5) secondary centrifugation (13,000× *g*, 4 °C, 5 min) for supernatant clarification. Dried residues were reconstituted in 300 μL methanol (0.1% formic acid) and filtered through 0.22 μm PTFE membranes (MilliporeSigma, MA, USA). Pooled quality control (QC) samples were generated by combining 30 μL aliquots from each specimen.

2.6.3. Chromatographic Conditions

Chromatographic separation utilized an Acquity UPLC BEH C18 column (100 mm × 2.1 mm, 1.8 μm; Waters, Milford, MA, USA) maintained at 35 °C. Mobile phases consisted of (A)

0.1% formic acid in water and (B) 0.1% formic acid in acetonitrile. The following gradient elution program was implemented: 5–20% B (0–2.0 min), 20–60% B (2.0–5.0 min), 60–99% B (5.0–6.0 min), 99% B (6.0–7.5 min), returning to 5% B (7.6–10.0 min) at 0.4 mL/min flow rate. The injection volume was 5 μL.

2.6.4. Mass Spectrometric Parameters

Data acquisition employed dual-polarity HESI mode with the following settings:

Positive ion mode: spray voltage 3.8 kV, capillary temperature 325 °C, vaporizer temperature 400 °C, sheath gas 50 arb, and auxiliary gas 10 arb; full-scan MS (m/z 100–1000) at 120,000 resolution; HCD fragmentation at normalized collision energies (15%, 30%, 45%) with 8 dependent scans; and negative ion mode: spray voltage 3.0 kV with identical thermal parameters. Mass axis calibration used leucine enkephalin ($[M+H]^+$: 556.2771; $[M-H]^-$: 554.2627). Preanalysis mass calibration employed FlexMix™ solution (Thermo Scientific).

2.6.5. Quality Assurance Protocol

System suitability testing involved (1) 10 blank (methanol) injections and (2) 10 consecutive QC injections for column equilibration. Experimental samples were analyzed in randomized order with QC injections every 10 samples. Data acquisition required QC peak intensity RSD < 15% and retention time drift < 0.1 min.

2.7. Gut Microbiota 16S rRNA Detection

The 16S rRNA gene sequencing analysis was conducted in collaboration with BGI Genomics (Shenzhen, China). Fecal DNA extraction was performed using the DNeasy PowerSoil Pro Kit (Qiagen Inc., Germantown, MD, USA), following the manufacturer's protocol with bead-beating homogenization (5 min at 30 Hz) to ensure microbial lysis efficiency. DNA purity and concentration were quantified using a NanoDrop 2000 spectrophotometer (Thermo Fisher Scientific Inc., Waltham, MA, USA), with A260/A280 ratios maintained between 1.8 and 2.0. DNA integrity was verified with 1% agarose gel electrophoresis (100 V, 40 min), demonstrating distinct bands > 15 kb.

A total of 30 ng of qualified genomic DNA samples and the corresponding fusion primers were taken to configure the PCR reaction system, and the PCR reaction parameters were set for PCR expansion. The PCR amplification products were purified using Agencourt AMPure XP magnetic beads (Beckman Coulter, Inc., Brea, CA, USA) and dissolved in elution buffer and labeled, completing the library construction. The fragment range and concentration of the library were detected using an Agilent 2100 Bioanalyzer (Agilent Technologies, Inc., Santa Clara, CA, USA). Qualified libraries are selected based on the size of the inserted fragments. Sequencing was performed on the HiSeq platform (Illumina, Inc., San Diego, CA, USA).

2.8. Data Analysis

2.8.1. Omics Data Preprocessing

Raw mass spectrometry data were processed using Progenesis QI software (v3.0, Waters Corporation, MA, USA) with a standardized workflow: (1) peak detection with adaptive sensitivity thresholds (minimum peak width = 0.1 min); (2) retention time alignment using a dynamic time warping algorithm; (3) baseline correction using asymmetric least squares smoothing; (4) spectral deconvolution with ApexTrack™ integration; and (5) intra-batch normalization based on total ion current. The three-dimensional matrix (m/z-retention time-peak intensity) was annotated against the Human Metabolome Database (HMDB, https://hmdb.ca/) (accessed on 15 September 2024) and LIPID MAPS® database (https://www.lipidmaps.org) (accessed on 20 October 2024) using the following dual-filter criteria: (i) mass accuracy tolerance $\leq$ 5 ppm and (ii) isotopic pattern similarity score >80%. Nonendogenous metabolites (pharmaceuticals, environmental xenobiotics, and dietary biomarkers) were systematically excluded with database cross-referencing and manual validation.

The raw sequencing data were processed as follows to obtain clean data: (1) for the reads that match the primers, the software cutadapt v2.6 was used to remove the primers and connectors to obtain the fragments of the target area; (2) the method of removing low-quality reads was performed, with the window length set as 30 bp. If the average quality value of the window is less than 20, the read end sequence starting from the window is removed, and reads with a final read length less than 75% of the original read length are excluded; (3) reads containing N were removed; (4) low-complexity reads (10 consecutive ATCGs) were removed to obtain the final clean data. The software USEARCH (v7.0.1090) was used to cluster the spliced Tags into OTUs. The main process is as follows: (1) clustering using UPARSE at a 97% similarity to obtain the representative OTU sequences; (2) using UCHIME (v4.2.40) to remove the chimeras generated by PCR amplification from the representative OTU sequences; and (3) using the usearch_global method to compare all tags with the OTU representative sequence and obtain the abundance statistics on OTUs for each sample.

2.8.2. Statistical Analysis

Continuous variables with a normal distribution were expressed as means ± standard deviations (SDs), whereas non-normally distributed data were reported as medians with interquartile ranges (IQRs). Categorical variables were summarized as frequencies with percentages (n (%)). For intergroup comparisons, independent two-group analyses of normally distributed data utilized Student's t-test with Levene's test for homogeneity of variance. Multi-group comparisons ($\geq$3 groups) employed one-way analysis of variance (ANOVA) with post hoc LSD tests for normally distributed data. Kruskal–Wallis test with Dunn's correction ($\geq$3 groups) was used for skewed distributions. Categorical variable comparisons were performed using Pearson's chi-square test or Fisher's exact test for small expected frequencies (<5). All statistical analyses were performed using SAS software (v.9.4; SAS Institute Inc.; Cary, NC, USA).

To explore the relationship between childhood obesity and metabolites, multivariate logistic regression analysis was performed using the OVOB group or the MUO group as the dependent variable. Independent variables included demographic characteristics, early nutritional factors, dietary behaviors with statistically significant differences in the univariate analysis, and differential metabolites obtained from the OPLS-DA analysis. For the independent variables identified in the multivariate analysis ($p < 0.05$), the random forest (RF) model was used to predict the importance of differential metabolites related to OVOB or MUO. In this study, the differential metabolites of the OPLS-DA analysis were taken as independent variables, and OVOB or MUO were taken as dependent variables. The importance of the variables was quantified based on the mean decrease in the Gini index, and the RF model was trained with 500 trees, and feature importance was validated using 10-fold cross-validation repeated 5 times to ensure stability. Permutation tests (n = 1000) were performed to assess significance of AUC values. The RF model was implemented using the "random forest" package (version 4.7-1.1) in R version 4.5.0 (R Foundation for Statistical Computing, Vienna, Austria). A graphical receiver operating characteristic (ROC) curve was generated, and the area under the ROC curve (AUC) was utilized as a performance metric to assess the model's effectiveness. A p value of less than 0.05, based on two-tailed test results, was considered statistically significant. All analyses were conducted using R version 4.5.0.

Metabolomic analysis was performed using MetaboAnalyst 6.0 (https://www.metaboanalyst.ca/) (accessed on 15 November 2024) to conduct multivariate statistical analysis and data visualization of sample differences. Principal component analysis (PCA) and partial least squares discriminant analysis (PLS-DA) were initially employed to characterize metabolic profile variations. Subsequently, orthogonal projections to latent structures discriminant analysis (OPLS-DA) was implemented for rigorous screening of differential metabolites between experimental groups. The following selection criteria were applied: variable importance in projection (VIP) score ≥ 1, false discovery rate (FDR) < 0.05, and significant fold change (FC) thresholds. Metabolic pathway enrichment analysis was subsequently conducted on the identified differential metabolites.

For gut microbiota characterization, α and β diversity analyses were performed using Prism 9.0 (GraphPad Software, Inc., San Diego, CA, USA). The α-diversity was assessed using four complementary indices: Ace (abundance-based coverage estimator), Chao1 (richness estimator), Shannon (diversity index), and Simpson (dominance index). Meanwhile, β diversity was determined using analysis of similarities (ANOSIM) based on Bray–Curtis distance matrices. We removed taxa existing in <10% of the samples to avoid the zero-inflated distributions, reducing the dataset from 389 to 209 genera (Table S1). Owing to the inherent sparsity and limited sample size of the data in our exploratory study, we used MaAsLin2 (version 1.22.0; Huttenhower Lab, Harvard T.H. Chan School of Public Health, Boston, MA, USA) to analyze the association between differential abundance and study groups. MaAsLin2 analysis was performed using total sum scaling (TSS) normalization with Log2 transformation to account for compositional data characteristics. The analysis method was performed using a linear model (LM). Covariates (fixed_effects: age, sex, and dietary) were included in the model to control for confounding effects, and multiple test corrections were performed using the Benjamini–Hochberg method (BH); associations with FDR < 0.10 were considered exploratory given the small sample size and should be interpreted with caution. Additionally, we have implemented random effects in our computational approach to more accurately capture between-individual and between-group variations, thereby enhancing the reliability of our results. The normalized microbial data were imported into R (version 4.5.0). Visualization was performed using ggplot2 (version 3.5.2). Finally, Spearman's rank correlation analysis ($p < 0.05$) was conducted to elucidate potential interactions between differential metabolites and discriminant bacterial taxa.

3. Results

3.1. Characteristics of Study Participants

The study comprised 285 children aged 5–7 years (73.2 $\pm$ 5.8 month; 164 boys (57.5%)), stratified into five BMIZ and metabolic phenotype-matched groups: WAS ($n = 55$), MHWH ($n = 54$), MUWH ($n = 67$), MHO ($n = 36$), and MUO ($n = 73$). Demographic characteristics revealed comparable age and gender distributions across groups ($p = 0.149$ and $p = 0.868$, respectively). However, significant intergroup variations emerged in geographic distribution (Henan/Guizhou), birth weight, breastfeeding ratio, and breastfeeding duration (all $p < 0.05$; Table 1).

	All (n = 285)	WAS (n = 55)	NOR			OVOB			F/χ^2	p
			MHWH (n = 54)	MUWH (n = 67)	All (n = 121)	MHO (n = 36)	MUO (n = 73)	All (n = 109)		
Age [a], m	73.2 ± 5.8	72.6 ± 5.7	72.9 ± 4.7	73.2 ± 4.8	73.1 ± 4.8	73.9 ± 6.2	71.7 ± 6.6	72.4 ± 6.5	1.772	0.149
Gender [b]										
Boy	164 (57.5)	30 (54.5)	30 (18.3)	38 (23.2)	68 (56.2)	20 (12.2)	46 (28)	66 (60.6)	1.261	0.868
Girl	121 (42.5)	25 (45.5)	24 (19.8)	29 (24)	53 (43.8)	16 (13.2)	27 (22.3)	43 (39.4)		
BMIZ [a,c]	0.276 ± 1.86	−2.35 ± 0.39	−0.37 ± 0.65	−0.12 ± 0.68	−0.23 ± 0.68	2.1 ± 1.11	2.18 ± 1.06	2.16 ± 1.08	298.987	<0.001
District [b]										
Henan	149 (100.0)	19 (12.8)	36 (24.2)	37 (24.8)	73 (49.0)	24 (16.1)	3 3(22.1)	57 (38.3)	16.098	0.003
Guizhou	136 (100.0)	36 (26.5)	18 (13.2)	30 (22.1)	48 (35.3)	12 (8.8)	40 (29.4)	52 (38.2)		
Nation [b]										
Han Chinese	207 (100)	33 (15.9)	44 (21.3)	53 (25.6)	97 (59.1)	27 (13)	50 (24.2)	77 47.0)	8.685	0.069
Ethnic minorities	78 (100)	22 (28.2)	10 (12.8)	14 (17.9)	24 (19.8)	9 (11.5)	23 (29.5)	32 (26.4)		
Birth weight [a], kg	3.29 ± 0.44	3.08 ± 0.47	3.25 ± 0.40	3.26 ± 0.43	3.26 ± 0.42	3.47 ± 0.36	3.41 ± 0.43	3.43 ± 0.41	3.225	0.024
Birth height [a], cm	50.24 ± 1.26	49.83 ± 1.29	50.09 ± 1.21	50.38 ± 1.39	50.25 ± 1.32	50.48 ± 1.26	50.41 ± 1.06	50.44 ± 1.13	0.918	0.433
Breast feeding [b]										
Yes	215 (86.0)	43 (93.5)	46 (90.2)	58 (87.9)	104 (88.9)	29 (93.5)	39 (69.6)	68 (78.2)	13.08	0.004
No	35 (14.0)	3 (6.5)	5 (9.8)	8 (12.1)	13 (11.1)	2 (6.5)	17 (30.4)	19 (21.8)		
Duration of breastfeeding [b], m										
≤6	54 (21.6)	7 (15.2)	11 (21.6)	11 (16.7)	22 (18.8)	6 (19.4)	19 (33.9)	25 (28.7)	35.06	<0.001
6–12	53 (21.2)	9 (19.6)	7 (13.7)	9 (13.6)	16 (13.7)	4 (12.9)	24 (42.9)	28 (32.2)		
≥12	143 (57.2)	30 (65.2)	33 (64.7)	46 (69.7)	79 (67.5)	21 (67.7)	13 (23.2)	34 (39.1)		

[a] Normal distribution is presented as mean ± standard deviation. One-way analysis of variance (ANOVA) was used to test for differences between groups. [b] Categorical or count data are expressed as proportions/rates. Chi-square test was used to analyze differences between groups. [c] BMIZ: body mass index Z-scores.

Birth weight demonstrated significant associations with subsequent weight status independent of metabolic health. The OVOB subgroup exhibited elevated birth weights compared to the NOR and WAS groups (3.43 ± 0.41 kg vs. 3.26 ± 0.42 kg for NOR and 3.08 ± 0.47 kg for WAS; $p < 0.001$). Similar patterns emerged when comparing metabolic phenotypes. MHO participants had higher birth weights than MHWH counterparts (3.54 ± 0.43 kg vs. 3.21 ± 0.39 kg, $p = 0.019$), whereas MUO subjects showed greater birth weights than MUWH peers (3.49 ± 0.41 kg vs. 3.32 ± 0.38 kg, $p = 0.046$). Notably, metabolic health status did not exhibit these associations (MHWH vs. MUWH: $p = 0.845$; MHO vs. MUO: $p = 0.536$). Breastfeeding patterns revealed striking disparities, particularly in the MUO group, which demonstrated substantially higher non-breastfeeding rates (35.4%) compared to other groups (6.5–12.1%). Short-term breastfeeding (≤6 months) predominated in MUO participants (33.9%) relative to the MHO (19.4%) and MUWH (16.7%) groups (Table 1). These findings suggest potential dual impacts of breastfeeding duration on both weight trajectories and metabolic health development. No significant between-group differences emerged in perinatal factors (preterm birth, delivery mode), family structure, or socioeconomic indicators (caregiver education, occupation, and household income; Table A1).

Serum biochemical profiles across metabolic phenotype groups are summarized in Table A2. The MUO group exhibited significantly elevated TG levels (1.67 ± 1.12 mmol/L) compared to other groups (overall $p < 0.001$). LDL-C levels differed significantly among groups ($p = 0.03$), with MHO individuals showing higher values (1.80 ± 0.37 mmol/L) than MUWH participants (1.50 ± 0.53 mmol/L; $p = 0.003$). FBG levels varied significantly across phenotypes ($p = 0.03$). Both MUO (5.61 ± 1.48 mmol/L) and MUWH (5.58 ± 1.71 mmol/L) groups had higher glucose concentrations than their metabolically healthy counterparts (MHO: 5.02 ± 0.93 mmol/L; MHWH: 5.06 ± 0.80 mmol/L; MUO vs. MHO: $p = 0.035$; MUWH vs. MHWH: $p = 0.036$); however, no significant differences were observed between metabolically concordant weight groups (MHO vs. MHWH: $p = 0.910$; MUO vs. MUWH: $p = 0.903$). Metabolic abnormality groups (MUO: 116.83 ± 9.87 mmHg; MUWH: 118.15 ± 8.47 mmHg) exhibited significantly higher SBP than metabolically normal groups (MHO: 107.47 ± 5.12 mmHg; MHWH: 109.20 ± 6.80 mmHg; all $p < 0.01$). Metabolically abnormal groups (MUO: 77.83 ± 8.21 mmHg; MUWH: 78.68 ± 7.76 mmHg) showed elevated DBP compared to metabolically normal groups (MHO: 67.47 ± 5.12 mmHg; MHWH: 69.20 ± 6.80 mmHg; all $p < 0.01$). No differences were observed between metabolically concordant weight groups (MHO vs. MHWH: SBP $p = 0.325$, DBP $p = 0.274$; MUO vs. MUWH: SBP $p = 0.546$, DBP $p = 0.502$). Furthermore, we also observed differences in biochemical outcomes related to obesity such as ADP, ALT, and CRP-H, as detailed in Table A2.

3.2. Metabolomic Characteristics

3.2.1. Metabolic Profile Characteristics

Initial metabolic profiling using principal component analysis (PCA) demonstrated robust analytical reliability. Tight clustering of quality control (QC) samples is observed (Figure A1), confirming system stability throughout the experimental workflow. Although preliminary PCA showed marginal intergroup separation in comparative analyses (OVOB vs. NOR, OVOB vs. WAS, and MUO vs, MHO), subsequent orthogonal partial least squares discriminant analysis (OPLS-DA) achieved effective metabolic profile discrimination across all paired groups: OVOB/NOR ($R^2Y = 0.81$, $Q^2 = 0.69$), OVOB/WAS ($R^2Y = 0.78$, $Q^2 = 0.65$), and MUO/MHO ($R^2Y = 0.73$, $Q^2 = 0.61$). Model validity was rigorously confirmed using permutation testing (200 iterations, $p < 0.001$), demonstrating resistance to overfitting (Figure 2 and Figure S2). These statistically robust OPLS-DA models establish a credible foundation for identifying biologically relevant differential metabolites between comparison groups.

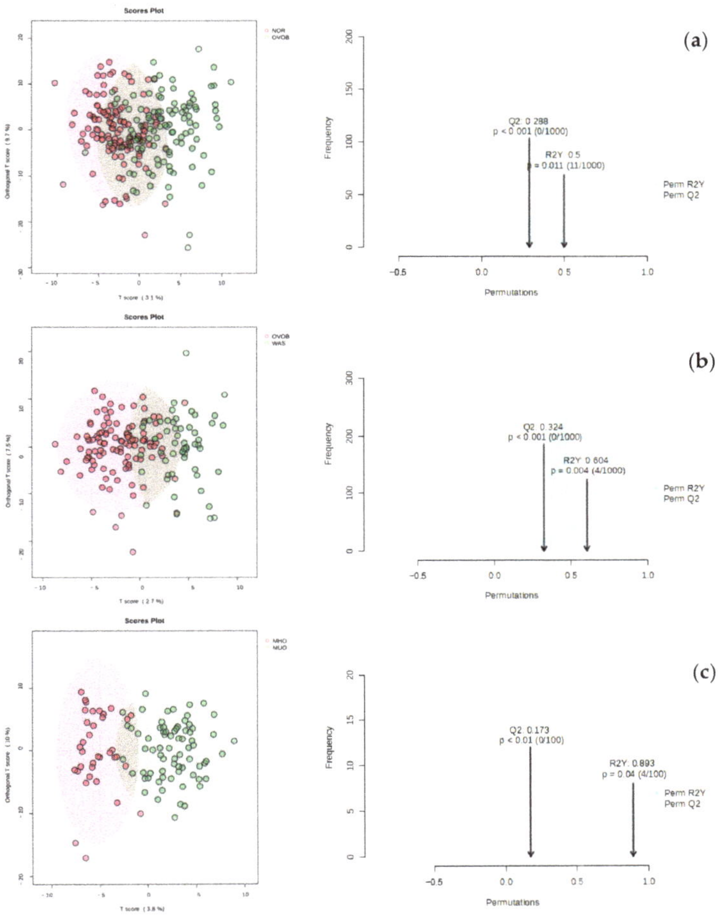

Figure 2. OPLS-DA model and permutation testing results of samples from comparison groups. Columns 1 and 2 are the results of metabolite group difference analysis using OPLS-DA and model permutation testing under positive ion modes, respectively. (**a**) Description of the results of the OPLS-DA and permutation tests for the OVOB/NOR comparison group; (**b**) description of the results of the OPLS-DA and permutation tests for the OVOB/WAS comparison group; (**c**) description of the results of the OPLS-DA and permutation tests for the MUO/MHO comparison group.

3.2.2. Classification of Differential Metabolites

Applying stringent bioinformatic thresholds (VIP $\geq$ 1.0, FDR < 0.05, and FC > 1.2/<0.83), we systematically identified 225 differential metabolites across comparative groups. The predominant metabolite classes included glycerophospholipids (44 metabolites, 19.4%), carboxylic acids and derivatives (43 metabolites, 18.9%), fatty acyls (33 metabolites, 14.5%), steroids and steroid derivatives (18 metabolites, 7.9%), and prenol lipids (16 metabolites, 7.0%). Comparative analysis revealed substantial intergroup heterogeneity in metabolite class distribution (Figure 3). The composition of differential metabolites in the OVOB/NOR group and the OVOB/WAS group is basically consistent with the top five category compositions of all differential metabolites, whereas the composition of differential metabolites in the MUO/MHO group is significantly different from that of other groups. Steroids and their derivatives (MUO/MHO: 2.12%; OVOB/NOR and OVOB/WAS: 7.9–14.1%) and terpene lipids (4.25% vs. 7.0–9.6%) were significantly lower in the MUO/MHO group compared with other groups.

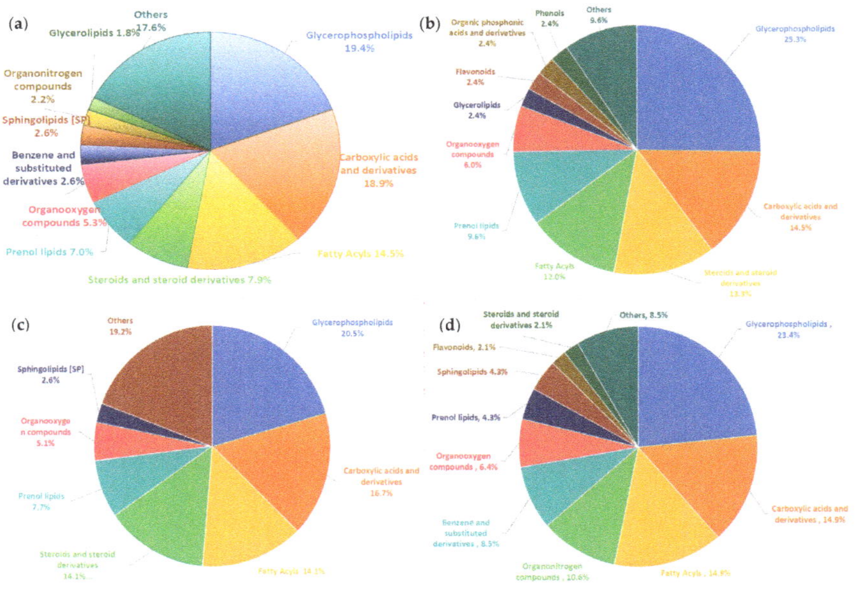

Figure 3. Class distribution of differential metabolites among comparative groups. Differential metabolites were analyzed using OPLS-DA and screened according to VIP $\geq$ 1, FDR < 0.05, FC > 1.2, or FC < 0.83. The primary classification of human metabolites was performed using The Human Metabolome Database (HMDB Version 5.0). (**a**) The distribution of differential metabolites in all groups; (**b**) the distribution of differential metabolites in the OVOB/NOR group; (**c**) the distribution of differential metabolites in the OVOB/WAS group; and (**d**) the distribution of differential metabolites in the MUO/MHO group.

3.2.3. Screening of Differential Metabolites and Pathway Enrichment Analysis

Heatmap visualization of metabolites surpassing stringent fold-change thresholds (FC > 1.5/<0.67) unveiled three distinct obesity-associated metabolic signatures across comparative groups (Figure 4). We observed that lysophosphatidylcholines, such as LysoPC (18:4) (FC = 2.23) and LysoPC (14:1) (FC = 2.16), and phosphatidylserines, such as PS (17:0/0:0) (FC = 1.72) and PS (16:0/16:0) (FC = 1.55), were upregulated in the OVOB group. Inositol 1,3,4-trisphosphate (FC = 0.58), inositol 1,4,5-trisphosphate (FC = 0.64), PE (24:0/14:0) (FC = 0.59), and PE (16:0/16:0) (FC = 0.39) were significantly downregulated in the OVOB group (FDR < 0.05). We also observed a similar situation based on the heatmaps. PS (17:0/0:0) (FC = 2.07), PS (16:0/16:0) (FC = 1.91), and LysoPC (20:5) (FC = 1.65) were enriched in the OVOB group, whereas PE (16:0/16:0) (FC = 51) and 1,3,4-trisphosphate (FC = 0.51) were enriched in the WAS group. Notably, different findings were observed in the MUO/MHO group. LysoPC (O-18:0/0:0) (FC = 1.45), LysoPC (16:1) (FC = 1.24), C16 sphinganine (FC = 1.27), sphinganine (FC = 1.24), phytosphingosine (FC = 1.24), neurine (FC = 1.24), and aminoadipic acid (FC = 1.28) were enriched in the MUO group. PE (16:0/20:4) (FC = 0.78), PI (P-16:0/15:0) (FC = 0.82), and PI (16:0/14:1) (FC = 0.81) were downregulated in the MUO group. Furthermore, we observed that metabolites such as 11-cis-retinol, retinyl beta-glucuronide, and vitamin A were also upregulated in obese children.

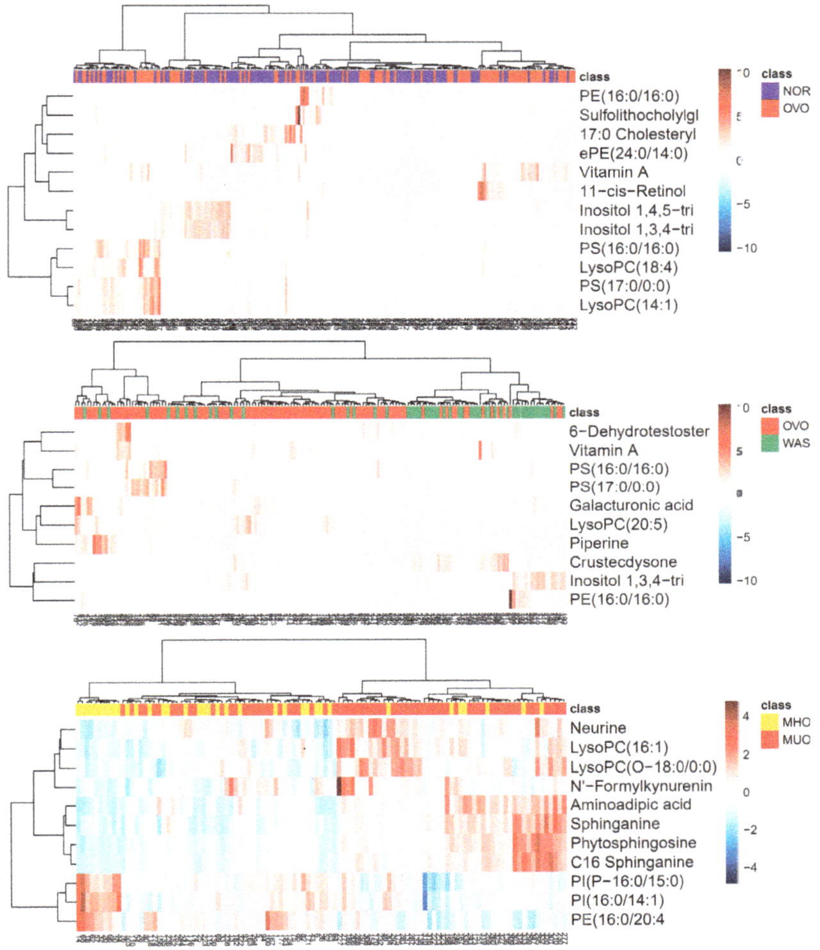

Figure 4. Heatmap analysis of different metabolites between comparative groups. Differential metabolites were screened for heatmap analysis across groups. Metabolites differentiating OVOB/NOR and OVOB/WAS were defined by an FC > 1.5 or FC < 0.67 (VIP $\geq$ 1, FDR < 0.05). Metabolites differentiating MUO/MHO were defined by an FC > 1.2 or FC < 0.83 (VIP $\geq$ 1, FDR < 0.05).

As noted in Figure 5, the differential metabolites in the OVOB/NOR and OVOB/WAS comparisons were co-enriched in glycerophospholipid metabolism and inositol phosphate metabolism. In addition to being enriched in glycerophospholipid metabolism, the differential metabolites of the MUO/MHO comparison also specifically activated ether lipid metabolism (p = 0.0065), sphingolipid metabolism pathways (p = 0.0163), and lysine degradation (pathway impact = 0.11), as detailed in Figure 5. In the MUO/MHO comparison, we found that, in addition to LysoPC (16:1/0:0), which was also identified in the glycerol phospholipid metabolic pathway in previous group comparisons, neurine and PE(16:0/20:4) were also enriched. Key differential metabolites involved in ether lipid metabolism included LysoPC (O-18:0/0:0), while phytosphingosine and sphinganine were enriched in the sphingolipid metabolism pathway. Additionally, aminoadipic acid was identified as the key differential metabolite of lysine degradation (Figure 5).

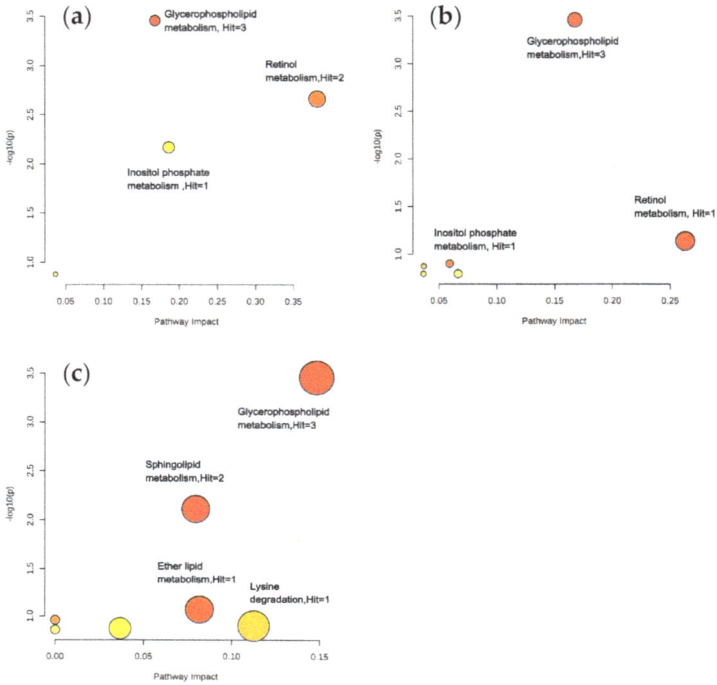

Figure 5. Pathway enrichment analysis of differential metabolites. Differential metabolites identified based on VIP $\geq$ 1, FDR < 0.05, and FC > 1.5/<0.67 were analyzed using MetaboAnalyst 6.0 to assess pathway enrichment. (**a**) Overview of metabolite enrichment sets and bubble diagram for OVOB/NOR, (**b**) OVOB/WAS, and (**c**) MUO/MHO.

3.2.4. Prediction of the Clinical Efficacy of Differential Metabolites

Integrated multivariate logistic regression models incorporating demographic characteristics, early-life nutritional factors, dietary behaviors, and physical activity patterns (Tables A2 and A3) identified statistically significant variables ($p < 0.05$). These variables were subsequently evaluated using random forest modeling to determine variable importance (Figures 6 and 7). The random forest algorithm quantified variable importance based on the mean decrease in the Gini index.

For OVOB/NOR (Figure 6), retinyl β-glucuronide, coroloside, 17:0 cholesteryl ester, cyclocalopin E, LysoPC(14:1), cortisone acetate, vitamin A, body weight, CRP-H, and sulfolithocholyl glycine were identified as top predictors. Diagnostic performance of selected biomarkers was assessed using receiver operating characteristic (ROC) curve analysis. ALT, CRP_H, and the identified metabolites predicted OVOB in children with an AUC of 0.888 (95% CI: 0.847, 0.928), a sensitivity of 76.0%, and a specificity of 86.2%, but external study is needed to confirm generalizability.

For MUO/MHO (Figure 7), PI (16:0/14:1), treosulfan, N′-formylkynurenine, LysoPE (16:0/0:0), elenaic acid, hexaethylene glycol, PS (P-20:0/0:0), ALT, and CRP_H were identified as critical discriminators. These potential biomarkers predicted MUO in obese children with an AUC of 0.967 (95% CI: 0.936, 0.998), a sensitivity of 88.9%, and a specificity of 95.9%.

The high AUC (0.967) in our internal validation suggests potential discriminative power, but external studies are needed to confirm generalizability.

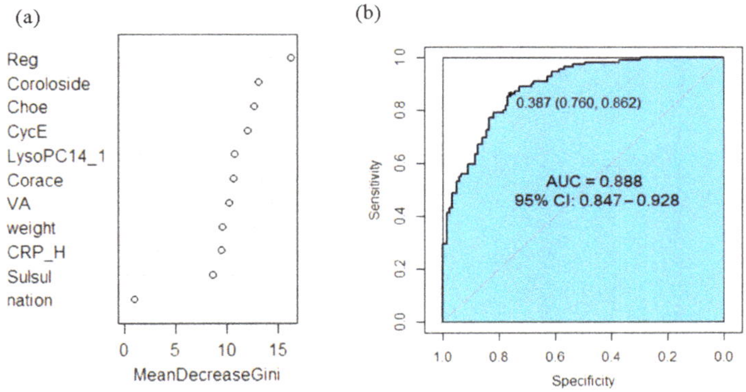

Figure 6. Importance ranking of differential metabolites and efficacy of predicting OVOB. (**a**) Random forest model for importance ranking of metabolites. The random forest algorithm quantified variable importance based on a mean decrease in the Gini index. (**b**) The combined efficacy of weight, nation, CRP_H, VA, and the identified metabolites in predicting OVOB in children had an AUC of 0.888 (95% CI: 0.847, 0.928), with a sensitivity of 76.0% and a specificity of 86.2%. CRP_H, C-reactive protein; Reg, retinyl beta-glucuronide; Choe, 17:0 cholesteryl ester; CycE, cyclocalopin E; LysoPC14_1, LysoPC (14:1); VA, vitamin A; Corace, cortisone acetate; Sulsul, sulfinpyrazone sulfide; weight, birth weight.

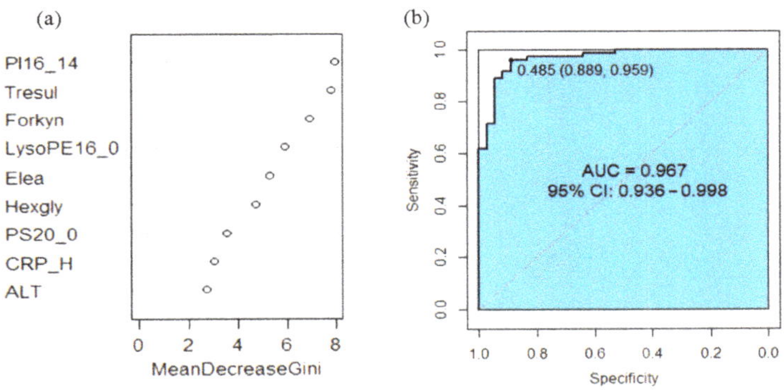

Figure 7. Importance ranking of differential metabolites and efficacy of predicting MUO. (**a**) Random forest model for importance ranking of metabolites. The random forest algorithm quantified variable importance based on a mean decrease in the Gini index. (**b**) The combined efficacy of ALT, CRP_H, and the metabolites in predicting MUO in obese children achieved an AUC of 0.967 (95% CI: 0.936, 0.998), with a sensitivity of 88.9% and a specificity of 95.9%. ALT, alanine aminotransferase; CRP_H, C-reactive protein; PI16_14, PI (16:0/14:1); Tresul, treosulfan; Forkyn, N′-formylkynurenine; LysoPE16_0, LysoPE (16:0/0:0); Elea, elenaic acid; Hexgly, hexaethylene glycol; PS20_0, PS (P-20:0/0:0).

3.3. *Gut Microbiome Characteristics*

3.3.1. Structural Characteristics of the Gut Microbiome

The gut microbiome analysis was performed for 42 children (median age: 76.6 months; 59.5% boys), with no significant differences in age, sex, delivery method, whether breastfeeding, and breastfeeding duration across WAS, NOR, and OVOB groups ($p > 0.05$). The diet survey showed that the energy intake of participants was 1320.4 (976.2,1637.5) kcal. Energy intake, grains and tubers, vegetables, fruits, meat, milk and dairy products, eggs, fish, snacks high in sugar and fat, and sugary drinks did not significantly differ among the WAS, NOR, and OVOB groups ($p > 0.05$). For details, please refer to Appendix A.4 (Table A4). In addition, 16S rRNA analysis showed that dominant phyla comprised Firmicutes (43.1%), Bacteroidetes (40.1%), and Actinobacteria (11.2%), with *Bacteroides* (24.4%) and *Prevotella* (14.4%) exhibiting genus-level dominance (Figure 8).

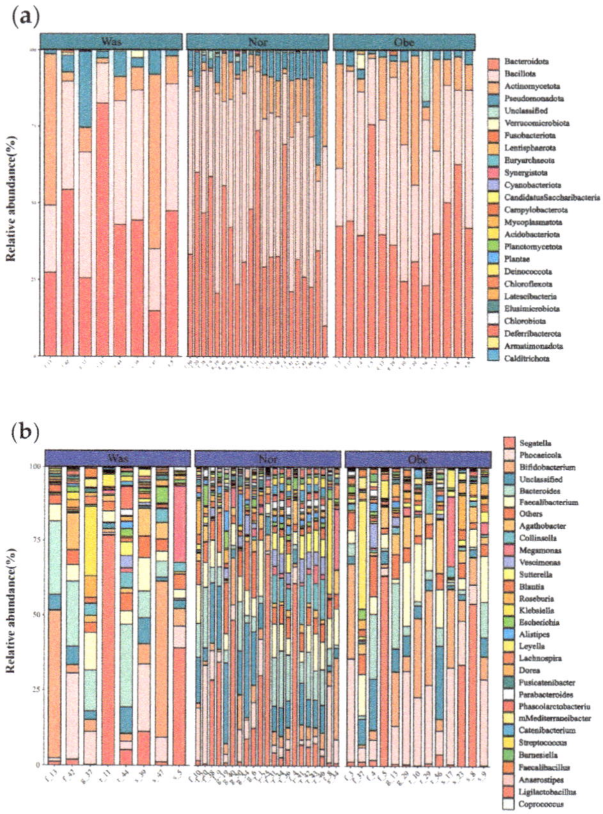

Figure 8. Relative abundance of gut microbiome in comparative groups. (**a**) Phylum level; (**b**) genus level.

Intergroup comparative analysis demonstrated two key structural divergences (Figure 9). The Firmicutes/Bacteroidetes ratio was elevated (2.07 in OVOB vs. 1.24 in NOR and 0.94 in WAS; $F = 7.86$, $p = 0.009$). In addition, Verrucomicrobia was depleted (0.04% in OVOB vs. 0.29% in NOR and 0.01% in WAS; $p = 0.0053$). The Verrucomicrobia abundance ranged from high to low in the following order: NOR (0.29%), OVOB (0.04%), and WAS group (0.01%). Pairwise comparisons showed statistically significant differences ($p = 0.005$).

3.3.2. Microbial Diversity Signatures

Comparative analysis revealed distinct α/β diversity patterns across different groups, and statistical differences in α/β diversity patterns were noted among the three groups (Figure 10). Pairwise comparison showed that, compared to NOR controls, obese children exhibited species richness reduction (Ace index: 395.25 ± 85.25 vs. 502.34 ± 92.17

(p = 0.0007), Chao1 index: 379.51 ± 75.78 vs. 490.39 ± 78.19 (p = 0.0013)) and a decline in community evenness (Shannon index: 2.96 ± 0.57 vs. 3.45 ± 0.62 (p = 0.03) and Simpson index: 0.12 ± 0.04 vs. 0.07 ± 0.05 (p = 0.01)). β diversity showed significant structural divergence (ANOSIM R = 0.114, p = 0.047). In addition, the Ace and Chao1 indices of children in the WAS group were lower than those in the NOR group (p values were < 0.0001 and 0.001, respectively); however, no statistically significant difference in the Shannon and Simpson indices (p > 0.05) were observed, indicating that the abundance of microbiota in emaciated children was lower than that of normal children (Figure 10).

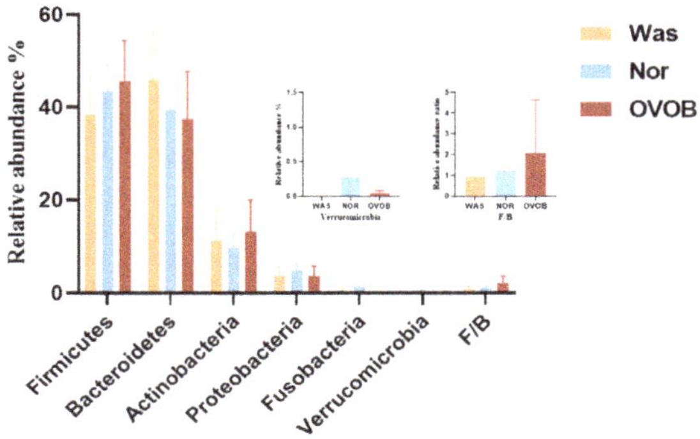

Figure 9. Analysis of relative abundance composition of gut microbiota in different groups. The Kruskal–Wallis test was used to analyze the difference in the F/B ratio and Verrucomicrobia abundance among the three groups.

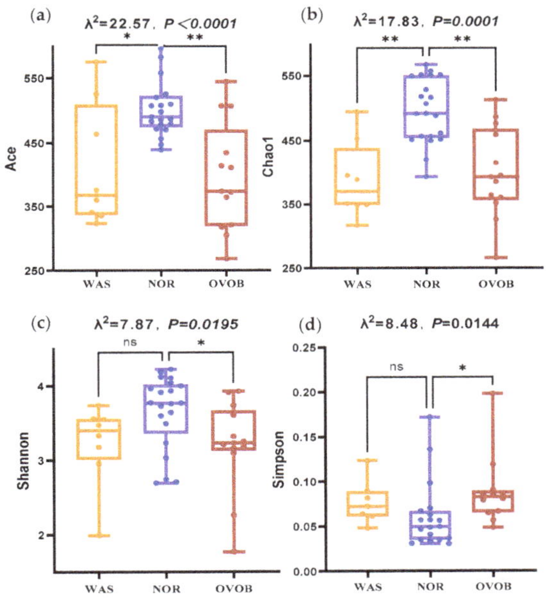

Figure 10. Box diagram of α diversity of gut microbiota in different groups. (**a**–**d**) represents the difference in the Ace, Chao1, Shannon, and Simpson indices among the three groups. respectively, and the difference was statistically significant among the three groups (p < 0.05). Kruskal–Wallis test was used to analyze the differences in the Ace, Chao1, Shannon, and Simpson indices. * indicates that the difference is statistically significant (p < 0.05), ** indicates that the difference is statistically significant (p < 0.01).

3.3.3. Differential Bacteria Screening

MaAsLin 2 analysis was performed to identify differentially abundant genera across groups. In the association analysis of the OVOB, WAS, and NOR groups, a total of 12 differential bacterial genera were identified (FDR < 0.10). As shown in Figure 11, compared with the NOR group, the OVOB group exhibited significant correlations with bacterial genera, including negative correlations with SCFA-producing bacterial genera, such as *Colidextribacter*, *Dysosmobacter*, *Intestinimonas*, *Longicatena*, and *Butyricimonas* (coefficients of −3.20, −3.03, −2.98, −1.04, and −2.92, respectively; FDR values of 0.02, 0.02, 0.02, 0.08, and 0.09, respectively). *Alistipes* were negatively correlated with children in the OVOB group (coefficients = −2.28 and FDR = 0.06). Associations with FDR < 0.10 were considered exploratory given the small sample size and should be interpreted with caution.

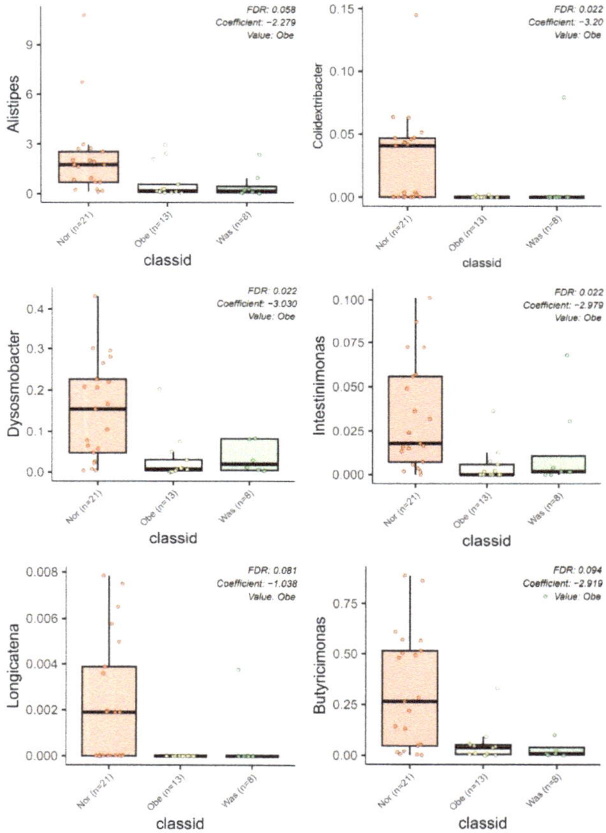

Figure 11. MaAsLin 2 analysis results of differential bacteria between comparative groups. The FDR of *Colidextribacter*, *Dysosmobacter*, and *Intestinimonas* was 0.02, 0.02, and 0.02, respectively; the FDR of *Alistipes*, *Longicatena*, and *Butyricimonas* was 0.06, 0.08, and 0.09, respectively. Associations with FDR < 0.10 were considered exploratory given the small sample size and should be interpreted with caution.

3.4. Correlation Analysis Between Differential Bacteria and Differential Metabolites

In the OVOB group, significant correlations were observed between differential metabolites and microbial genera (Figure 12). PE (16:0/16:0) demonstrated positive correlations with multiple genera, including *Butyricimonas* ($r = 0.448$, $p = 0.008$), *Dysosmobacter* (r = 0.483, p = 0.003), *Intestinimonas* (r = 0.411, p = 0.015), *Longicatena* (r = 0.386, p = 0.024), and *Alistipes* (r = 0.422, p = 0.012). Methyl sorbate was positively associated with *Butyricimonas* (r = 0.432, p = 0.011) and *Intestinimonas* (r = 0.413, p = 0.015), whereas deacetylnomilin displayed negative correlations with *Intestinimonas* (r = −0.349, p = 0.043) and *Alistipes* (r = −0.399, p = 0.019).

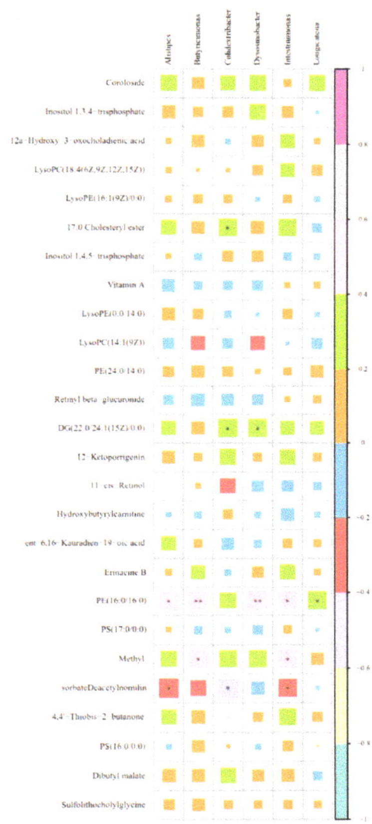

Figure 12. Spearman association between different metabolites and different bacteria in the OVOB/NOR group comparison. Square size represents the absolute value of the correlation coefficient (larger size = stronger association). * indicates that the correlation is statistically significant ($p < 0.05$), ** indicates that the correlation is statistically significant ($p < 0.01$).

4. Discussion

This multi-omics study explored the metabolic and gut microbiota characteristics associated with the weight and metabolic phenotypes of obese children and analyzed the associations between different metabolites and different bacterial genera. These findings provide a new perspective for understanding the heterogeneity in childhood obesity. However, it is necessary to note the limitations of the study population. Our study included children from four districts and counties in central and western China. The population characteristics were relatively simple (such as similar diet, cultural background, and environmental exposure). Although this improved the comparability of the results, it also limited the universality of the conclusions. The correlation between the gut microbiome and obesity is also influenced by multiple factors such as race, age, region, diet, and environmental exposure [24]. Yan He found that the influence of regional factors on the microbiota was significantly greater than that of other factors such as age, disease, and lifestyle [34]. The influence of different geographical locations on the composition of gut microbiota may stem from differences in lifestyle and dietary culture. For instance, a "geographical gradient" is noted among the gut microbiota of European infants, which is manifested in the higher abundance of Bifidobacterium and Clostridium in infants from Northern Europe (such as Denmark, Sweden, and the United Kingdom). In Southern Europe (such as Spain and Portugal), the abundance of Lactobacillus and Bacteroides in the intestines of infants is relatively high [35]. Meanwhile, the dietary patterns of different ethnic groups and different regions vary greatly, and dietary patterns affect the structural characteristics of the gut microbiota [26]; these differences have a significant impact on the association between the gut microbiota and obesity [18,24,36]. Therefore, the results of this study need to be further verified in populations representing other races and regions.

Our findings reaffirm the fetal origins of obesity [10], with elevated birth weight independently predicting adiposity (OVOB: 3.43 vs. NOR: 3.26 kg, $p < 0.001$), aligning with the fetal overnutrition hypothesis. Breastfeeding duration emerged as a dual modifier, reducing both obesity risk (MHO short-term breastfeeding: 19.4% vs. MUO: 33.9%) and metabolic dysregulation (MUO non-breastfeeding rate: 35.4% vs. <12% in other groups). The systematic review revealed that, compared with formula-fed or mixed-fed children, children who were exclusively breastfed from 3 to 12 months of age exhibited lower BMI trajectories or a reduced likelihood of following a high BMI trajectory. Furthermore, the results indicated that an extended duration of breastfeeding was associated with a progressively lower BMI trajectory until the age of 18 [37].

We found that the abundance of steroid derivatives and terpenoids in children with MUO decreased. A study involving 191 obese children aged 5 to 18 show that childhood obesity, especially prepubertal obesity, is associated with several steroid changes caused by excessive weight [15]. They defined childhood obesity as a "steroid-related complex disease", and the metabolomics characteristics of urinary steroids in obese children revealed the targeted characteristics of 31 steroid metabolites [38]. Studies have shown that the lipid marker LysoPC promotes adipocyte proliferation through PPARγ activation in vitro [39], and the upregulation of LysoPC may be related to the downregulation of genes and proteins related to lipid transport and decomposition (PPARγ) [40]. This mechanism is consistent with the increase in LysoPC observed in obese children in our study. It is worth noting that downregulation of PI (16:0/14:1) in the MUO/MHO model has important significance. PI (16:0/14:1) is an anti-inflammatory phosphatidylinositol, and its depletion may impair the membrane anchoring ability of the insulin signaling pathway [41], which is directly related to the insulin resistance phenotype in children with MUO [42]. This molecule promotes the membrane localization of glucose transporter GLUT4 by binding to the PH domain of IRS-1, and its deletion may lead to impaired glucose uptake in skeletal muscle [43]. The high predictive power of the ROC curve (MUO AUC of 96.7%) suggests that a combination of metabolic markers (e.g., PI (16:0/14:1) and treosulfan) and liver function markers (ALT) can effectively distinguish MHO and MUO obesity. However, this research result still requires external verification.

The observed "low diversity-high Firmicutes/Bacteroidetes ratio" pattern in obese children mirrors obesity-associated dysbiosis [18]. As a bridge between obesity and intestinal homeostasis, SCFAs are closely related to the pathogenesis of obesity and related metabolic diseases [44]. Studies indicated that depletion of SCFA-producing genera in obese children may compromise intestinal barrier function and energy regulation [27], and we also found a reduced abundance of SCFA-producing genera in the OVOB group. We found a positive correlation between PE (16:0/16:0) and SCFA-producing genera, which is consistent with the finding that phosphatidylethanolamines enhance butyrate production in animal models [45]. However, cross-sectional data cannot determine whether microbial activity directly influences PE levels or whether shared dietary factors (e.g., fiber intake) independently affect both variables. Lysophospholipids, such as LysoPE, are known to modulate membrane permeability and inflammatory responses [46]; however, whether these correlations reflect microbial modulation of host lipid metabolism or vice versa remains unclear. Similarly, the negative correlation between deacetylnomilin and *Alistipes* parallels reports linking *Alistipes* to reduced secondary bile acid metabolism [47]. However, mechanistic studies are needed to clarify this relationship. Thus, our exploratory findings nominate multi-omics signatures for further validation as potential stratification tools, pending replication in larger cohorts.

5. Innovations and Limitations

This study innovatively combines metabolic phenotyping with multi-omics profiling in a pediatric cohort. The identification of terpenoid/steroid deficiencies and sphingolipid alterations in MUO children provides potential biomarkers for distinguishing high-risk subgroups.

However, this study also has limitations that should be noted: (1) the cross-sectional design precludes causal inferences; longitudinal cohorts are needed to track metabolite–microbiota dynamics during MUO progression. (2) The microbiome sample size (n = 42) may be underpowered to detect rare genera and increase overfitting risk; independent validation is essential. Subsequent studies can integrate multi-omics techniques (such as metagenomics, metabolomics, and epigenome) to further verify the regulatory effects of key metabolic pathways and functional targets of the microbiota.

6. Conclusions

This multi-omics study characterized the preliminary metabolic and gut microbial profiles of Chinese children aged 5–7 years with obesity and metabolic heterogeneity phenotypes. Our data suggest that MUO children may exhibit alterations in ether lipid metabolism and sphingolipid metabolism pathways, showed tentative associations with elevated LysoPCs, and reduced PEs/PIs. Obese children displayed reduced microbial diversity, an elevated Firmicutes/Bacteroidetes ratio, along with apparent reductions in certain SCFA-producing genera. Observed correlations between specific bacterial taxa and phospholipid metabolites could indicate microbial–host metabolic interactions, though alternative explanations, including shared dietary influences, cannot be excluded.

These exploratory results contribute to the growing understanding of metabolic heterogeneity in childhood obesity but should be interpreted with appropriate caution until replicated in more diverse populations and supported by functional validation.

Supplementary Materials: The following supporting information can be downloaded at: https://www.mdpi.com/article/10.3390/nu17111876/s1, Figure S1: Spearman association between all different metabolites and different bacteria in OVOB/NOR group; Figure S2: OPLS-DA model and permutation testing results of samples from comparison groups. Table S1: Genera retained after filtering.

Author Contributions: Article idea, Z.X. and J.H.; methodology, Y.L., J.Y. and Z.X.; questionnaire survey and physical measurements, J.S. and T.L.; biological sample collection, Z.G. and Y.L.; untargeted metabolomics detection, Z.X., S.S. and Y.Y.; 16S rRNA sequencing, L.W. and Z.G.; biochemical indicators and vitamin tests, T.L. and Z.X.; formal analysis, J.Y.; resources, J.H. and Y.Y.; data analysis and visualization, Z.X. and Y.Y.; writing—original draft preparation, Z.X.; project administration, T.L. and Z.G.; funding acquisition, J.H. All authors have read and agreed to the published version of the manuscript.

Funding: This research was funded by the Public Health Emergency Project Nutrition Health and Healthy Diet Campaign (Grant No. 102393220020070000012), and the APC was waived.

Institutional Review Board Statement: This study was conducted in accordance with the Declaration of Helsinki and approved by the Ethics Committee of the National Institute of Nutrition and Health, Chinese Center for Disease Control and Prevention (Approval No. 2018-017; 20 July 2018).

Informed Consent Statement: Informed consent was obtained from all subjects involved in the study.

Data Availability Statement: The original contributions presented in this study are included in the article. Further inquiries can be directed to the corresponding author.

Conflicts of Interest: The authors declare no conflicts of interest.

Abbreviations

The following abbreviations are used in this manuscript:

AAAs	Aromatic amino acids
ADP	Adiponectin
ALT	Alanine transaminase
AST	Aspartate aminotransferase
AUC	Area under the curve
BCAAs	Branched chain amino acids
BMI	Body mass index
BMIZ	Body mass index Z-scores
CI	Confidence interval
CRP-H	High-sensitivity C-reactive protein
DBP	Diastolic blood pressure
F/B	Firmicutes/Bacteroidetes
FBG	Fasting blood glucose
FC	Fold change
FDR	False discovery rate
GLUT4	Glucose transporter type 4
HDLC	High-density lipoprotein cholesterol
IRS-1	Insulin receptor substrate 1
LDL-C	Low-density lipoprotein cholesterol
LEfSe	Linear discriminant analysis effect size
LPC	Lysophosphatidylcholine
LysoPE	Lysophosphatidylethanolamine
MHO	Metabolically healthy obesity
MHWH	Metabolically healthy and normal weight
mTORC1	Mechanistic target of rapamycin complex 1
MUO	Metabolically unhealthy obesity
MUWH	Metabolically unhealthy and normal weight
NOR	Normal weight
OPLS-DA	Orthogonal projections to latent structures-discriminant analysis
OVOB	Overweight and obesity
PC	Phosphatidylcholine
PCA	Principal component analysis
PE	Phosphatidylethanolamine
PI	Phosphatidylinositol
PLS-DA	Partial least squares discriminant analysis
PPARγ	Peroxisome proliferator-activated receptor gamma
PRS	Polygenic risk score
PS	Phosphatidylserine
QC	Quality control
ROC	Receiver operating characteristic

SBP	Systolic blood pressure
SCFA	Short-chain fatty acid
SCL	Short-chain fatty acid-linked
TC	Total cholesterol
TG	Triglycerides
TLR4	Toll-like receptor 4
VIP	Variable importance in projection
WAS	Wasting

Appendix A

Appendix A.1. Characteristics of Study Participants in the Metabolomics Analysis

Table A1 shows no significant differences in gender distribution among the three groups (p = 0.420 and p = 0.706 for respective comparisons). The prevalence rates of WAS, NOR, and OVOB in Henan Province were 12.8%, 49.0%, and 38.2%, respectively. In Guizhou Province, the rates were 26.5%, 35.3%, and 38.2%, revealing statistically significant regional variations (p = 0.006). Ethnic disparities were also evident: the Han population exhibited prevalence rates of 15.9% (WAS), 46.9% (NOR), and 37.2% (OVOB), while minority groups showed rates of 28.2% (WAS), 30.8% (NOR), and 41.0% (OVOB) (p = 0.018). The OVOB group demonstrated a significantly higher mean birth weight compared to both the WAS and NOR groups (F = 11.2, $p < 0.001$). No associations were found between parental education level, occupation, household income, and the distribution of WAS/NOR/OVOB categories (all $p > 0.05$). Breastfeeding prevalence differed significantly across groups: 93.5% (WAS), 88.9% (NOR), and 78.2% (OVOB) ($\chi^2 = 7.39$, p = 0.025). Regarding breastfeeding duration, 21.6% (n = 54) of infants were breastfed $\leq$ 6 months, 21.2% (n = 53) for 6–12 months, and 57.2% (n = 143) $\geq$12 months. Notably, the proportion of breastfeeding $\leq$ 6 months varied among groups (WAS: 15.2%, NOR: 18.8%, OVOB: 28.7%), with significant intergroup differences ($\chi^2 = 19.17$, $p < 0.001$). No significant associations were detected among preterm birth, delivery mode, singleton status, primary caregiver, or caregiver's occupation/cultural background and the three categories (all $p > 0.05$).

Table A1. Early life birth and feeding information of children with different nutritional status.

	WAS (n = 55)	NOR (n = 121)	OVOB (n = 109)	All (n = 285)	F/χ^2	p
ge [a], m	72.6 ± 5.7	73.1 ± 4.8	72.4 ± 6.5	73.2 ± 5.8	1.202	0.420
ender [b]						
Boy	30 (54.5)	68 (56.2)	66 (60.6)	164 (57.5)	0.70	0.706
Girl	25 (45.5)	53 (43.8)	43 (39.4)	121 (42.5)		
eight [a], cm	114.32 ± 5.02	116.75 ± 5.4	119.47 ± 5.47	117.33 ± 5.67	18.082	<0.001
'eight [a], kg	16.45 ± 1.63	20.57 ± 2.45	27.76 ± 4.99	22.54 ± 5.64	217.396	<0.001
MIZ [a]	−2.35 ± 0.39	−0.23 ± 0.68	2.16 ± 1.08	0.276 ± 1.86	594.642	<0.001
istrict [b]						
Henan	19 (12.8)	73 (49.0)	57 (38.3)	149 (100)	10.08	0.006
Guizhou	36 (26.5)	48 (35.3)	52 (38.2)	136 (100)		
ation [b]						
Han Chinese	33 (15.9)	97 (59.1)	77 (47.0)	207 (100)	8.09	0.018
Ethnic minorities	22 (28.2)	24 (19.8)	32 (26.4)	78 (100)		
rth weight [a], g	3077 ± 467	3256 ± 415	3434 ± 407	3285 ± 440	11.2	<0.001

Table A1. *Cont.*

	WAS (n = 55)	NOR (n = 121)	OVOB (n = 109)	All (n = 285)	F/χ^2	p
Birth length [a], cm	49.83 ± 1.29	50.25 ± 1.32	50.44 ± 1.13	50.24 ± 1.26	3.62	0.028
Breast feeding [b]						
Yes	43 (93.5)	104 (88.9)	68 (78.2)	215 (86.0)	7.39	0.025
No	3 (6.5)	13 (11.1)	19 (21.8)	35 (14.0)		
Duration of breastfeeding [b], m						
≤6	7 (15.2)	22 (18.8)	25 (28.7)	54 (21.6)	19.17	0.001
6–12	9 (19.6)	16 (13.7)	28 (32.2)	53 (21.2)		
≥12	30 (65.2)	79 (67.5)	34 (39.1)	143 (57.2)		
Premature delivery [b]						
Yes	2 (4.3)	3 (2.6)	2 (2.3)	7 (2.8)	0.509	0.776
No	44 (95.7)	114 (97.4)	85 (97.7)	243 (97.2)		
Delivery methods [b]						
Vaginal delivery	31 (67.4)	69 (59)	43 (49.4)	143 (57.2)	4.25	0.119
Cesarean section	15 (32.6)	48 (41)	44 (50.6)	107 (42.8)		
Only child [b]						
Yes	3 (6.5)	22 (18.8)	15 (17.2)	40 (16.0)	4.60	0.331
No	41 (89.1)	93 (79.5)	70 (80.5)	204 (81.6)		
Primary caregiving [b]						
Parental care	33 (71.7)	87 (74.4)	61 (70.1)	181 (72.4)	0.462	0.794
Non-parental care	13 (28.3)	30 (25.6)	26 (29.9)	69 (27.6)		
Educational level of caregivers [b]						
Primary and below	15 (32.6)	38 (32.5)	24 (27.6)	77 (30.8)	3.90	0.420
Junior and senior high school	26 (56.5)	53 (45.3)	47 (54)	126 (50.4)		
Above university level	5 (10.9)	26 (22.2)	16 (18.4)	47 (18.8)		
Occupation of caregivers [b]						
Housework	25 (54.3)	71 (60.7)	51(58.6)	147(58.8)	0.549	0.760
Agriculture related	21 (45.7)	46 (39.3)	36(41.4)	103(41.2)		
Annual household economic income [b] (RMB/year)						
<6	13 (46.43)	63 (64.29)	30 (57.7%)	106 (59.55)	3.04	0.39
≥6	15 (53.57)	35 (35.71)	22 (42.3%)	72 (40.45)		

[a] Data conforming to a normal distribution are presented as mean ± standard deviation. One-way analysis of variance (ANOVA) with post hoc LSD test was used to test for differences between groups. [b] Categorical or count data are expressed as proportions/rates. Chi-square test was used to analyze differences between groups.

In addition to the relevant indicators of the MUO/MHO classified criteria expressed in the main text, we also observed that serum ADP levels (14.07 ± 5.95 μg/mL) differed significantly based on metabolic status (p = 0.033). The MHWH group demonstrated the highest ADP concentrations (15.88 ± 5.31 μg/mL), surpassing MUWH (14.10 ± 5.83 μg/mL; p = 0.039), MHO (12.31 ± 5.31 μg/mL; p = 0.005), and MUO (13.56 ± 6.53 μg/mL; p = 0.029). MUO participants displayed elevated ALT levels (14.03 ± 10.91 U/L) compared to MHWH (10.43 ± 4.32 U/L; p = 0.005) and MUWH (10.21 ± 3.56 U/L; p = 0.002).

Abnormal-weight groups (MHO: 2.96 ± 6.78 mg/L; MUO: 1.64 ± 2.72 mg/L) showed significantly higher CRP-H levels than normal-weight groups (MHWH: 0.73 ± 1.24 mg/L; MUWH: 0.90 ± 1.84 mg/L; both $p = 0.003$).

Table A2. Serum biochemical profiles across metabolic phenotype groups.

	MHW (n = 54)	MUWH (n = 67)	MHO (n = 36)	MUO (n = 73)	ALL (n = 230)	F	p
HO [a], mmol/L	4.24 ± 0.69	4.22 ± 0.8	4.44 ± 0.48	4.27 ± 0.98	4.27 ± 0.8	0.664	0.575
[a], mmol/L	0.99 ± 0.31	1.09 ± 0.47	1.06 ± 0.33	1.67 ± 1.12	1.25 ± 0.76	13.097	<0.001
DL-C [a], mmol/L	1.63 ± 0.28	1.52 ± 0.57	1.62 ± 0.27	1.46 ± 0.48	1.54 ± 0.45	1.878	0.134
DL-C [a], mmol/L	1.65 ± 0.39	1.5 ± 0.53	1.8 ± 0.37	1.64 ± 0.54	1.63 ± 0.49	3.037	0.030
U [a], mmol/L	5.06 ± 0.8	5.58 ± 1.71	5.02 ± 0.93	5.61 ± 1.48	5.38 ± 1.37	3.033	0.030
DP [a], μg/mL	15.88 ± 5.31	14.1 ± 5.83	12.31 ± 5.31	13.56 ± 6.53	14.07 ± 5.95	2.973	0.033
T [a], U/L	10.43 ± 4.32	10.21 ± 3.56	12.3 ± 4.64	14.03 ± 10.91	11.81 ± 7.19	4.31	0.006
T [a], U/L	27.87 ± 5.95	26.76 ± 4.82	26.77 ± 5.18	28.74 ± 13.07	27.66 ± 8.59	0.76	0.518
RP-H [a], mg/L	0.73 ± 1.24	0.9 ± 1.84	2.96 ± 6.78	1.64 ± 2.72	1.42 ± 3.36	4.064	0.008
[a], g/dL	136.09 ± 9.55	137.12 ± 9.63	138.78 ± 8.96	140.71 ± 7.16	138.29 ± 8.92	3.388	0.019
P, mmHg	109.2 ± 6.8	118.15 ± 8.47	107.47 ± 5.12	116.83 ± 9.87	113.91 ± 9.25	22.362	<0.001
BP, mmHg	69.2 ± 6.8	78.68 ± 7.76	67.47 ± 5.12	77.83 ± 8.21	74.38 ± 8.73	32.357	<0.001

[a] Data conforming to a normal distribution are presented as mean ± standard deviation. One-way analysis of variance (ANOVA) was used to test for differences between groups. Pairwise comparisons were made using the LSD method.

Appendix A.2. Multivariate Logistic Regression Analysis of Differential Metabolites

Variables demonstrating statistical significance in univariate analyses ($p < 0.05$), including ethnicity, geographic region, breastfeeding status, breastfeeding duration, and serum biochemical parameters (ADP, ALT, vitamin A, vitamin D, and Hb), were included as covariates in the multivariate logistic regression model. The analysis identified Han ethnicity, elevated birth weight, high serum vitamin A, elevated CRP-H, LysoPC (14:1(9Z)), retinyl β-glucuronide, and cortisone acetate as independent risk factors for pediatric OVOB. Conversely, sulfolithocholyl glycine, 17:0 cholesteryl ester, and cycloflavin E emerged as protective factors against OVOB (Table A3).

Table A3. Multivariate logistic regression between the OVOB and NOR groups.

riables	β	S.E.	Wald	p	OR (95% CI)
ation	1.234	0.475	6.756	0.009	3.434 (1.355–8.708)
rth weight	0.002	0.001	17.534	<0.001	1.002 (1.001–1.003)
tamin A	0.004	0.002	8.019	0.005	1.004 (1.001–1.007)
RP-H	0.260	0.088	8.803	0.003	1.297 (1.092–1.540)
oroloside	−0.008	0.003	6.161	0.013	0.992 (0.986–0.998)
:0 Cholesteryl ester	−0.001	0.000	14.201	<0.001	0.999 (0.998–0.999)
soPC(14:1)	0.000	0.000	5.115	0.024	1.000 (1.000–1.001)
tinyl beta-glucuronide	0.004	0.002	5.169	0.023	1.004 (1.001–1.007)
lfolithocholyl glycine	−0.003	0.001	6.320	0.012	0.997 (0.995–0.999)
clocalopin E	−0.001	0.000	13.516	<0.001	0.999 (0.998–0.999)
ortisone acetate	0.002	0.001	8.141	0.004	1.002 (1.000–1.003)

Multi-factor logistic regression analysis incorporating clinically relevant covariates (adjusted for demographic characteristics, early feeding patterns, dietary behaviors, and physical activity levels) identified differential metabolites across the OVOB/NOR groups.

The multivariate analysis demonstrated that ALT, elaidic acid, LysoPE(16:0/0:0), N′-formylkynurenine, and PS(P-20:0/0:0) were identified as independent risk factors for MUO. Conversely, CRP-H, hexaethylene glycol and PI (16:0/14:1(9Z)) emerged as protective factors against this condition (Table A4).

Table A4. Multivariate logistic regression between the MUO and MHO groups.

Variables	β	S.E.	Wald	*p*	OR (95% CI)
ALT	0.123	0.059	4.384	0.036	1.131 (1.008–1.269)
CRP-H	−0.219	0.080	7.396	0.007	0.804 (0.686–0.941)
Hexaethylene glycol	−0.002	0.001	7.344	0.007	0.998 (0.997–1.000)
Elenaic acid	0.004	0.002	6.782	0.009	1.004 (1.001–1.007)
Treosulfan	0.001	0.000	13.968	<0.001	1.001 (1.001–1.002)
LysoPE (16:0/0:0)	0.000	0.000	11.078	0.001	1.000 (1.000–1.000)
N′-Formylkynurenine	0.009	0.003	8.768	0.003	1.009 (1.003–1.015)
PS (P-20:0/0:0)	0.007	0.002	12.149	<0.001	1.007 (1.003–1.011)
PI (16:0/14:1)	−0.005	0.001	13.201	<0.001	0.995 (0.993–0.998)

Multi-factor logistic regression analysis incorporating clinically relevant covariates (adjusted for demographic characteristics, early feeding patterns, dietary behaviors, and physical activity levels) identified differential metabolites across the MUO/MHO groups.

Appendix A.3. Metabolomics Quality Control Results

As shown in Figure A1, PCA scores of positive and negative ion detection and QC samples generally clustered together, indicating that the system has good repeatability, and the collected data can be further studied.

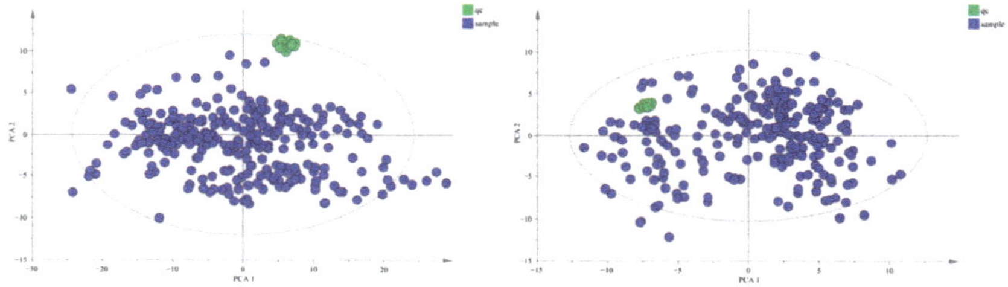

Figure A1. PCA scores for positive and negative (**left** and **right**, respectively) ion modes (including QC).

Appendix A.4. Characteristics of Study Participants in the Gut Microbiota

Table A5 shows the gut microbiome analysis of 42 children (median age: 77.9 months; 59.5% boys). Significant differences in age, sex, delivery methods, whether breastfeeding, and the duration of breastfeeding were not observed across different groups ($p > 0.05$). The daily food intake of grains and tubers, vegetables, fruits, meat, red meat, milk and dairy products, fish, eggs, snacks high in sugar fat, sugary drinks, and energy for children in the WAS, NOR, and OVOB groups were r 195.9 (109.4, 267.6) g, 53.6 (17.9, 166.2) g, 72 (32, 193.9) g, 40.8 (20.7, 100.8) g, 24.6 (9.2, 67.9) g, 71.4 (0, 184.4) g, 26.8 (10, 38.6) g, 0 (0, 0) g, 35.7 (9.6, 56.7) g, 78.6 (0, 121.4) mL, and 1320.4 (976.2, 1637.5) kcal, respectively, and there were no statistically significant differences among the different groups ($p > 0.05$).

Table A5. Analysis of the potential covariates of gut microbiome abundance in the research subjects.

	ALL (n = 42)	NOR (n = 21)	OVOB (n = 13)	WAS (n = 8)	χ^2	p
ge [a], m	76.6 ± 5.21	77.04 ± 4.66	76 ± 6.02	76.4 ± 5.8	0.159	0.853
ender [b]						
Boy	24 (57.1)	11 (52.4)	8 (61.5)	5 (62.5)	0.10	0.950
Girl	18 (42.9)	10 (47.6)	5 (38.5)	3 (37.5)		
rth weight [a], g	3.33 ± 0.42	3.30.43 ± 0.31	3.53 ± 0.57	3.09 ± 0.24	3.146	0.054
elivery methods [b]						
Vaginal delivery	20 (58.2)	8 (50.0)	7 (63.6)	5 (71.4)	1.08	0.580
esarean section	14 (41.2)	8 (50.0)	4 (36.4)	2 (28.6)		
east feeding [b]						
Yes	31 (73.8)	16 (76.2)	9 (69.2)	6 (75.0)	0.21	0.90
No	11 (26.2)	5 (23.8)	4 (30.8)	2 (25.0)		
uration of eastfeeding [b], m	12 (10–15)	12 (10–15)	11.5 (10–18)	13 (12–15)	0.23	0.89
rains and tubers [ac], g	195.9 (109.4, 267.6)	200.4 (127.6, 273.4)	168.4 (67.9, 255.6)	172.8 (74.6, 254.9)	1.382	0.501
egetables [ac], g	53.6 (17.9, 166.2)	64.3 (15.3, 169.1)	57.1 (26.3, 193.8)	26.8 (9.4, 129.7)	1.520	0.468
uits [ac], g	72 (32, 193.9)	107.1 (37, 226.2)	71.4 (38.8, 150.4)	36.6 (19.3, 140.5)	1.941	0.379
eat [ac], g	40.8 (20.7, 100.8)	34.7 (15.5, 113.5)	67.3 (23.8, 112.7)	38.1 (14.7, 100)	0.463	0.793
ed meat [ac], g	24.6 (9.2, 67.9)	22.3 (7.7, 87.1)	35.7 (8.7, 93.8)	21.7 (11.6, 56.7)	0.094	0.954
ilk and dairy oducts [ac], g	71.4 (0, 184.4)	66.7 (0, 197.3)	89.3 (23.8, 281.8)	83.3 (24.6, 141.1)	0.742	0.690
ggs [ac], g	26.8 (10, 38.6)	26.8 (11.1, 41.9)	26.8 (9.5, 38.8)	29 (10.1, 37.7)	0.190	0.909
sh [ac], g	0 (0, 0)	0 (0, 0)	0 (0, 4.5)	0 (0, 12.1)	1.893	0.388
acks high in sugar d fat [ac], g	35.7 (9.6, 56.7)	50 (10.7, 62.1)	17.1 (4.3, 39.6)	46.4 (21.1, 59.5)	4.029	0.133
gary drinks [ac], mL	78.6 (0, 121.4)	42.9 (0, 201.8)	28.6 (0, 91.1)	107.1 (32.1, 237.5)	3.391	0.183
ergy intake [ac], Kcal	1320.4 (976.2, 1637.5)	1320.6 (1137.7, 1743.9)	1309.6 (558.7, 1493.1)	1376.9 (684.5, 1609.5)	1.226	0.542

[a] Non-normally distributed data were reported as median with interquartile range (IQR, 25–75). Kruskal–Wallis test was used to test for differences between groups. [b] Categorical or count data are expressed as proportions/rates, n (%). Chi-square test was used to analyze differences between groups and Fisher's exact test for small expected frequencies. [c] The dietary survey of the research subjects was conducted using the semi-quantitative food frequency questionnaire (FFQ).

ferences

Tumas, N.; López, S.R. Double burden of underweight and obesity: Insights from new global evidence. *Lancet* **2024**, *403*, 998–999. [CrossRef] [PubMed]

GBD 2021 Adult BMI Collaborators. Global, regional, and national prevalence of adult overweight and obesity, 1990–2021, with forecasts to 2050: A forecasting study for the Global Burden of Disease Study 2021. *Lancet* **2025**, *405*, 813–838. [CrossRef] [PubMed]

Wang, Y.; Zhao, L.; Gao, L.; Pan, A.; Xue, H. Health policy and public health implications of obesity in China. *Lancet Diabetes Endocrinol.* **2021**, *9*, 446–461. [CrossRef] [PubMed]

Dong, Y.; Lau, P.W.C.; Dong, B.; Zou, Z.; Yang, Y.; Wen, B.; Ma, Y.; Hu, P.; Song, Y.; Ma, J.; et al. Trends in physical fitness, growth, and nutritional status of Chinese children and adolescents: A retrospective analysis of 1·5 million students from six successive national surveys between 1985 and 2014. *Lancet Child Adolesc. Health* **2019**, *3*, 871–880. [CrossRef]

Pan, X.F.; Fang, Z.Z. Obesity in China: What we know and what we can do. *Lancet Public Health* **2024**, *9*, E1000–E1001. [CrossRef]

Lister, N.B.; Baur, L.A. Child and adolescent obesity. *Nat. Rev. Dis. Primers* **2023**, *9*, 24. [CrossRef]

7. Schulze, M.B.; Stefan, N. Metabolically healthy obesity: From epidemiology and mechanisms to clinical implications. *Nat. Endocrinol.* **2024**, *20*, 633–646. [CrossRef]
8. Gaikwad, S.; Bhavnagarwala, A. American Academy of Pediatrics, 2023: Guideline for the Evaluation and Treatment of Chil and Adolescents With Obesity. *Indian Pediatr* **2023**, *60*, 759–761. [CrossRef]
9. Woldemariam, S.; Dorner, T.E.; Wiesinger, T.; Stein, K.V. Multi-omics approaches for precision obesity management: Potent and limitations of omics in precision prevention, treatment and risk reduction of obesity. *Wien Klin Wochenschr* **2023**, *135*, 113– [CrossRef]
10. Voruganti, V.S. Precision Nutrition: Recent Advances in Obesity. *Physiology* **2023**, *38*, 0. [CrossRef]
11. Abiri, B.; Valizadeh, M.; Amini, S.; Kelishadi, R.; Hosseinpanah, F. Risk factors, cutoff points, and definition of metabolica healthy/unhealthy obesity in children and adolescents: A scoping review of the literature. *Obes. Rev.* **2023**, *24*, e13548. [CrossR [PubMed]
12. Ramos-Lopez, O.; Riezu-Boj, J.I.; Milagro, F.I. Genetic and epigenetic nutritional interactions influencing obesity risk and adipo outcomes. *Curr. Opin. Clin. Nutr. Metab. Care* **2022**, *25*, 235–240. [CrossRef] [PubMed]
13. Liang, Y.; Pan, C.; Yin, T.; Wang, L.; Gao, X.; Wang, E.; Quang, H.; Huang, D.; Tan, L.; Xiang, K.; et al. Branched-Chain Am Acid Accumulation Fuels the Senescence-Associated Secretory Phenotype. *Adv. Sci.* **2024**, *11*, e2303489. [CrossRef] [PubMed]
14. Siddik, M.A.B.; Shin, A.C. Recent Progress on Branched-Chain Amino Acids in Obesity, Diabetes, and Beyond. *Endocrinol. Me* **2019**, *34*, 234–246. [CrossRef]
15. Sumińska, M.; Podgórski, R. The Impact of Obesity on the Excretion of Steroid Metabolites in Boys and Girls: A Comparison w Normal-Weight Children. *Nutrients* **2023**, *15*, 1734. [CrossRef]
16. Huang, Y.; Sulek, K.; Stinson, S.E. Lipid profiling identifies modifiable signatures of cardiometabolic risk in children a adolescents with obesity. *Nat. Med.* **2025**, *31*, 294–305. [CrossRef]
17. Robinson, T.N.; Armstrong, S.C. Treatment Interventions for Child and Adolescent Obesity: From Evidence to Recommendati to Action. *JAMA* **2024**, *332*, 201–203. [CrossRef]
18. Borrego-Ruiz, A.; Borrego, J.J. Human gut microbiome, diet, and mental disorders. *Int. Microbiol.* **2025**, *28*, 1–15. [CrossRef]
19. Wang, J.; Zhuang, P.; Lin, B.; Li, H.; Zheng, J.; Tang, W.; Ye, W.; Chen, X.; Zheng, M. Gut microbiota profiling in obese child from Southeastern China. *BMC Pediatr.* **2024**, *24*, 193. [CrossRef]
20. Ma, T.; Wu, Z.; Lin, J.; Shan, C.; Abasijiang, A.; Zhao, J. Characterization of the oral and gut microbiome in children with obe aged 3 to 5 years. *Front. Cell. Infect. Microbiol.* **2023**, *13*, 1102650. [CrossRef]
21. Chen, X.; Sun, H.; Jiang, F.; Shen, Y.; Li, X.; Hu, X.; Shen, X.; Wei, P. Alteration of the gut microbiota associated with childhc obesity by 16S rRNA gene sequencing. *PeerJ* **2020**, *8*, e8317. [CrossRef] [PubMed]
22. Niu, H.; Zhou, M.; Zogona, D.; Xing, Z.; Wu, T.; Chen, R.; Cui, D.; Liang, F.; Xu, X. Akkermansia muciniphila: A poten candidate for ameliorating metabolic diseases. *Front. Immunol.* **2024**, *15*, 1370658. [CrossRef]
23. Yang, Y.; Chen, J.; Gao, H.; Cui, M.; Zhu, M.; Xiang, X.; Wang, Q. Characterization of the gut microbiota and fecal and blc metabolomes under various factors in urban children from Northwest China. *Front. Cell. Infect. Microbiol.* **2024**, *14*, 1374 [CrossRef]
24. Sankararaman, S.; Noriega, K.; Velayuthan, S.; Sferra, T.; Martindale, R. Gut Microbiome and Its Impact on Obesity a Obesity-Related Disorders. *Curr. Gastroenterol. Rep.* **2023**, *25*, 31–44. [CrossRef]
25. Murga-Garrido, S.M.; Ulloa-Pérez, E.J. Virulence Factors of the Gut Microbiome Are Associated with BMI and Metabolic Blc Parameters in Children with Obesity. *Microbiol. Spectr.* **2023**, *11*, e0338222. [CrossRef] [PubMed]
26. Tang, M.; Marroquin, E. The role of the gut microbiome in the intergenerational transmission of the obesity phenotype: narrative review. *Front. Med.* **2022**, *9*, 1057424. [CrossRef]
27. Mann, E.R.; Lam, Y.K. Short-chain fatty acids: Linking diet, the microbiome and immunity. *Nat. Rev. Immunol.* **2024**, *24*, 577– [CrossRef] [PubMed]
28. Wu, X.; Xia, Y.; He, F.; Zhu, C.; Ren, W. Intestinal mycobiota in health and diseases: From a disrupted equilibrium to clini opportunities. *Microbiome* **2021**, *9*, 60. [CrossRef]
29. Damanhoury, S.; Newton, A.S.; Rashid, M.; Hartling, L.; Byrne, J.L.S.; Ball, G.D.C. Defining metabolically healthy obesity children: A scoping review. *Obes. Rev.* **2018**, *19*, 1476–1491. [CrossRef]
30. *WS/T 424-2013;* Anthropometric measurements method in health surveillance. National Health Commission: Beijing, China, 20
31. Flynn, J.T.; Kaelber, D.C.; Baker-Smith, C.M.; Blowey, D.; Carroll, A.E.; Daniels, S.R.; de Ferranti, S.D.; Dionne, J.M.; Falkner, Flinn, S.K.; et al. Clinical Practice Guideline for Screening and Management of High Blood Pressure in Children and Adolesce *Pediatrics* **2017**, *140*, e20171904. [CrossRef]
32. *WS/T 553-2017;* Method for Vitamin A Deficiency Screening. National Health Commission: Beijing, China, 2017.
33. *WS/T 677-2020;* Method for Vitamin D Deficiency Screening. National Health Commission: Beijing, China, 2020.

He, Y.; Wu, W.; Zheng, H.M.; Li, P.; McDonald, D.; Sheng, H.F.; Chen, M.X.; Chen, Z.H.; Ji, G.Y.; Zheng, Z.D.; et al. Regional variation limits applications of healthy gut microbiome reference ranges and disease models. *Nat. Med.* **2018**, *24*, 1532–1535. [CrossRef] [PubMed]

Fallani, M.; Young, D.; Scott, J.; Norin, E.; Amarri, S.; Adam, R.; Aguilera, M.; Khanna, S.; Gil, A.; Edwards, C.A.; et al. Intestinal microbiota of 6-week-old infants across Europe: Geographic influence beyond delivery mode, breast-feeding, and antibiotics. *J. Pediatr. Gastroenterol. Nutr.* **2010**, *51*, 77–84. [CrossRef] [PubMed]

Bliesner, A.; Eccles-Smith, J.; Bates, C.; Hayes, O.; Ho, J.Y.; Martins, C.; Truby, H.; Nitert, M.D. Impact of Food-Based Weight Loss Interventions on Gut Microbiome in Individuals with Obesity: A Systematic Review. *Nutrients* **2022**, *14*, 1953. [CrossRef]

Dewey, K.G.; Güngör, D. Breastfeeding and risk of overweight in childhood and beyond: A systematic review with emphasis on sibling-pair and intervention studies. *Am. J. Clin. Nutr.* **2021**, *114*, 1774–1790. [CrossRef]

Sumińska, M.; Podgórski, R.; Fichna, P.; Fichna, M. Steroid Metabolism in Children and Adolescents With Obesity and Insulin Resistance: Altered SRD5A and 20α/20βHSD Activity. *Front. Endocrinol.* **2021**, *12*, 759971. [CrossRef]

Gaich, G.; Chien, J.Y.; Fu, H.; Glass, L.C.; Deeg, M.A.; Holland, W.L.; Kharitonenkov, A.; Bumol, T.; Schilske, H.K.; Moller, D.E. The effects of LY2405319, an FGF21 analog, in obese human subjects with type 2 diabetes. *Cell Metab.* **2013**, *18*, 333–340. [CrossRef] [PubMed]

Xie, P.; Xie, J.B.; Xiao, M.Y.; Guo, M.; Qi, Y.S.; Li, F.F.; Piao, X.L. Liver lipidomics analysis reveals the anti-obesity and lipid-lowering effects of gypnosides from heat-processed Gynostemma pentaphyllum in high-fat diet fed mice. *Phytomedicine* **2023**, *115*, 154834. [CrossRef]

Barker, C.J.; Tessaro, F.H.G.; Ferreira, S.S.; Simas, R.; Ayala, T.S.; Köhler, M.; Rajasekaran, S.S.; Martins, J.O.; Darè, E.; Berggren, P.O. XPR1 Mediates the Pancreatic β-Cell Phosphate Flush. *Diabetes* **2021**, *70*, 111–118. [CrossRef]

Telle-Hansen, V.H.; Christensen, J.J.; Formo, G.A.; Holven, K.B.; Ulven, S.M. A comprehensive metabolic profiling of the metabolically healthy obesity phenotype. *Lipids Health Dis.* **2020**, *19*, 90. [CrossRef]

Inthanon, K.; Wong, A.N.N.; Dheeranupattana, S.; Guerra, A.G.; Davies, N.M.; Kesornpun, C.; Sangher, S.; Kittakoop, P. Regulation of adipocyte differentiation and lipid metabolism by novel synthetic chromenes exploring anti-obesity and broader therapeutic potential. *Sci. Rep.* **2025**, *15*, 4051. [CrossRef]

You, H.; Tan, Y.; Yu, D.; Qiu, S.; Bai, Y.; He, J.; Cao, H.; Che, Q.; Guo, J.; Su, Z. The Therapeutic Effect of SCFA-Mediated Regulation of the Intestinal Environment on Obesity. *Front. Nutr.* **2022**, *9*, 886902. [CrossRef] [PubMed]

Vance, J.E.; Tasseva, G. Formation and function of phosphatidylserine and phosphatidylethanolamine in mammalian cells. *Biochim. Biophys. Acta* **2013**, *1831*, 543–554. [CrossRef] [PubMed]

Prabutzki, P.; Schiller, J.; Engel, K.M. Phospholipid-derived lysophospholipids in (patho)physiology. *Atherosclerosis* **2024**, *398*, 118569. [CrossRef] [PubMed]

Lin, J.; Liu, H.; Sun, Y.; Zou, J.; Nie, Q.; Nie, S. Arabinoxylan Alleviates Obesity by Regulating Gut Microbiota and Bile Acid Metabolism. *J. Agric. Food Chem.* **2024**, *72*, 23295–23305. [CrossRef]

nutrients

Article

Phthalate Metabolites and Their Relationship with Abdominal and General Obesity: Evidence from the Aragon Workers' Health Study (AWHS)

Jordan Akritidis [1], Diana María Mérida [1,2,3], Carolina Torrijo-Belanche [4], Belén Moreno-Franco [4,5,6], Sofía Gimeno-Ruiz [7], Jimena Rey-García [8], María Morales-Suarez-Varela [2,9] and Pilar Guallar-Castillón [1,2,10,*]

1 Department of Preventive Medicine and Public Health, School of Medicine, Universidad Autónoma de Madrid, Arzobispo Morcillo 4, 28029 Madrid, Spain; dianamerida26@gmail.com (D.M.M.)
2 CIBERESP (CIBER of Epidemiology and Public Health), 28029 Madrid, Spain; maria.m.morales@uv.es
3 Fundación Teófilo Hernando, Las Rozas de Madrid, 28290 Madrid, Spain
4 Department of Preventive Medicine and Public Health, Universidad de Zaragoza, 50009 Zaragoza, Spain; carolinatorrijob@gmail.com (C.T.-B.); belenmorenofranco@gmail.com (B.M.-F.)
5 Instituto de Investigación Sanitaria Aragón, Hospital Universitario Miguel Servet, 50009 Zaragoza, Spain
6 CIBERCV (CIBER de Enfermedades Cardiovasculares), 28029 Madrid, Spain
7 Veterinary School, Universidad de Zaragoza, 50013 Zaragoza, Spain; gimenoruizsofia@gmail.com
8 Department of Internal Medicine, Hospital Universitario Rey Juan Carlos, Instituto de Investigación Sanitaria-Fundación Jiménez Díaz (IIS-FJD), 28933 Móstoles, Spain; jimena.reygarcia@gmail.com
9 Departament de Medicina Preventiva i Salut Pública, Ciències d'Alimentació, Toxicologia i Medicina Legal, Universitat de València, 46003 Valencia, Spain
10 Instituto Madrileño de Estudios Avanzados en Alimentación (IMDEA)-Food Institute, Campus de Excelencia Internacional Universidad Autónoma de Madrid + Consejo Superior de Investigaciones Científicas (CEI UAM + CSIC), Carretera de Cantoblanco 8, 28049 Madrid, Spain
* Correspondence: mpilar.guallar@uam.es

Abstract: Background/Objectives: Phthalates are endocrine-disrupting chemicals that are commonly used in plastic consumer products and food packaging, with growing evidence suggesting that they have a potential role in obesity. This study aimed to investigate the association between urinary concentrations of phthalate metabolites and both general and abdominal obesity among adult males in Spain. Methods: We analysed data from 1124 male participants of the Aragon Workers' Health Study (AWHS) collected between 2011 and 2014 in Zaragoza, Spain. Eleven urinary phthalate metabolites were measured and adjusted for creatinine levels. Multivariate logistic regression models were used to evaluate associations between phthalate exposure and general and abdominal obesity, controlling for dietary and lifestyle factors. Dose–response relationships were explored using restricted cubic spline models. Results: Higher urinary concentrations of di(2-ethylhexyl) phthalate (∑DEHP) and two of its metabolites—mono-(2-ethyl-5-oxohexyl) phthalate (MEOHP) and mono-(2-ethyl-5-hydroxyhexyl) phthalate (MEHHP)—were significantly associated with general obesity. The adjusted odds ratios were: ∑DEHP [OR = 1.26; 95% CI: 1.01, 1.58], MEOHP [OR = 1.24; 95% CI: 1.00, 1.53], and MEHHP [OR = 1.26; 95% CI: 1.03, 1.55]. In contrast, mono-isobutyl phthalate (MiBP) was inversely associated with abdominal obesity [OR = 0.73; 95% CI: 0.57, 0.93]. Conclusions: These findings suggest a positive association between exposure to DEHP and its metabolites and general obesity. This highlights the potential importance of environmental exposures as modifiable factors in obesity prevention and supports the need for further investigation in nutritional and public health contexts.

Keywords: phthalates; abdominal obesity; general obesity; DEHP; environmental epidemiology; nutritional epidemiology

1. Introduction

Obesity is a multifactorial condition associated with an elevated risk of many chronic diseases and all-cause mortality [1]. While excessive caloric intake and insufficient physical activity are key risk factors for obesity, environmental exposure to endocrine disruptors such as phthalates may also play an important role. Phthalates are organic lipophilic compounds used mainly as additives to soften plastics in food packaging [2], vinyl flooring [3], medical equipment [4], water bottles [5], and personal care products [6]. Since they do not covalently bind to plastic, phthalates easily leak into surrounding air, water, and food resulting in inhalation, ingestion, and dermal absorption [7]. Subsequently, they are quickly metabolised and excreted via urine and faeces.

Phthalate exposure is ubiquitous and industrial use is extensive with between 6 and 8 million tons of phthalates being manufactured globally each year [8]. This exposure has been linked to type 2 diabetes [9], metabolic syndrome [10], thyroid function [11], low birthweight [12], attention deficit hyperactivity disorder [13], endometriosis [14], decreased testosterone [15], decreased anogenital distance [16], and hearing disorders [17]. Infants and children in particular appear to be most susceptible to the endocrine-disrupting properties of phthalates especially during early growth [18,19]. Consequently, attempts have been made to limit the use of several phthalates in children's toys in many countries including China, the world's largest producer and consumer of phthalate-containing products [20,21].

Phthalate exposure may play a key role in the development of obesity, although its association differs significantly between males and females, as well as between childhood and adulthood [22,23]. The National Health and Nutrition Examination Survey (NHANES) conducted in the United States provides key data on the association between phthalate exposure and obesity in the general population [22,24–26]. While among children, studies show that prenatal phthalate exposure is positively associated with higher body mass index (BMI) and waist circumference (WC) [27–29], the effects of chronic exposure among adults is less clear due to a lack of longitudinal studies, high heterogeneity between studies, and inconsistent results. For instance, specifically among men, several NHANES studies found that certain phthalates of high molecular weight were significantly associated with either abdominal or general obesity [24,25,30], while other large studies reported non-significant or inverse associations between phthalates and body weight outcomes in men [23,31].

Epidemiological studies including NHANES have reported positive associations between di(2-ethylhexyl) phthalate (DEHP) metabolites and obesity in men [22,24,25]. Among women, DEHP has also demonstrated positive associations with obesity and body weight outcomes in several studies [31–33]. Exposure to DEHP is high in the general population as it is found in high quantities in plastic food packaging [20] and personal care products [34]. Phthalates including DEHP likely act by interfering with energy metabolism and adipose tissue structure [35], which in turn contributes to the development of obesity.

Given the widespread exposure of the general population to phthalates and the conflicting evidence in the current scientific literature, further research into the obesogenic effects of phthalates in adults is clearly warranted. We hypothesise that phthalates are positively associated with both abdominal and general obesity. This study aims to investigate the association between urinary phthalate metabolite concentrations and abdominal and general obesity in adult Spanish males.

2. Materials and Methods

2.1. Study Design and Participants

This is a cross-sectional study using data from the Aragon Workers' Health Study (AWHS), whose design and methodology has been detailed elsewhere [36]. The AWHS is a prospective cohort study, based on data from the annual physical examinations of

5678 workers in a large car assembly plant in Figueruelas, Zaragoza, Spain, aimed to investigate the determinants of the development and progression of subclinical atherosclerosis. From 2011 to 2014, participants aged 39–59 years (95.0% men) underwent subclinical atherosclerosis imaging and an interview with questionnaires on diet, behaviour and lifestyle factors. The current study utilises data from 2133 participants with blood and urine samples. We excluded females (n = 114), those with a personal history of cardiovascular disease (n = 27), those without urinary creatinine measurements (n = 837), those with extremely diluted or concentrated urinary creatinine (less than 30 mg/dL or more than 300 mg/dL) (n = 30), and those with a BMI of <18.5 kg/m^2 (n = 1). The final analyses included 1124 participants. We report these findings in line with the Strengthening the Reporting of Observational Studies in Epidemiology (STROBE) guidelines [37].

2.2. Endpoints

There were two endpoints in this study. (1) Abdominal obesity, which in males is defined as having a WC of >102 cm (42 inches) [38]; and (2) general obesity, defined as having a BMI of $\geq$30.0 kg/m^2 [39]. Anthropometric data (WC, weight, and height) were measured by trained physicians and nurses using standardised procedures. A total of 40 participants had missing values for WC but had recorded BMI.

2.3. Urinary Phthalate Metabolite Measurements

Phthalate metabolites were quantified in urine using high-performance liquid chromatography in tandem with mass spectrometry (LC-MS/MS) and expressed in ng/mL. Valid urinary concentrations were obtained for 11 phthalate metabolites: monoethyl phthalate (MEP); mono-isobutyl phthalate (MiBP); mono-n-butyl phthalate (MnBP); monobenzyl phthalate (MBzP); mono-(2-ethyl-5-oxohexyl) phthalate (MEOHP); mono-(2-ethyl-5-carboxypentyl) phthalate (MECPP); mono-(2-ethyl-5-hydroxyhexyl) phthalate (MEHHP); mono(2-carboxymethylhexyl) phthalate (MCMHP); mono-carboxy isononyl phthalate (cx-MiDP); mono-hydroxy-isodecyl phthalate (OH-MiDP); and mono-hydroxy-isononyl phthalate (OH-MiNP). The limit of detection (LOD) was established at 0.5 ng/mL for MEP, MBzP, MEOHP, MECPP, MEHHP, and MCMHP, and 1.0 ng/mL for MiBP, MnBP, cx-MiDP, OH-MiDP, and OH-MiNP. Nine of the eleven phthalate metabolites were detected in all 1124 participants, while cx-MiDP and OH-MiDP were detected in 981 (87.3%) and 977 (86.9%) participants, respectively. Values below the LOD were estimated by dividing the LOD by the square root of two [40]. In line with previous research [12,41], we excluded three phthalate metabolites with more than 75% of measurements below the LOD: mono-cyclohexyl phthalate (MCHP), mono-n-pentyl phthalate (MnPP), and mono-n-octyl phthalate (MnOP). The molar sum of DEHP metabolites ($\sum$DEHP) was calculated from the sum of each metabolite divided by its molecular weight: MEOHP/292.33 + MECPP/308.33 + MEHHP/294.34 + MCMHP/308.33.

2.4. Creatinine Correction

We corrected urinary phthalate metabolite (in µg/g creatinine) and $\sum$DEHP (in µmol/g creatinine) concentrations for creatinine to account for urine dilution. The sample median was 151.25 mg/dL. We converted phthalate metabolite values from ng/mL to µg/dL by multiplying by 0.1, and creatinine values from mg/dL to g/dL by multiplying by 0.001. As a result, to obtain phthalate metabolite values, we divided each phthalate metabolite by creatinine and then multiplied each concentration by 100. To obtain DEHP values, we divided $\sum$DEHP by creatinine concentration and multiplied by 100.

2.5. Data Collection and Covariates

Demographic data and smoking status were collected via questionnaires. A 136-item semi-quantitative food frequency questionnaire (FFQ) [42] validated in Spain assessed dietary intake over the previous year to obtain alcohol and energy intake. Physical activity data were collected via the validated Spanish-language version of the physical activity questionnaire from the Nurses' Health Study and Health Professionals' Follow-up Study [43]. Hypertension was defined by having systolic blood pressure $\geq$ 140 mmHg or diastolic blood pressure $\geq$ 90 mmHg, or by taking hypertension medication [44]. Dyslipidaemia was defined by having total blood cholesterol $\geq$ 240 mg/dL, triglycerides $\geq$ 150 mg/dL, LDL $\geq$ 160 or HDL < 40 mg/dL, or by taking dyslipidaemia medication [45]. Diabetes was defined by having blood glucose $\geq$ 126 mg/dL, or by taking diabetes medication [44]. Participants were classified according to work type, as sedentary work (office) or manual labour (assembly line). Participants worked one of four shift schedules. There were two rotating shifts: morning–evening (06:00–14:00 and 14:00–22:00), and morning–evening–night (06:00–14:00, 14:00–22:00, and 22:00–06:00). There were two fixed shifts: central (08:00–16:00), and night (22:00–06:00). Workers on rotating shifts changed on a weekly basis.

2.6. Statistical Analysis

All eleven phthalate metabolites and ∑DEHP were categorised into quartiles and analysed by comparing successive quartiles to the first quartile using multivariate logistic regression. To calculate *p*-test for linear trend, quartiles were considered as a continuous variable. Correlations between each phthalate metabolite concentration were calculated using Spearman's rank correlation test. Phthalate metabolites were also analysed as continuous variables after ln-transformation to improve normality. To assess dose–response between the metabolites and abdominal and general obesity, we depicted restricted cubic spline models (RCS). In alternative (sensitivity) analyses to correct for urinary dilution, we repeated the logistic models with ln-phthalate metabolites as dependent variables and adjusted for urinary creatinine. Data were analysed using STATA v18 [46] and *p*-values of <0.05 were considered significant.

2.7. Ethics and Consent

This study was approved by the Clinical Research Ethics Committee of Aragon (CEICA) (PI07/09). Informed consent was granted by participants in the AWHS who allowed the use of their data collected via the annual health exam, additional questionnaires on cardiovascular and lifestyle risk factors, and blood and urine samples collected for the study biobank. All participants belong to the AWHS cohort; therefore, prior to their inclusion, they signed a written consent form.

3. Results

3.1. Participant Characteristics

All participants were males of Spanish origin with an average age of 50.7 years (±3.7 years). Alcohol intake (g/day) was significantly higher among those with greater urinary concentrations of MEHHP and ∑DEHP, while energy intake (kcal/day) was significantly higher among those with greater urinary concentrations of MEOHP, MEHHP, and ∑DEHP. Most participants were manual labourers (87.5%) and worked the rotating morning–afternoon shift (61.3%). Greater urinary concentrations of MEOHP, MEHHP, and ∑DEHP were observed for manual workers in morning–afternoon shifts (Table 1).

Table 1. Summary of participant characteristics (Aragon Workers' Health Study, 2011–2014) N = 1124.

Characteristic	N = 1124	MEOHP			MEHHP			∑DEHP *		
		Q1	Q4	*p*-Value	Q1	Q4	*p*-Value	Q1	Q4	*p*-Value
Urinary creatinine concentration (mg/dL)	154.4 (57.1)	152.5 (62.4)	152.0 (54.6)	0.803	150.9 (60.7)	155.7 (55.9)	0.481	153.4 (62.4)	153.3 (54.9)	0.898
Age (years), mean (SD)	50.7 (3.66)	50.7 (3.63)	50.9 (3.74)	0.541	50.6 (3.68)	50.8 (3.69)	0.565	50.7 (3.68)	50.7 (3.75)	0.732
Alcohol (g/day)	22.5 (21.3)	21.1 (20.7)	24.0 (22.7)	0.081	19.9 (19.6)	24.5 (22.9)	**0.005**	21.0 (20.5)	24.0 (22.5)	**0.046**
Physical activity (total METs/week)	35.3 (21.5)	36.2 (21.5)	34.3 (21.0)	0.612	35.2 (21.4)	35.7 (21.5)	0.971	35.9 (21.8)	35.7 (22.0)	0.853
Energy intake (kcal/day)	2945.1 (764.9)	2850.1 (795.3)	3011.9 (754.2)	**0.022**	2862.8 (832.8)	2980.4 (724.9)	**0.046**	2855.1 (787.0)	2976.4 (736.1)	**0.045**
Smoking status, *n* (%)				0.071			**0.034**			0.115
No smoker	255 (22.7)	83 (32.6)	54 (21.2)		84 (32.9)	53 (20.8)		78 (30.6)	49 (19.2)	
Former smoker	487 (43.3)	110 (22.6)	123 (25.3)		105 (21.6)	129 (26.5)		108 (22.2)	130 (26.7)	
Current smoker	382 (34.0)	88 (23.0)	104 (27.2)		92 (24.1)	99 (25.9)		95 (24.9)	102 (26.7)	
Hypertension				0.870			0.662			0.913
No hypertension	682 (60.7)	170 (24.9)	173 (25.4)		172 (25.2)	176 (25.8)		170 (24.9)	173 (25.34)	
Hypertension	442 (39.3)	111 (25.1)	108 (24.4)		109 (24.7)	105 (23.8)		111 (25.1)	108 (24.4)	
Dyslipidaemia				**0.029**			0.145			0.136
No dyslipidaemia	390 (34.7)	86 (22.1)	110 (28.2)		94 (24.1)	107 (27.4)		87 (22.3)	108 (27.7)	
Dyslipidaemia	734 (65.3)	195 (26.6)	171 (23.3)		187 (25.5)	174 (23.7)		194 (26.4)	173 (23.6)	
Diabetes				0.635			0.722			0.906
No diabetes	1064 (94.7)	268 (25.2)	271 (25.5)		268 (25.2)	271 (25.5)		267 (25.1)	269 (25.3)	
Diabetes	60 (5.34)	13 (21.7)	10 (16.7)		13 (21.7)	10 (16.7)		14 (23.3)	12 (20.0)	
Work type				**0.007**			**0.018**			**0.001**
Sedentary work (office)	141 (12.5)	42 (29.8)	24 (17.0)		39 (27.7)	25 (17.7)		41 (29.1)	18 (12.8)	
Manual labour (assembly line)	983 (87.5)	239 (24.3)	257 (26.1)		242 (24.6)	256 (26.0)		240 (24.4)	263 (26.8)	
Work shift				**0.045**			**0.041**			**0.010**
Rotating: morning–afternoon	689 (61.3)	168 (24.4)	186 (27.0)		167 (24.2)	185 (26.9)		167 (24.2)	190 (27.6)	
Rotating: morning–afternoon–night	241 (21.4)	51 (21.2)	55 (22.8)		53 (22.0)	56 (23.2)		52 (21.6)	54 (22.4)	
Central	96 (8.54)	31 (32.3)	17 (17.7)		27 (28.1)	17 (17.7)		31 (32.3)	13 (13.5)	
Night	98 (8.72)	31 (31.6)	23 (23.5)		34 (34.7)	23 (23.5)		31 (31.6)	24 (24.5)	

Bolded *p*-values are statistically significant according to linear regression for continuous variables and logistic regression for categorical variables the exception of smoking status and work shift (Pearson's chi-squared test). * ∑DEHP: sum of MEOHP, MEHHP, MECPP, and MCMHP.

3.2. *Urinary Phthalate Metabolites*

MEP had the highest median urinary concentration in our sample (100.9 μg/g creatinine). We also detected MiBP (16.3 μg/g creatinine), MnBP (13.5 μg/g creatinine),

MBzP (5.5 μg/g creatinine), MEOHP (6.38 μg/g creatinine), MECPP (13.0 μg/g creatinine), MEHHP (12.2 μg/g creatinine), MCMHP (2.79 μg/g creatinine), OH-MiNP (8.16 μg/g creatinine), cx-MiDP (1.30 μg/g creatinine), and OH-MiDP (1.60 μg/g creatinine). Correlations between the four metabolites of DEHP (MEOHP, MECPP, MEHHP, and MCMHP) were high (Rho > 0.80), as was the correlation between cx-MiDP and OH-MiDP (Rho = 0.83). All other phthalate metabolites were weakly or non-correlated (Table 2).

Table 2. Correlations (Spearman) between urinary phthalate metabolites concentrations.

	∑DEHP *	MEP	MiBP	MnBP	MBzP	MEOHP	MECPP	MEHHP	MCMHP	OH-MiNP	cx-MiDP	OH-MiDP
∑DEHP	1.000											
MEP	0.128	1.000										
MiBP	0.010	0.054	1.000									
MnBP	0.004	0.010	0.048	1.000								
MBzP	0.115	0.090	0.115	0.023	1.000							
MEOHP	**0.979**	0.111	0.082	0.000	0.091	1.000						
MECPP	**0.982**	0.151	0.120	0.005	0.128	**0.933**	1.000					
MEHHP	**0.996**	0.118	0.096	0.004	0.114	**0.973**	**0.970**	1.000				
MCMHP	**0.912**	0.107	0.090	0.003	0.134	**0.878**	**0.893**	**0.899**	1.000			
OH-MiNP	0.081	0.051	0.047	−0.004	0.146	0.058	0.103	0.078	0.063	1.000		
cx-MiDP	0.036	0.009	0.027	−0.002	0.081	0.019	0.054	0.0300	0.046	0.219	1.000	
OH-MiDP	0.068	0.035	0.046	0.005	0.142	0.046	0.088	0.065	0.064	0.319	**0.826**	1.000

Bolded values signify Rho > 0.800. * ∑DEHP: molar sum of MEOHP, MEHHP, MECPP, and MCMHP.

3.3. Phthalate Metabolites and Abdominal Obesity

In total, 29.2% (317/1084) had abdominal obesity. In multivariate logistic regression analysis, MiBP showed an inverse and significant association with abdominal obesity when comparing extreme quartiles. We obtained consistent results when MiBP was considered as a continuous variable.

MEOHP was significantly higher in the second [OR = 1.99 (95% CI: 1.33–2.96)] and fourth [OR = 1.53 (95% CI: 1.02–2.30)] quartiles compared with the first quartile adjusted for covariates (p-test for linear trend = 0.249). We obtained consistent results when MEOHP was considered as a continuous variable.

MBzP was significantly higher in the second quartile compared with the first quartile adjusted for covariates, but this association did not hold for the fourth quartile and the p-test for linear trend was not significant.

When the dose–response relationship was depicted using RCS, a positive but non-linear association was observed between ln-MEOHP and ln-MEHHP with abdominal obesity (Figure 1).

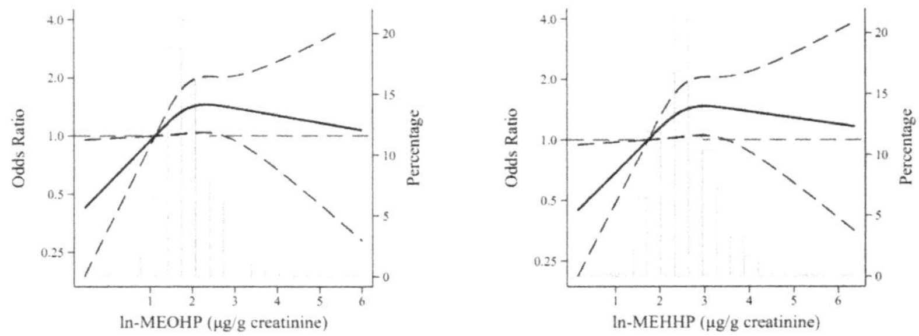

(a) (b)

Figure 1. Adjusted restricted cubic spline models for the association between abdominal obesity and (**a**) ln-MEOHP and (**b**) ln-MEHHP in the AWHS cohort (N = 1084). Models adjusted for age, alcohol intake, physical activity, energy intake, smoking status, hypertension, dyslipidaemia, diabetes, work type, and work shift. The solid and long-dashed lines represent the estimated odds ratios and their 95% confidence intervals, respectively.

∑DEHP was marginally associated with abdominal obesity. The association was approximately 50% higher when the fourth quartile was compared to the first one. When considered as a continuous variable, the association was 26% higher for each unit increase in ln-∑DEHP (Table 3). In sensitivity analyses, similar but more conservative results were obtained (Table S1).

Table 3. Odds ratios (95% CI) of urinary creatinine-corrected concentrations (μg/g creatinine) of phthalate metabolites and ΣDEHP in relation to abdominal obesity in the AWHS cohort (N = 1084).

Phthalate Metabolites as Continuous ^			Phthalate Metabolites in Quartiles				
Phthalate Metabolites (μg/g Creatinine)	OR (95% CI) for Every 1-ln Increase	*p*-Value	Q1 OR (95% CI)	Q2 OR (95% CI)	Q3 OR (95% CI)	Q4 OR (95% CI)	*p*-Test for Line Trend
MEP							
	Events/*n*	317/1084		88/272	70/270	69/272	90/270
	Crude model	1.02 (0.92, 1.15)	0.678	1 (Ref.)	0.73 (0.50, 1.06)	0.71 (0.49, 1.03)	1.05 (0.73, 1.50
	Adjusted model *	1.03 (0.91, 1.15)	0.682	1 (Ref.)	0.70 (0.47, 1.04)	0.69 (0.46, 1.03)	1.03 (0.70, 1.51
MiBP							
	Events/*n*	317/1084		98/271	77/272	79/271	63/270
	Crude model	0.68 (0.54, 0.86)	**0.001**	1 (Ref.)	0.68 (0.49, 1.00)	0.73 (0.51, 1.04)	**0.54 (0.37, 0.78**
	Adjusted model	0.73 (0.57, 0.93)	**0.010**	1 (Ref.)	0.73 (0.49, 1.07)	0.81 (0.55, 1.19)	**0.55 (0.37, 0.83**
MnBP							
	Events/*n*	317/1084		82/269	86/70	72/273	77/272
	Crude model	0.89 (0.73, 1.09)	0.269	1 (Ref.)	1.07 (0.74, 1.53)	0.82 (0.56, 1.19)	0.90 (0.62, 1.30
	Adjusted model	0.92 (0.74, 1.14)	0.442	1 (Ref.)	1.17 (0.79, 1.73)	0.84 (0.56, 1.25)	0.95 (0.64, 1.42
MBzP							
	Events/*n*	317/1084		73/272	93/271	81/273	70/268
	Crude model	0.99 (0.84, 1.18)	0.953	1 (Ref.)	1.42 (0.99, 2.06)	1.15 (0.79, 1.67)	0.96 (0.66, 1.41
	Adjusted model	1.02 (0.85, 1.22)	0.861	1 (Ref.)	**1.53 (1.04, 2.27)**	1.26 (0.84, 1.87)	0.99 (0.66, 1.49
MEOHP							
	Events/*n*	317/1084		65/273	99/268	72/271	81/272
	Crude model	1.09 (0.91, 1.31)	0.342	1 (Ref.)	**1.87 (1.29, 2.72)**	1.16 (0.79, 1.71)	1.36 (0.93, 1.99
	Adjusted model	1.17 (0.96, 1.42)	0.119	1 (Ref.)	**1.99 (1.33, 2.96)**	1.24 (0.82, 1.88)	**1.53 (1.02, 2.30**
MECPP							
	Events/*n*	317/1084		73/274	88/270	72/268	84/272
	Crude model	1.11 (0.92, 1.34)	0.274	1 (Ref.)	1.33 (0.92, 1.93)	1.01 (0.69, 1.48)	1.23 (0.85, 1.78
	Adjusted model	1.14 (0.93, 1.40)	0.204	1 (Ref.)	1.27 (0.86, 1.88)	0.97 (0.65, 1.46)	1.28 (0.86, 1.90

Table 3. *Cont.*

Phthalate Metabolites as Continuous ^			Phthalate Metabolites in Quartiles				
Phthalate Metabolites (µg/g Creatinine)	OR (95% CI) for Every 1-ln Increase	*p*-Value	Q1 OR (95% CI)	Q2 OR (95% CI)	Q3 OR (95% CI)	Q4 OR (95% CI)	*p*-Test for Linear Trend
MEHHP							
	Events/*n*	317/1084		70/273	87/270	78/269	82/272
	Crude model	1.10 (0.91, 1.31)	0.324	1 (Ref.)	1.38 (0.95, 2.00)	1.18 (0.81, 1.73)	1.25 (0.86, 1.82)
	Adjusted model	1.18 (0.97, 1.43)	0.096	1 (Ref.)	1.42 (0.95, 2.11)	1.24 (0.82, 1.86)	1.43 (0.96, 2.13)
MCMHP							
	Events/*n*	317/1084		77/272	91/268	65/273	83/271
	Crude model	1.01 (0.82, 1.24)	0.950	1 (Ref.)	1.30 (0.90, 1.88)	0.81 (0.55, 1.18)	1.12 (0.77, 1.62)
	Adjusted model	1.05 (0.84, 1.31)	0.686	1 (Ref.)	1.44 (0.97, 2.14)	0.86 (0.57, 1.29)	1.19 (0.80, 1.77)
∑DEHP †							
	Events/*n*	317/1084		72/274	88/269	73/268	84/273
	Crude model	1.10 (0.91, 1.34)	0.320	1 (Ref.)	1.36 (0.94, 1.98)	1.05 (0.72, 1.54)	1.25 (0.86, 1.81)
	Adjusted model	1.16 (0.95, 1.43)	0.152	1 (Ref.)	1.46 (0.98, 2.16)	1.04 (0.69, 1.56)	1.40 (0.94, 2.09)
cx-MiDP							
	Events/*n*	317/1084		78/273	74/272	87/270	78/269
	Crude model	1.04 (0.87, 1.25)	0.642	1 (Ref.)	0.93 (0.64, 1.36)	1.19 (0.82, 1.71)	1.02 (0.70, 1.48)
	Adjusted model	1.06 (0.87, 1.29)	0.578	1 (Ref.)	0.94 (0.63, 1.41)	1.17 (0.79, 1.73)	1.00 (0.67, 1.49)
OH-MiDP							
	Events/*n*	317/1084		73/272	83/271	80/269	81/272
	Crude model	1.03 (0.87, 1.22)	0.722	1 (Ref.)	1.20 (0.83, 1.75)	1.15 (0.79, 1.68)	1.16 (0.80, 1.68)
	Adjusted model	1.12 (0.93, 1.35)	0.224	1 (Ref.)	1.31 (0.88, 1.95)	1.19 (0.79, 1.77)	1.36 (0.91, 2.04)
OH-MiNP							
	Events/*n*	317/1084		82/273	67/269	83/269	85/273
	Crude model	1.08 (0.94, 1.24)	0.280	1 (Ref.)	0.77 (0.53, 1.13)	1.04 (0.72, 1.50)	1.05 (0.73, 1.52)
	Adjusted model	1.10 (0.95, 1.28)	0.205	1 (Ref.)	0.80 (0.53, 1.20)	1.06 (0.71, 1.57)	1.12 (0.76, 1.65)

OR: odds ratio; CI: confidence interval. Bolded *p*-values < 0.05. * Adjusted for age, alcohol intake, physical activity, energy intake, smoking status, hypertension, dyslipidaemia, diabetes, work type and work shift. ^ log-transformed phthalate metabolites. † ∑DEHP: molar sum of MEOHP, MEHHP, MECPP, and MCMHP.

3.4. Phthalate Metabolites and General Obesity

In total, 21.9% (246/1124) had general obesity. In multivariate logistic regression analysis, MEOHP was significantly higher in the second [OR = 1.79 (95% CI: 1.15–2.76)] and fourth [OR = 1.70 (95% CI: 1.09–2.64)] quartiles compared with the first quartile and the *p*-test for linear trend was marginally significant (*p*-test for linear trend = 0.088). Additionally, we obtained an OR of 1.24 (95% CI: 1.00, 1.53; $p = 0.047$) for each unit increase in ln-MEOHP.

For MECPP, we obtained marginally statistically significant results when studied in quartiles [OR = 1.53 (95% CI: 0.98–2.32)] comparing the fourth with the first quartile (*p*-test for linear trend = 0.112). When considered as a continuous variable [OR = 1.23 (95% CI: 0.99–1.53; $p = 0.062$)] was obtained for each unit increase in ln-MECPP.

MEHHP was positively associated with general obesity, with an OR of 1.63 (95% CI: 1.06–2.52) when comparing the fourth quartile to the first quartile. This association was monotonic (*p*-test for linear trend = 0.041). Additionally, an OR of 1.26 (95% CI: 1.03–1.55; $p = 0.027$) was obtained for each unit increase in ln-MEHHP.

∑DEHP was marginally associated with abdominal obesity when studied in quartiles [OR = 1.54 (95% CI: 0.99–2.37)] when comparing the fourth with the first quartile (*p*-test for linear trend = 0.075). Similar results were obtained when considered as a continuous variable; an OR of 1.26 (95% CI: 1.01, 1.58; $p = 0.038$) was observed for each unit increase in ln-∑DEHP.

The remaining seven phthalate metabolites did not show significant associations with general obesity in these analyses (Table 4). In sensitivity analyses, similar results were obtained however MECPP reached statistical significance [OR = 1.63 (95% CI: 1.00–2.66)] when comparing the fourth with the first quartile (p-test for linear trend = 0.101) (Table S2).

Table 4. Odds ratios (95% CI) of urinary creatinine-corrected concentrations (μg/g creatinine) of phthalate metabolites and ΣDEHP in relation to general obesity in the AWHS cohort (N = 1124).

Phthalate Metabolites as Continuous ^			Phthalate Metabolites in Quartiles				
Phthalate Metabolites (μg/g-Creatinine)	OR (95% CI) for Every 1-ln Increase	p-Value	Q1 OR (95% CI)	Q2 OR (95% CI)	Q3 OR (95% CI)	Q4 OR (95% CI)	p-Test for Line Trend
MEP							
Events/n	246/1124		65/281	57/281	54/281	70/281	
Crude model	1.06 (0.94, 1.19)	0.376	1 (Ref.)	0.85 (0.57, 1.26)	0.79 (0.53, 1.19)	1.10 (0.75, 1.62	
Adjusted model *	1.07 (0.95, 1.22)	0.272	1 (Ref.)	0.86 (0.56, 1.31)	0.78 (0.51, 1.21)	1.13 (0.74, 1.70	
MiBP							
Events/n	246/1124		73/281	62/281	59/281	52/281	
Crude model	0.85 (0.67, 1.08)	0.178	1 (Ref.)	0.81 (0.55, 1.19)	0.76 (0.51, 1.12)	**0.65 (0.43, 0.97**	
Adjusted model	0.91 (0.71, 1.17)	0.485	1 (Ref.)	0.87 (0.57, 1.31)	0.85 (0.56, 1.29)	0.68 (0.44, 1.04	
MnBP							
Events/n	246/1124		64/281	60/281	57/281	65/281	
Crude model	0.97 (0.79, 1.19)	0.765	1 (Ref.)	0.92 (0.62, 1.37)	0.86 (0.58, 1.29)	1.02 (0.69, 1.51	
Adjusted model	0.97 (0.78, 1.21)	0.788	1 (Ref.)	0.95 (0.62, 1.45)	0.87 (0.57, 1.34)	1.03 (0.68, 1.58	
MBzP							
Events/n	246/1124		62/281	61/281	58/281	65/281	
Crude model	1.06 (0.88, 1.26)	0.557	1 (Ref.)	0.98 (0.66, 1.46)	0.92 (0.61, 1.38)	1.06 (0.72, 1.58	
Adjusted model	1.06 (0.88, 1.29)	0.523	1 (Ref.)	0.96 (0.63, 1.47)	0.95 (0.62, 1.46)	1.03 (0.68, 1.58	
MEOHP							
Events/n	246/1124		48/281	73/281	58/281	67/281	
Crude model	1.17 (0.96, 1.43)	0.110	1 (Ref.)	**1.70 (1.13, 2.57)**	1.26 (0.83, 1.93)	**1.52 (1.00, 2.30**	
Adjusted model	1.24 (1.00, 1.53)	**0.047**	1 (Ref.)	**1.79 (1.15, 2.76)**	1.29 (0.82, 2.03)	**1.70 (1.09, 2.64**	
MECPP							
Events/n	246/1124		53/281	64/281	57/281	72/281	
Crude model	1.21 (0.99, 1.48)	0.066	1 (Ref.)	1.27 (0.84, 1.91)	1.09 (0.72, 1.66)	1.48 (0.99, 2.21	
Adjusted model	1.23 (0.99, 1.53)	0.062	1 (Ref.)	1.20 (0.78, 1.86)	1.03 (0.66, 1.60)	1.51 (0.98, 2.32	
MEHHP							
Events/n	246/1124		51/281	64/281	62/281	69/281	
Crude model	1.19 (0.98, 1.45)	0.075	1 (Ref.)	1.33 (0.88, 2.01)	1.28 (0.84, 1.93)	1.47 (0.98. 2.21	
Adjusted model	1.26 (1.03, 1.55)	**0.027**	1 (Ref.)	1.32 (0.86, 2.06)	1.28 (0.82, 1.99)	**1.63 (1.06, 2.52**	
MCMHP							
Events/n	246/1124		64/281	62/281	52/281	68/281	
Crude model	1.01 (0.80, 1.26)	0.961	1 (Ref.)	0.96 (0.65, 1.43)	0.77 (0.51, 1.16)	1.08 (0.73, 1.60	
Adjusted model	1.08 (0.85, 1.37)	0.551	1 (Ref.)	1.07 (0.70, 1.64)	0.84 (0.54, 1.30)	1.20 (0.79, 1.83	
ΣDEHP †							
Events/n	246/1124		52/281	62/281	64/281	68/281	
Crude model	1.21 (0.98, 1.48)	0.071	1 (Ref.)	1.25 (0.83, 1.88)	1.30 (0.86, 1.96)	1.41 (0.94, 2.11	
Adjusted model	1.26 (1.01, 1.58)	**0.038**	1 (Ref.)	1.31 (0.85, 2.03)	1.27 (0.82, 1.96)	1.54 (0.99, 2.37	
cx-MiDP							
Events/n	246/1124		70/281	56/281	63/281	57/281	
Crude model	0.90 (0.73, 1.10)	0.287	1 (Ref.)	0.75 (0.50, 1.12)	0.87 (0.59, 1.29)	0.77 (0.52, 1.14	
Adjusted model	0.87 (0.70, 1.09)	0.233	1 (Ref.)	0.76 (0.50, 1.17)	0.82 (0.54, 1.25)	0.70 (0.46, 1.08	

Table 4. *Cont.*

Phthalate Metabolites as Continuous ^			Phthalate Metabolites in Quartiles				
Phthalate Metabolites g/g-Creatinine)	OR (95% CI) for Every 1-ln Increase	*p*-Value	Q1 OR (95% CI)	Q2 OR (95% CI)	Q3 OR (95% CI)	Q4 OR (95% CI)	*p*-Test for Linear Trend
OH-MiDP							
	Events/*n*	246/1124		59/281	59/281	64/281	64/281
	Crude model	1.01 (0.84, 1.22)	0.892	1 (Ref.)	1.00 (0.67, 1.50)	1.11 (0.74, 1.66)	1.11 (0.74, 1.66)
	Adjusted model	1.05 (0.86, 1.28)	0.649	1 (Ref.)	1.03 (0.67, 1.59)	1.11 (0.72, 1.69)	1.15 (0.75, 1.77)
ohminp							
	Events/*n*	246/1124		63/281	53/281	65/281	65/281
	Crude model	1.10 (0.94, 1.28)	0.227	1 (Ref.)	0.80 (0.53, 1.21)	1.04 (0.70, 1.54)	1.04 (0.70, 1.54)
	Adjusted model	1.10 (0.94, 1.29)	0.251	1 (Ref.)	0.81 (0.53, 1.25)	1.02 (0.67, 1.56)	1.04 (0.68, 1.58)

OR: odds ratio; CI: confidence interval. Bolded *p*-values < 0.05. * Adjusted for age, alcohol intake, physical activity, energy intake, smoking status, hypertension, dyslipidaemia, diabetes, work type, and work shift. ^ log-transformed phthalate metabolites. † ∑DEHP: molar sum of MEOHP, MEHHP, MECPP, and MCMHP.

When the dose–response relationship was depicted using RCS, a positive but non-linear association was observed between ln-MEOHP and ln-MEHHP with general obesity (Figure 2).

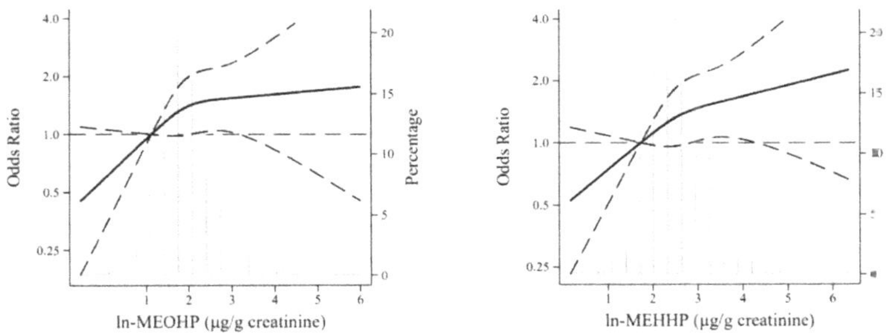

(**a**) (**b**)

Figure 2. Adjusted restricted cubic spline models for the association between general obesity and (**a**) ln-MEOHP and (**b**) ln-MEHHP in the AWHS cohort (N = 1124). Models adjusted for age, alcohol intake, physical activity, energy intake, smoking status, hypertension, dyslipidaemia, diabetes, work type, and work shift. The solid and long-dashed lines represent the estimated odds ratios and their 95% confidence intervals, respectively.

4. Discussion

In this study conducted among Spanish adult males, we observed that urinary concentrations of MEOHP, MEHHP and ∑DEHP were associated with an increased prevalence of general obesity. Only MEHHP showed a monotonic trend, indicating a linear dose–response relationship on a logarithmic scale. In addition, MiBP was inversely associated with abdominal obesity. As expected, due to their high correlation as downstream metabolites of DEHP (Rho = 0.97), results for MEOHP and MEHHP were similar.

Our findings align with other key cross-sectional studies assessing the relationship between urinary phthalate metabolite concentrations and obesity among adults [22,24,25]. The positive association that we observed between MEOHP and MEHHP and general obesity is in keeping with NHANES (2007–2010) by Buser et al. [25] in which MEOHP and MEHHP were both associated with general obesity in males and female aged $\geq$ 20 years. Moreover, Li et al. [47] found a positive association between MEOHP and general obesity among Chinese males aged $\geq$ 60 years old, while in a comprehensive meta-analysis by Wu et al. [48], MEHHP showed a positive correlation with general obesity among adults. Furthermore, NHANES (1999–2002) by Hatch et al. [22] demonstrated a positive relationship between both MEOHP and MEHHP and BMI among 20- to 59-year-old American males. Our findings provide supporting evidence for this association.

Notwithstanding this, these findings were not corroborated by some studies. For example, the Shanghai Food Consumption Survey (SHFCS) (2012–2014) by Dong et al. [23] reported a positive association between both MEOHP and MEHHP and general obesity among women, but not among men. This result was replicated for MEHHP among males aged $\geq$ 19 years old in the Korean National Environmental Health Survey (KoNEHS) (2012–2014) by Kang et al. [31]. Another discrepancy between our findings and those of previous studies is that we did not find an association between MEOHP and MEHHP and abdominal obesity, while results from NHANES (1999–2002) by Stahlhut et al. [24] reported higher WC among males with greater urinary concentrations of these two metabolites. The conflicting results could be due to methodological differences; for example, some studies adjust for different covariates or apply creatinine correction to phthalate metabolites after principal analyses. Furthermore, variations between different age groups, sex, and race may increase heterogeneity [24,30,49]. This cumulative evidence highlights the important role of demographic differences and distinct study designs when assessing these exposures and associations.

DEHP is found in high quantities in plastic-packaged food products, especially fatty foods [50]. Foods containing a high content of fat (for example, meat and dairy) are more likely to absorb phthalates from packaging [20]. Our study found that those with higher urinary concentrations of ∑DEHP and its metabolites had a significantly higher calorie intake, suggesting that high-calorie food (especially ultra-processed food) could be the source of consumption. Even after adjustment for calorie intake and physical activity, the association with obesity was significant, indicating potentially obesogenic effects beyond energy balance.

The remaining two DEHP metabolites in our study, MECPP and MCMHP, showed positive associations with general obesity but failed to reach statistical significance (p = 0.062 and p = 0.551, respectively). Dong et al. [23] and Buser et al. [25] reported significant positive associations between MECPP and abdominal and general obesity, respectively, as shown in NHANES (2013–2014) by Zhang et al. [26] among Americans aged $\geq$ 20 years. In our dataset, these phthalate metabolites were highly correlated with ∑DEHP (Rho for MECPP = 0.9822; Rho for MCMHP = 0.9123) and maintained positive associations with general obesity. One possible explanation for this discrepancy is the variation in sample sizes between our study and that of NHANES. Regarding MCMHP, to our knowledge, its association with obesity in adults has not been assessed in previous research, except for its inclusion in the molar sum of DEHP in Dong et al. [23].

∑DEHP (weighted molar sum of urinary metabolites of DEHP) was positively associated with general obesity in this study. Results from NHANES (2007–2010) by Buser et al. [25] were similar, in that ∑DEHP was significantly associated with general obesity in older males ($\geq$60 years). Furthermore, NHANES (2001–2010) by James-Todd et al. [51] also showed a positive relationship between ∑DEHP and abdominal obesity in 20- to 59-year-old American males. Previous studies have shown that DEHP exhibits anti-androgenic associations, and higher DEHP exposure in males has been linked to lower free testosterone levels [52], which in turn are associated with an increase in adiposity in males [53]. A further study found that, in humans, DEHP also significantly elevated leptin levels and interfered with fatty acid metabolism and lipid storage [54].

Contrary to our findings, NHANES (2013–2016) by Zhang et al. [55] showed that the sum of MEOHP, MEHHP, and MECPP was negatively associated with general obesity in the general US population. The variable used resembles ∑DEHP in our study (except lacking MCMHP). These mixed results should be interpreted with caution because of differences in phthalate metabolite concentration levels and the inclusion of both sexes in the NHANES study.

The inverse association observed between urinary MiBP levels and abdominal obesity may be influenced by specific occupational or behavioural factors rather than indicating a true protective effect. In our cohort of male car assembly plant workers, MiBP was the second most prevalent phthalate metabolite. It is a metabolite of diisobutyl phthalate (DiBP), a substance commonly found in industrial coatings, adhesives, and polymer-based materials. According to the European Chemicals Agency (ECHA) [56], DiBP can be released during industrial processes, particularly from materials with a high emission potential, such as tyres and brake pads. In this occupational context, therefore, workplace exposure could contribute to the overall phthalate burden. Differences in job type or the use of personal care products could influence exposure patterns. These variations may reflect underlying socioeconomic, lifestyle, or hygiene-related behaviours, which may also correlate with obesity prevalence. Additionally, like other endocrine-disrupting chemicals, MiBP may exhibit non-monotonic dose–response relationships, whereby different exposure levels produce different biological effects. Together, these factors may help to explain the inverse association observed, which warrants further investigation in future studies.

This study has several strengths. Firstly, because phthalate metabolites are produced in the human body, the samples collected could not have been contaminated by additional exposure to plastics. Second, the sample size was relatively large, with more than 1000 participants. Thirdly, the sample was well characterised for cardiovascular risk factors, including obesity, which was assessed using standardised methods. Finally, the study population is relatively homogeneous, consisting of male adults of similar age, origin and socio-economic background, which enhances the control of confounding factors.

This study also presents some limitations. Firstly, the cross-sectional design does not allow for establishing causal or temporal relationships. Secondly, the lipophilic properties of phthalates suggest that fat mass may be a more accurate physiological measure than WC and BMI. Thirdly, phthalates are rapidly metabolised by the human body, so it is possible that the urinary concentrations may only reflect short-term exposure. Finally, non-linear associations were found between some phthalate metabolites and obesity. A cautious interpretation is needed since they may reflect causal effects; however, we cannot rule out the existence of co-exposure.

5. Conclusions

In conclusion, this study provides supportive evidence for the potential obesogenic effects of DEHP and its metabolites (MEOHP and MEHHP) in adult males. These findings suggest that phthalates may contribute to the development of obesity and highlight the need for policy interventions to restrict the industrial use of these chemicals. Future research should focus on elucidating the mechanisms by which DEHP and its metabolites influence obesity beyond energy balance. Given that exposure to phthalates is largely unintentional and, due to their ubiquity, affects virtually all human populations. regulatory action to reduce unintentional exposure to these potentially harmful substances is both necessary and urgent.

Supplementary Materials: The following supporting information can be downloaded at: https://www.mdpi.com/article/10.3390/nu17111869/s1, Table S1. Sensitivity analysis of the association between phthalate metabolites and abdominal obesity. Table S2. Sensitivity analysis of the association between phthalate metabolites and general obesity.

Author Contributions: Conceptualisation and methodology: P.G.-C. and B.M.-F.; data curation and formal analysis: J.A., P.G.-C. and D.M.M.; project administration: P.G.-C. and B.M.-F.; supervision: P.G.-C.; validation and visualisation: J.A., S.G.-R., J.R.-G. and C.T.-B.; writing—original draft: J.A.; writing—review and editing: P.G.-C., D.M.M., B.M.-F., S.G.-R., J.R.-G., C.T.-B. and M.M.-S.-V. All authors have read and agreed to the published version of the manuscript.

Funding: This study was supported by the following grants: Health Research Fund FIS PI20-144 and PI23-240 (State Secretary of R + D and FEDER/FSE. Instituto de Salud Carlos III. Spain).

Institutional Review Board Statement: This study was approved by the Clinical Research Ethics Committee of Aragon (CEICA). Reference: CEICA 09/2007 (code: PI07/09, date on 23 May 2007). All procedures were performed in compliance with relevant laws and institutional guidelines and have been approved by the appropriate institutional committee(s).

Informed Consent Statement: Informed consent was obtained from all subjects involved in the study.

Data Availability Statement: Data are available for research purposes upon specific request.

Conflicts of Interest: The authors declare no conflicts of interest.

Abbreviations

The following abbreviations are used in this manuscript:

AWHS	Aragon Workers' Health Study
BMI	Body mass index
cx-MiDP	Mono-carboxy isononyl phthalate
DEHP	Di(2-ethylhexyl) phthalate
DIBP	Diisobutyl phthalate
MBzP	Monobenzyl phthalate
MCMHP	Mono(2-carboxymethylhexyl) phthalate
MECPP	Mono-(2-ethyl-5-carboxypentyl) phthalate
MEHHP	Mono-(2-ethyl-5-hydroxyhexyl) phthalate
MEOHP	Mono-(2-ethyl-5-oxohexyl) phthalate
MEP	Monoethyl phthalate
MiBP	Mono-isobutyl phthalate
MnBP	Mono-n-butyl phthalate
NHANES	National Health and Nutrition Examination Survey
OH-MiDP	Mono-hydroxy-isodecyl phthalate
OH-MiNP	Mono-hydroxy-isononyl phthalate
WC	Waist circumference

References

1. Berrington De Gonzalez, A.; Hartge, P.; Cerhan, J.R.; Flint, A.J.; Hannan, L.; MacInnis, R.J.; Moore, S.C.; Tobias, G.S.; Anton-Cul H.; Freeman, L.B.; et al. Body-Mass Index and Mortality among 1.46 Million White Adults. *N. Engl. J. Med.* **2010**, *363*, 2211–2 [CrossRef]
2. Fierens, T.; Servaes, K.; Van Holderbeke, M.; Geerts, L.; De Henauw, S.; Sioen, I.; Vanermen, G. Analysis of phthalates in fo products and packaging materials sold on the Belgian market. *Food Chem. Toxicol.* **2012**, *50*, 2575–2583. [CrossRef] [PubMed]
3. Liang, Y.; Xu, Y. Emission of Phthalates and Phthalate Alternatives from Vinyl Flooring and Crib Mattress Covers: The Influe of Temperature. *Environ. Sci. Technol.* **2014**, *48*, 14228–14237. [CrossRef] [PubMed]
4. Huygh, J.; Clotman, K.; Malarvannan, G.; Covaci, A.; Schepens, T.; Verbrugghe, W.; Dirinck, E.; Van Gaal, L.; Jorens, Considerable exposure to the endocrine disrupting chemicals phthalates and bisphenol—A in intensive care unit (ICU) patie *Environ. Int.* **2015**, *81*, 64–72. [CrossRef]
5. Luo, Q.; Liu, Z.H.; Yin, H.; Dang, Z.; Wu, P.X.; Zhu, N.W.; Lin, Z.; Liu, Y. Migration and potential risk of trace phthalates bottled water: A global situation. *Water Res.* **2018**, *147*, 362–372. [CrossRef] [PubMed]
6. Guo, Y.; Kannan, K. A Survey of Phthalates and Parabens in Personal Care Products from the United States and Its Implicati for Human Exposure. *Environ. Sci. Technol.* **2013**, *47*, 14442–14449. [CrossRef]

Dewalque, L.; Charlier, C.; Pirard, C. Estimated daily intake and cumulative risk assessment of phthalate diesters in a Belgian general population. *Toxicol. Lett.* **2014**, *231*, 161–168. [CrossRef]

Sahoo, T.P.; Kumar, M.A. Remediation of phthalate acid esters from contaminated environment—Insights on the bioremedial approaches and future perspectives. *Heliyon* **2023**, *9*, 14945. [CrossRef]

Sun, Q.; Cornelis, M.C.; Townsend, M.K.; Tobias, D.K.; Eliassen, A.H.; Franke, A.A.; Hauser, R.; Hu, F.B. Association of Urinary Concentrations of Bisphenol A and Phthalate Metabolites with Risk of Type 2 Diabetes: A Prospective Investigation in the Nurses' Health Study (NHS) and NHSII Cohorts. *Environ. Health Perspect.* **2014**, *122*, 616–623. [CrossRef]

Mérida, D.M.; Moreno-Franco, B.; Marquès, M.; León-Latre, M.; Laclaustra, M.; Guallar-Castillón, P. Phthalate exposure and the metabolic syndrome: A systematic review and meta-analysis. *Environ. Pollut.* **2023**, *333*, 121957. [CrossRef]

Huang, H.B.; Pan, W.H.; Chang, J.W.; Chiang, H.C.; Guo, Y.L.; Jaakkola, J.J.K.; Huang, P.-C. Does exposure to phthalates influence thyroid function and growth hormone homeostasis? The Taiwan Environmental Survey for Toxicants (TEST) 2013. *Environ. Res.* **2017**, *153*, 63–72. [CrossRef] [PubMed]

Jin, S.; Cui, S.; Xu, J.; Zhang, X. Associations between prenatal exposure to phthalates and birth weight: A meta-analysis study. *Ecotoxicol. Environ. Saf.* **2023**, *262*, 115207. [CrossRef]

Oh, J.; Kim, K.; Kannan, K.; Parsons, P.J.; Mlodnicka, A.; Schmidt, R.J.; Schweitzer, J.B.; Hertz-Picciotto, I.; Bennett, D.H. Early childhood exposure to environmental phenols and parabens, phthalates, organophosphate pesticides, and trace elements in association with attention deficit hyperactivity disorder (ADHD) symptoms in the CHARGE study. *Environ. Health* **2024**, *23*, 27. [CrossRef]

Yi, H.; Wu, H.; Zhu, W.; Lin, Q.; Zhao, X.; Lin, R.; Luo, Y.; Wu, L.; Lin, D. Phthalate exposure and risk of ovarian dysfunction in endometriosis: Human and animal data. *Front. Cell Dev. Biol.* **2023**, *11*, 1154923. [CrossRef]

Chang, W.H.; Li, S.S.; Wu, M.H.; Pan, H.A.; Lee, C.C. Phthalates might interfere with testicular function by reducing testosterone and insulin-like factor 3 levels. *Hum. Reprod.* **2015**, *30*, 2658–2670. [CrossRef] [PubMed]

Bustamante-Montes, L.P.; Hernández-Valero, M.A.; Flores-Pimentel, D.; García-Fábila, M.; Amaya-Chávez, A.; Barr, D.B.; Borja-Aburto, V.H. Prenatal exposure to phthalates is associated with decreased anogenital distance and penile size in male newborns. *J. Dev. Orig. Health Dis.* **2013**, *4*, 300–306. [CrossRef]

Shiue, I. Urinary heavy metals, phthalates, perchlorate, nitrate, thiocyanate, hydrocarbons, and polyfluorinated compounds are associated with adult hearing disturbance: USA NHANES, 2011–2012. *Environ. Sci. Pollut. Res.* **2015** *22*, 20306–20311. [CrossRef] [PubMed]

Chou, Y.Y.; Huang, P.C.; Lee, C.C.; Wu, M.H.; Lin, S.J. Phthalate Exposure in Girls During Early Puberty. *J. Pediatr. Endocrinol. Metab.* **2009**, *22*, 69–77. [CrossRef]

Dong, R.; Zheng, J.; Zhang, M.; Chen, J.; Zhang, H.; Gao, X.; Wang, Y.; Wu, M.; Li, S.; Chen, B. The concentrations and cumulative risk assessment of phthalates in general population from Shanghai: The comparison between groups with different ages. *Sci. Total Environ.* **2018**, *637–638*, 871–880. [CrossRef]

Wang, Y.; Qian, H. Phthalates and Their Impacts on Human Health. *Healthcare* **2021**, *9*, 603. [CrossRef]

Bu, S.; Wang, Y.; Wang, H.; Wang, F.; Tan, Y. Analysis of global commonly-used phthalates and non-dietary exposure assessment in indoor environment. *Build. Environ.* **2020**, *177*, 106853. [CrossRef]

Hatch, E.E.; Nelson, J.W.; Stahlhut, R.W.; Webster, T.F. Association of endocrine disruptors and obesity: Perspectives from epidemiological studies. *Int. J. Androl.* **2010**, *33*, 324–332. [CrossRef] [PubMed]

Dong, R.; Zhou, T.; Chen, J.; Zhang, M.; Zhang, H.; Wu, M.; Li, S.; Zhang, L.; Chen, B. Gender- and Age-Specific Relationships Between Phthalate Exposures and Obesity in Shanghai Adults. *Arch. Environ. Contam. Toxicol.* **2017**, *73*, 431–441. [CrossRef]

Stahlhut, R.W.; Van Wijngaarden, E.; Dye, T.D.; Cook, S.; Swan, S.H. Concentrations of Urinary Phthalate Metabolites Are Associated with Increased Waist Circumference and Insulin Resistance in Adult U.S. Males. *Environ. Health Perspect.* **2007**, *115*, 876–882. [CrossRef]

Buser, M.C.; Murray, H.E.; Scinicariello, F. Age and sex differences in childhood and adulthood obesity association with phthalates: Analyses of NHANES 2007–2010. *Int. J. Hyg. Environ. Health* **2014**, *217*, 687–694. [CrossRef]

Zhang, Y.; Dong, T.; Hu, W.; Wang, X.; Xu, B.; Lin, Z.; Hofer, T.; Stefanoff, P.; Chen, Y.; Wang, X.; et al. Association between exposure to a mixture of phenols, pesticides, and phthalates and obesity: Comparison of three statistical models. *Environ. Int.* **2019**, *123*, 325–336. [CrossRef]

Perez-Diaz, C.; Uriz-Martínez, M.; Ortega-Rico, C.; Leno-Duran, E.; Barrios-Rodríguez, R.; Salcedo-Bellido, I.; Arrebola, J.P.; Requena, P. Phthalate exposure and risk of metabolic syndrome components: A systematic review. *Environ. Pollut.* **2024**, *340*, 122714. [CrossRef] [PubMed]

Golestanzadeh, M.; Riahi, R.; Kelishadi, R. Association of exposure to phthalates with cardiometabolic risk factors in children and adolescents: A systematic review and meta-analysis. *Environ. Sci. Pollut. Res.* **2019**, *26*, 35670–35686. [CrossRef] [PubMed]

Zarean, M.; Poursafa, P.; Amin, M.M.; Kelishadi, R. Association of Endocrine Disrupting Chemicals, Bisphenol A and Phthalates, with Childhood Obesity: A Systematic Review. *J. Pediatr. Rev.* **2017**, *6*, 1. [CrossRef]

30. Hatch, E.E.; Nelson, J.W.; Qureshi, M.M.; Weinberg, J.; Moore, L.L.; Singer, M.; Webster, T.F. Association of urinary phthal metabolite concentrations with body mass index and waist circumference: A cross-sectional study of NHANES data, 1999–20 *Environ. Health* **2008**, *7*, 27. [CrossRef]
31. Kang, Y.; Park, J.; Youn, K. Association between urinary phthalate metabolites and obesity in adult Korean population: Kor National Environmental Health Survey (KoNEHS), 2012–2014. *Ann. Occup. Environ. Med.* **2019**, *31*, 23. [CrossRef] [PubMed]
32. Díaz Santana, M.V.; Hankinson, S.E.; Bigelow, C.; Sturgeon, S.R.; Zoeller, R.T.; Tinker, L.; Manson, J.A.E.; Calafat, A.M.; Meli J.R.; Reeves, K.W. Urinary concentrations of phthalate biomarkers and weight change among postmenopausal women: prospective cohort study. *Environ. Health* **2019**, *18*, 20. [CrossRef] [PubMed]
33. Haggerty, D.K.; Flaws, J.A.; Li, Z.; Strakovsky, R.S. Phthalate exposures and one-year change in body mass index across menopausal transition. *Environ. Res.* **2021**, *194*, 110598. [CrossRef]
34. Martínez-Razo, L.D.; Martínez-Ibarra, A.; Vázquez-Martínez, E.R.; Cerbón, M. The impact of Di-(2-ethylhexyl) Phthalate a Mono(2-ethylhexyl) Phthalate in placental development, function, and pathophysiology. *Environ. Int.* **2021**, *146*, 106 [CrossRef] [PubMed]
35. Heindel, J.J.; Howard, S.; Agay-Shay, K.; Arrebola, J.P.; Audouze, K.; Babin, P.J.; Barouki, R.; Bansal, A.; Blanc, E.; Cave, M.C.; e Obesity II: Establishing causal links between chemical exposures and obesity. *Biochem. Pharmacol.* **2022**, *199*, 115015. [CrossR
36. Casasnovas, J.A.; Alcaide, V.; Civeira, F.; Guallar, E.; Ibañez, B.; Borreguero, J.J.; Laclaustra, M.; León, M.; Peñalvo, J.L.; Ordov J.M.; et al. Aragon workers' health study—Design and cohort description. *BMC Cardiovasc. Disord.* **2012**, *12*, 45. [CrossRef]
37. Von Elm, E.; Altman, D.G.; Egger, M.; Pocock, S.J.; Gøtzsche, P.C.; Vandenbroucke, J.P. The Strengthening the Reporting Observational Studies in Epidemiology (STROBE) statement: Guidelines for reporting observational studies. *Lancet* **20** *370*, 1453–1457. [CrossRef]
38. Rayner, B.; Charlton, K.E.; Derman, W.; Jones, E. *Comprehensive Clinical Nephrology*, 4th ed.; Johnson, R.J., Feehally, J., Floege Eds.; Saunders Elsevier: Philadelphia, PA, USA, 2010; pp. 428–435.
39. Nuttall, F.Q. Body Mass Index: Obesity, BMI, and Health A Critical Review. *Nutr. Today* **2015**, *50*, 117–128. [CrossRef]
40. Hornung, R.W.; Reed, L.D. Estimation of Average Concentration in the Presence of Nondetectable Values. *Appl. Occup. Envi Hyg.* **1990**, *5*, 46–51. [CrossRef]
41. Ferguson, K.K.; Loch-Caruso, R.; Meeker, J.D. Exploration of Oxidative Stress and Inflammatory Markers in Relation to Urin Phthalate Metabolites: NHANES 1999–2006. *Environ. Sci. Technol.* **2012**, *46*, 477–485. [CrossRef]
42. De La Fuente-Arrillaga, C.; Vázquez Ruiz, Z.; Bes-Rastrollo, M.; Sampson, L.; Martinez-González, M.A. Reproducibility of FFQ validated in Spain. *Public Health Nutr.* **2010**, *13*, 1364–1372. [CrossRef] [PubMed]
43. Martínez-González, M.A.; López-Fontana, C.; Varo, J.J.; Sánchez-Villegas, A.; Martinez, J.A. Validation of the Spanish versior the physical activity questionnaire used in the Nurses' Health Study and the Health Professionals' Follow-up Study. *Public He Nutr.* **2005**, *8*, 920–927. [CrossRef] [PubMed]
44. Pearson, T.A.; Palaniappan, L.P.; Artinian, N.T.; Carnethon, M.R.; Criqui, M.H.; Daniels, S.R.; Fonarow, G.C.; Fortmann, S Franklin, B.A.; Galloway, J.M.; et al. American Heart Association Guide for Improving Cardiovascular Health at the Commur Level, 2013 Update: A Scientific Statement for Public Health Practitioners, Healthcare Providers, and Health Policy Mak *Circulation* **2013**, *127*, 1730–1753. [CrossRef]
45. National Cholesterol Education Program (NCEP) Expert Panel on Detection, Evaluation, and Treatment of High Blood Choleste in Adults. Third Report of the National Cholesterol Education Program (NCEP) Expert Panel on Detection, Evaluation, a Treatment of High Blood Cholesterol in Adults (Adult Treatment Panel III) Final Report. *Circulation* **2002**, *106*, 3143–34 [CrossRef]
46. StataCorp. *Stata Statistical Software: Release 18*, version 18; StataCorp LLC.: College Station, TX, USA, 2023.
47. Li, Y.L.; Lv, J.; Du, Z.P.; Feng, S.; Sheng, J.; Jin, Z.X.; Liu, K.-Y.; Gao, H.; Li, X.-D.; Cao, H.-J.; et al. The levels of phthalate expos and associations with obesity in an elderly population in China. *Ecotoxicol. Environ. Saf.* **2020**, *201*, 110749. [CrossRef]
48. Wu, Q.; Li, G.; Zhao, C.Y.; Na, X.L.; Zhang, Y.B. Association between phthalate exposure and obesity risk: A meta-analysis observational studies. *Environ. Toxicol. Pharmacol.* **2023**, *102*, 104240. [CrossRef]
49. Lind, P.M.; Roos, V.; Rönn, M.; Johansson, L.; Ahlström, H.; Kullberg, J.; Lind, L. Serum concentrations of phthalate metabol are related to abdominal fat distribution two years later in elderly women. *Environ. Health* **2012**, *11*, 21. [CrossRef]
50. Cirillo, T.; Fasano, E.; Esposito, F.; Prete, E.D.; Cocchieri, R.A. Study on the influence of temperature, storage time and packag type on di-n-butylphthalate and di(2-ethylhexyl)phthalate release into packed meals. *Food Addit. Contam. Part A* **2013**, *30*, 403–4 [CrossRef] [PubMed]
51. James-Todd, T.M.; Huang, T.; Seely, E.W.; Saxena, A.R. The association between phthalates and metabolic syndrome: The Natio Health and Nutrition Examination Survey 2001–2010. *Environ. Health* **2016**, *15*, 52. [CrossRef]
52. Pan, G.; Hanaoka, T.; Yoshimura, M.; Zhang, S.; Wang, P.; Tsukino, H.; Inoue, K.; Nakazawa, H.; Tsugane, S.; Takahashi Decreased Serum Free Testosterone in Workers Exposed to High Levels of Di-n-butyl Phthalate (DBP) and Di-2-ethylhe Phthalate (DEHP): A Cross-Sectional Study in China. *Environ. Health Perspect.* **2006**, *114*, 1643–1648. [CrossRef]

Ma, H.; Sun, J.; Wu, X.; Mao, J.; Han, Q. Percent body fat was negatively correlated with Testosterone levels in male. *PLoS ONE* **2024**, *19*, 0294567. [CrossRef] [PubMed]
Schaedlich, K.; Gebauer, S.; Hunger, L.; Beier, L.S.; Koch, H.M.; Wabitsch, M.; Fischer, B.; Ernst, J. DEHP deregulates adipokine levels and impairs fatty acid storage in human SGBS-adipocytes. *Sci. Rep.* **2018**, *8*, 3447. [CrossRef] [PubMed]
Zhang, J.; Gu, W.; Zhai, S.; Liu, Y.; Yang, C.; Xiao, L.; Chen, D. Phthalate metabolites and sex steroid hormones in relation to obesity in US adults: NHANES 2013–2016. *Front. Endocrinol.* **2024**, *15*, 1340664. [CrossRef] [PubMed]
European Chemicals Agency. Diisobutyl Phthalate (EC No. 201-553-2; CAS No. 84-69-5). ECHA Substance Information. Available online: https://echa.europa.eu/substance-information/-/substanceinfo/100.001.412 (accessed on 27 May 2025).

nutrients

MDPI

Article

Association Between the Healthy Eating Index and the Body Mass Index of Older Adults: An Analysis of Food Frequency and Preferences

Andres Fontalba-Navas [1,2,3,*], Ruth Echeverria [4,5], Cristina Larrea-Killinger [5,6,7,8,9], Mabel Gracia-Arnaiz [10], Claudia Soar [11] and Juan Pedro Arrebola [12,13,14,*]

1 Antequera Hospital, Northern Málaga Integrated Healthcare Area, 29200 Antequera, Spain
2 Department of Public Health and Psychiatry, University of Málaga, 29010 Málaga, Spain
3 Group BE-21, Institute of Biomedical Research in Málaga (IBIMA Plataforma BIONAND), 29010 Málaga, Spain
4 Fundación para la Investigación Biomédica del Hospital Universitario 12 de Octubre (FIBH12O), Instituto de Investigación Sanitaria Hospital 12 de Octubre (imas12), 28041 Madrid, Spain; recheverria.imas12@h12o.es
5 "Toxic Body" Interdisciplinary Network, Department of Social Anthropology, University of Barcelona, 08001 Barcelona, Spain; larrea@ub.edu
6 Department of Social Anthropology, University of Barcelona, 08001 Barcelona, Spain
7 Research Group Anthropology of Crisis and Contemporary Transformations (CRITS), Department of Social Anthropology, University of Barcelona, 08001 Barcelona, Spain
8 INSA-UB (Nutrition and Food Safety Research Institute) María de Maeztu Unit of Excellence, University of Barcelona, 08921 Santa Coloma de Gramanet, Spain
9 CIBER de Epidemiología y Salud Pública (CIBERESP), 28029 Madrid, Spain
10 Department of Anthropology, Philosophy and Social Work, Universitat Rovira i Virgili, 43002 Tarragona, Spain; mabel.gracia@urv.cat
11 Nutrition Post-Graduate Program, Department of Nutrition, Federal University of Santa Catarina, Florianopolis 88040-900, Brazil; claudia.soar@ufsc.br
12 Department of Preventive Medicine and Public Health, Pharmacy School, Universidad de Granada, Campus de Cartuja s/n, 18071 Granada, Spain
13 Instituto de Investigación Biosanitaria (ibs.GRANADA), Avda. de Madrid, 15. Pabellón de Consultas Externas 2, 2a Planta, 18012 Granada, Spain
14 Consortium for Biomedical Research in Epidemiology and Public Health (CIBERESP), Instituto de Salud Carlos III, C/ Monforte de Lemos 3-5, Pabellón 11. Planta 0, 28029 Madrid, Spain
* Correspondence: afontalba@uma.es (A.F.-N.); jparrebola@ugr.es (J.P.A.)

Abstract: Background/Objectives: The nutritional habits of older adults are increasingly relevant to public health, particularly given the rising prevalence of obesity and its associated chronic diseases. This study aims to analyze the relationship between the Healthy Eating Index (IASE) and Body Mass Index (BMI) in older adults in Spain, focusing on food frequency, dietary preferences, and socioeconomic factors influencing nutritional security. **Methods:** The study is part of the Eating Matters project, assessing food (in)security in older adults across Andalusia and Catalonia between April 2022 and January 2024. A cross-sectional survey was conducted among 190 participants (≥65 years), recruited in primary healthcare centers. The questionnaire included three blocks: food insecurity assessment (FIES scale), diet quality with the Healthy Eating Index for the Spanish Population (IASE), and sociodemographic factors. Data analysis involved descriptive statistics, Pearson correlations, and logistic regression models to identify associated factors with overweight and obesity. **Results:** The average BMI was 28.5 kg/m^2 (SD = 4.29), with 46.3% of participants classified as overweight and 32.1% as obese. A significant negative correlation (r = −0.79, $p < 0.05$) was found between healthy food consumption and BMI, while personal income showed a moderate positive correlation with adherence to a healthy diet (r = 0.42, $p < 0.05$). Logistic regression indicated that frequent consumption of processed meats and confectionery was a significant identify associated factors with overweight/obesity, with a model accuracy of 68% and sensitivity of 95%. **Conclusions:** Older adults with lower incomes and higher consumption of ultra-processed foods exhibited a higher risk of obesity. These findings highlight the need for public policies promoting food accessibility and targeted nutrition education for older adults, including guidance on balanced diets, adequate protein intake, and the prevention of sarcopenia, to encourage healthier dietary patterns in aging populations.

Keywords: Healthy Eating Index; Body Mass Index; older adults; food security; obesity; ultra-processed foods

1. Introduction

In Spain, the nutrition of older adults is an issue of growing research interest, given the progressive aging of the population and the challenges this poses in terms of public health [1]. With rising life expectancy, which by 2022 had reached 80.7 years in the European Union and 83.2 years in Spain [2], it is essential to pay close attention to the eating habits of the elderly, and to devise and apply public policies to promote safe, fair, adequate, healthy, and sustainable nutrition, in view of its importance in preventing chronic diseases and improving the quality of life.

People in this age group are subject to overweight and obesity. The phenomenon of increasing obesity among older people is not exclusive to Spain, but has been observed worldwide, as demonstrated by various population studies. The problem affects both men and women, although it is observed more frequently in the latter [3–5], and is present in many regions, spurred by demographic, socioeconomic, and lifestyle factors, further complicating the health status of older adults.

Numerous studies have recorded a strong association between obesity and the consumption of ultra-processed, high-calorie foods (UPFs) [6,7]. These products, which often contain high levels of added sugars, saturated fats, and sodium and lack essential nutrients, are designed to be highly palatable and appetizing, thus stimulating overconsumption. Moreover, UPFs tend to displace healthier options, contributing to high caloric intake without providing a corresponding nutritional input. High consumption of UPFs by older people can also aggravate health problems such as type 2 diabetes, cardiovascular disease, and other metabolic disorders that are closely linked to obesity [8,9].

Vulnerable older people, especially those with economic, physical, or social limitations, may be predisposed to consume UPFs for several reasons. First, these foods are usually more accessible and affordable than fresh alternatives, making them attractive to people with limited means. Furthermore, the ease of preparation of these products is of great importance for people with a physical or cognitive impairment, and also for older people who live alone, since cooking fresh foods can be more difficult and laborious. In addition, the mass distribution of UPFs and their ready availability in local stores facilitate their consumption by older adults, especially in areas with poor accessibility to fresh foods [9].

Among the UPFs most commonly consumed in Spain are confectionery and processed meats. The latter, such as sausages, chorizo, and cooked ham, are industrial foods that contain additives, preservatives, and large amounts of added salt and fats. Baker's confectionery products (such as biscuits, pastries, and cakes) include refined flours, added sugars, and hydrogenated vegetable oils. They are easily accessible, low-cost foods, which are often consumed by older people with dental problems or difficulties in chewing [10]. These factors, together with the decreased sense of taste often experienced in later age, make UPFs such as processed meats and confectionery very popular, with markedly negative consequences for the health of vulnerable older people [11,12].

In the present article, we analyze the dietary patterns of older adults in Spain, their relationship with overweight/obesity, and the resulting implications for public health and wellbeing among this population group. Our research goal is to provide evidence on key determinants of food security and nutritional habits in an elderly population, a group traditionally regarded as vulnerable to health-related factors. By leveraging the findings of this study, we seek to inform policies and health promotion programs, thus improving wellbeing and reducing the risks of chronic disease among this population, whilst promoting sustainability and fairness in the food system.

2. Materials and Methods

2.1. Study Goals: The 'Eating Matters' Project

The main objective of this study was to conduct a detailed survey of food (in)security in people aged over 65 years in the Spanish autonomous communities of Andalusia and Catalonia, between April 2022 and January 2024.

This research is part of a larger project, called Eating Matters, whose main goal is to investigate food (in)security problems affecting older people in Spain, via qualitative and quantitative methods applied to the population over 65 years of age in rural and urban areas of Andalusia, Catalonia, and the Valencian Community in the Spanish Mediterranean area [13–15]. The study has been approved by the Ethics Committees of the University of Barcelona, the Rovira i Virgili University, the Jordi Gol Foundation in Catalonia, and Northern Malaga Healthcare Area in Andalusia, corroborating its compliance with ethical standards and confidentiality requirements.

2.2. Recruitment of Participants and Sample Size

Participants were recruited from primary healthcare centers in Andalusia and Catalonia, specifically in the provinces of Málaga, Tarragona, and Barcelona. These centers provided an ideal setting due to their accessibility and the high level of trust patients place in healthcare staff, which helped minimize response bias. Eligible participants were individuals aged 65 years or older, residing in Spain for at least 40 years, and capable of providing informed consent. Those with severe cognitive impairments, language barriers, or who declined participation were excluded. Recruitment followed a randomized selection process using predefined lists at each site to ensure a representative sample across geographic and sociodemographic profiles. The required sample size was calculated assuming a food insecurity prevalence in vulnerable older adults, with a 95% confidence level and a 6% margin of error. A minimum of 171 participants was needed. To account for potential non-response, the final target was increased to 200. This strategy ensured sufficient statistical power and robustness for data analysis [16].

2.3. Questionnaire Design

The questionnaire was designed to address key aspects of nutrition in older people, and is divided into three distinct blocks:

- Block 1: Assessment of food insecurity using the Food Insecurity Experience Scale (FIES), an internationally validated tool, composed of eight questions [17];
- Block 2: Assessment of diet quality was conducted using the Healthy Eating Index for the Spanish Population (IASE, Spanish initials). This validated instrument includes nine items that measure the frequency of consumption of key food groups and is aligned with national dietary recommendations. The SCORE IASE refers to the total score obtained from the IASE, which quantifies adherence to healthy dietary patterns—higher scores indicate better diet quality. The IASE was selected for this study as it provides a straightforward and culturally appropriate assessment of diet

quality within the Spanish context, and it has been previously used and validated in populations aged over 65 years [18–20];

- Block 3: Sociodemographic data, medical history, diet and exposure to contaminants in food and food contact materials, sources of food supply, and perceptions of food (in)security. This block, exploratory in nature, was internally validated by a group of experts after implementing a pilot survey with 10 participants, a process which enabled any adjustments in the wording and sequence of the questions that might be necessary.

To ensure the validity and applicability of the questionnaire, a pilot study was conducted with 10 participants aged 65 years and older. The pilot tested content and face validity, evaluating the clarity, relevance, and understanding of all items. Based on the feedback received, minor modifications were made to improve question wording and sequencing. This process ensured that the final questionnaire was suitable for the target population and facilitated accurate data collection.

In older adults, the interpretation of Body Mass Index (BMI) differs from that of the general adult population due to age-related physiological changes such as reduced muscle mass and altered fat distribution. Evidence suggests that a BMI between 22 and 27 kg/m^2 is associated with better outcomes and lower mortality in the elderly. Therefore, the classification in this population is typically as follows: underweight is defined as a BMI less than 22 kg/m^2, normal weight ranges from 22 to 27 kg/m^2, overweight is considered between 27 and 30 kg/m^2, and obesity is defined as a BMI greater than 30 kg/m^2. These thresholds are recommended by geriatric and nutritional societies such as the European Society for Clinical Nutrition and Metabolism (ESPEN) and are supported by research showing that slightly higher BMI values in older individuals may have a protective effect against frailty and mortality [21]. Income data included individual and household monthly earnings from all sources, such as pensions, rental income, and investment returns, as reported by the participants.

2.4. Data Collection and Quality

The study data were collected in a quiet environment at the Health Centre, where participants' comfort was assured, and explanations could be provided when necessary. The interviewers, who were staff members at the Health Centre, carried out regular quality control exercises to ensure the consistency and integrity of the data collected, and a member of the research team supervised the purging of the database.

To ensure patient confidentiality, each participant was pseudonymized using a unique code. Printed data were destroyed once transferred to the digital database, which was stored following open science protocols. This database will be deposited in the Social Science Database (ARCES, Spanish initials) managed by the Centre for Sociological Research, within the Ministry for the Presidency, Relations with Parliament and Democratic Memory, in accordance with open science and transparency requirements.

2.5. Data Analysis

When data collection was complete, a descriptive statistical analysis was made of each of the three questionnaire blocks. Of the 199 surveys returned, 9 did not meet the inclusion/exclusion criteria and were discarded. A preliminary analysis of the remaining 190 included the identification of trends and possible problems in data quality, such as the tendency of participants to give homogeneous answers to the questions in the third block. For future application of the survey, this potential problem was resolved by changing the order of the blocks.

Statistical analyses included bivariate tests (Chi-square and Fisher's exact test) to explore the relationships between the variables of the three blocks, as well as multivariable logistic regression to identify associated factors with obesity. Given the skewed distribution of many of the variables, non-parametric approaches were applied to ensure the robustness of the statistical analyses. The aim of these analyses was to enable evidence-based recommendations for the design of public policies addressing the nutritional challenges of older people within a context of growing social inequality. All these analyses were performed using the R statistical software package (Version 4.4.1) [22].

3. Results

The sample population was composed of 190 participants with a mean age of 77.3 years (SD = 7.37). With respect to anthropometric characteristics, the average Body Mass Index (BMI) was 28.5 kg/m^2 (SD = 4.29). A total of 46.3% of participants were classified as overweight, 32.1% as obese, and 21.6% as normal weight. The average weight was 74.5 kg (SD = 12.77) and the average height, 161.6 cm (SD = 8.14) (Table 1).

Table 1. Sociodemographic, economic, and BMI data.

	Andalusia		**Catalonia**		**TOTAL**	
Participants (*n*)	91	47.9%	99	52.1%	190	100.0%
Women	59	64.8%	40	40.4%	99	52.1%
Men	32	35.2%	59	59.6%	91	47.9%
Spanish nationality	90	98.9%	94	94.9%	184	96.8%
Median age (years) (P25–P75)	77.2 (70.0–83.9)		76.8 (72.4–80.8)		77.1 (71.8–82.5)	
	Residence					
Residence in urban setting	39	42.9%	54	54.5%	93	48.9%
Residence in semi-rural/rural setting	52	57.1%	45	45.5%	97	51.1%
Home owner	86	94.5%	86	86.9%	172	90.5%
Median co-habitants (*n*) (P25–P75)	2 (1–2)		2 (1.5–2)		2 (1–2)	
	Education					
Primary education—none or incomplete	30	33.0%	24	24.2%	54	28.4%
Primary education	38	41.8%	52	52.5%	90	47.4%
Secondary education: High school/Initial vocational training	17	18.7%	20	20.2%	37	19.5%
University education/Advanced vocational training	6	6.6%	3	3.0%	9	4.7%
	Finance					
Median per capita monthly income (€)—(P25–P75)	800 (700–1100)		1000 (664.50–1350)		850 (700–1300)	
Median household monthly income (€)—(P25–P75)	1500 (1000–2100)		1600 (1200–2000)		1557.50 (1100–2000)	
	Health					
Median BMI (kg/m^2)—(P25–P75)	28.9 (25.7–31.2)		28.1 (25.5–30.5)		28.4 (25.6–30.8)	
Median monthly healthcare spending (€)—(P25–P75)	10 (0–30)		0 (0–16.5)		4.5 (0–23.75)	
Median daily consumption of medicaments (*n*) (P25–P75)	4 (2–7)		4 (3–6)		4 (2–6)	

Responses to the 'Healthy diet' questionnaire showed that 123 participants (68.3%) believe their diet "needs changes", acknowledging that their current eating habits and nutritional health are sub-optimal. Four persons (2.2%) indicated that their current diet was "unhealthy" and might be significantly contributing to the risk of overweight or obesity. By contrast, 53 participants (29.4%) claimed to have a "healthy" diet.

The relationship between BMI and the frequency of healthy food consumption was assessed using Spearman's correlation coefficient. A significant negative correlation was observed (rho = −0.79, $p < 0.05$), indicating that individuals who consume healthy foods more frequently—such as fruits and vegetables—tend to have lower BMI values. This result suggests that a balanced diet rich in nutritious foods is associated with a reduced risk of overweight and obesity, emphasizing the importance of promoting consistent healthy eating patterns within this population.

The SCORE IASE is a validated index that measures adherence to the Mediterranean diet based on the frequency of consumption of key food groups such as fruits, vegetables, legumes, whole grains, fish, and olive oil, while limiting red meat and processed foods.

Our analyses also examined the relationship between personal income levels and the score obtained on the IASE healthy eating scale. Using the Spearman correlation coefficient, a moderate positive correlation was found between these variables (rho = 0.42, $p < 0.05$). This suggests that participants with higher incomes tend to obtain higher scores on the IASE scale, indicating greater access and adherence to healthy eating patterns. This result reinforces the idea that income plays an important role in the ability to maintain health-promoting eating habits, although other factors may also influence this relationship.

The association between the SCORE IASE and body mass index (BMI) was examined using Spearman's rank correlation. The analysis revealed a statistically significant but weak negative correlation (rho = −0.089, $p = 0.021$), indicating that greater adherence to the Mediterranean diet was only modestly associated with lower BMI. Although statistically significant, the strength of this association is limited and should be interpreted with caution. Nevertheless, this finding suggests a potential inverse relationship between healthy dietary patterns and body weight status in the studied population.

Similarly, the relationship between individual income level and adherence to the Mediterranean diet was also assessed using Spearman's rank correlation. The analysis showed a weak but statistically significant positive correlation (rho = 0.062, $p = 0.039$), suggesting that higher income levels were associated with better adherence to the Mediterranean dietary pattern

Table 2 shows the variables significantly associated with increased Body Mass Index (BMI), based on a multivariable logistic regression model. The analysis revealed a consistent relationship between lower dietary quality scores and higher odds of being overweight. Specifically, lower scores for vegetable consumption—which indicate a reduced intake of vegetables—were significantly associated with increased likelihood of being overweight (OR = 0.887; 95% CI: 0.790–0.997; $p = 0.045$). Likewise, lower scores on the confectionery and processed meats indices, which reflect greater consumption of sweets and processed meats, were also significantly associated with higher odds of overweight (SCORE.CONFECTIONERY: OR = 0.923; 95% CI: 0.843–0.999; $p = 0.049$; SCORE.PROCESSED MEATS: OR = 0.905; 95% CI: 0.825–0.993; $p = 0.037$).

Table 2. Variables associated with increased BMI. Multivariable logistic regression model.

Variable	Odds Ratio (OR)	95% CI (Lower–Upper)	*p*-Value
SCORE VEGETABLES	0.887	0.790–0.997	0.045
SCORE CONFECTIONERY	0.923	0.843–0.999	0.049
SCORE PROCESSED MEATS	0.905	0.843–0.999	0.037

Adjusted R-squared: 0.2698.

These findings indicate that lower dietary quality scores—characterized by lower vegetable intake and higher consumption of confectionery and processed meats—are associated with increased BMI.

4. Discussion

The results of this study align with prior research indicating a direct association between unbalanced diets and the prevalence of obesity in older adults, particularly in Western societies where ultra-processed foods (UPFs) are widely accessible and often more affordable than healthier alternatives [7]. The high consumption of these foods among participants reflects earlier findings that identified processed meats (e.g., chorizo, ham, sausages) and bakery products (e.g., biscuits, pastries) as the primary UPFs consumed by older populations in these regions [10,12]. The low percentage of participants reporting a healthy diet underscores the urgent need for targeted interventions aimed at improving nutritional quality. Such strategies should not only focus on reducing UPF consumption but also emphasize the inclusion of fresh, nutrient-dense foods in older adults' diets. Nutrition education campaigns tailored to this demographic, alongside public policies that enhance access to healthy foods, could substantially reduce obesity rates in this vulnerable group [23]. Our analysis revealed a strong inverse relationship between the frequency of healthy food consumption and BMI. Participants who reported regular intake of fruits and vegetables had notably lower BMI values compared to those with infrequent or no consumption. This underscores the pivotal role of a balanced diet in weight regulation and suggests that fostering healthier eating behaviors among older adults could be a key strategy in improving health outcomes and lowering the risk of chronic, diet-related conditions [24].

Conversely, low socioeconomic status appears to negatively affect dietary quality and, consequently, BMI. Individuals with limited financial resources often face barriers to accessing fresh and nutritious food, leading to reliance on cheaper, calorie-dense UPFs high in fat, sugar, and sodium. Economic hardship may also induce stress that influences food choices, driving consumption of comfort foods that are typically less nutritious—contributing to long-term metabolic health risks [25,26].

These findings highlight the necessity of implementing preventive nutritional policies that go beyond dietary education to address broader social determinants of health, including income, education level, and geographic accessibility to healthy food sources [27–29]. Moreover, lifelong dietary patterns significantly influence food choices in later life. Habits formed in early and middle adulthood often persist into older age, reinforcing both healthy and unhealthy behaviors. As such, preventive efforts should extend across the life course, promoting nutritional literacy from a young age to establish sustainable and health-supportive eating practices over time [30].

This study has some limitations. Although detailed information on income, education level, and household composition was collected, the present analysis focused specifically on dietary patterns and their association with body mass index. Future analyses will explore the influence of other sociodemographic variables. Income and education are often closely correlated and represent overlapping aspects of socioeconomic status. In this study, we focused on income as a more direct proxy for food accessibility, while acknowledging that the independent effect of education could not be fully isolated due to potential multicollinearity. Additionally, the cross-sectional design limits the ability to establish causal relationships. Longitudinal studies are needed to better understand the complex interplay between socioeconomic factors, dietary habits, and obesity in older adults. Another limitation of this study is the reliance on self-reported food questionnaires, which are inherently subject to recall bias and possible misreporting of dietary intake. While the instruments used (FIES and IASE) are internationally validated, their use depends on participants' memory and subjective perception, which may affect data accuracy. Prospective methods or direct observation could provide more precise dietary information but were not feasible in this context.

Finally, social and familial contexts play a critical role in dietary adherence among older adults. Evidence suggests that strong social support networks are associated with better adherence to healthy diets, while social isolation correlates with higher risks of malnutrition and obesity [31,32]. Community-based programs that involve family members, caregivers, and local institutions have shown greater effectiveness than individual-focused interventions. When integrated with policies that subsidize fresh produce and regulate the availability of UPFs, such initiatives have the potential to yield broader and more sustainable public health benefits.

Overall, this study underscores the importance of a multidimensional and integrated approach to nutritional health in older adults—one that simultaneously addresses economic, educational, and environmental barriers to healthy eating.

5. Conclusions

The nutrition of older people is a major public health issue in Spain, which has an ageing population subject to increasing levels of obesity. According to our study results, factors such as economic limitations and the consumption of ultra-processed foods, like pastries, biscuits, and processed meats, contribute to unhealthy dietary patterns that increase the risk of obesity and hence chronic disease. These results underline the need for preventive public policies with a multidimensional approach aimed at promoting a more balanced and accessible diet, thus improving the quality of life and reducing the health risks associated with overweight and obesity in old age.

Author Contributions: A.F.-N. contributed to the study design, data analysis, and manuscript drafting. R.E. coordinated the research methodology and supervised the statistical analysis. C.L.-K. provided expertise in conceptualization and critical revision of the manuscript. M.G.-A. contributed to data collection and interpretation. C.S. assisted in literature review, data analysis, and manuscript editing. J.P.A. provided supervision, contributed to the discussion, and revised the final version of the manuscript. All authors have read and agreed to the published version of the manuscript.

Funding: The research projects I + D + I 2019 were: Eating Matters: Precarization and (In) secure Food Itineraries in Later Life (IP: M.G.-A.), Coordination: Universitat Rovira i Virgili. Code 10.13039/5011000011033/PID2019-104253RB-C21, Ministry of Science and Innovation, Spain and Research Project R + D + I 2019: Eating Matters: Environmental Risks and Dietary Uncertainties in Later Life. (IP: C.L.-K.). Coordination: University of Barcelona, Code 10.13039/5011000011033/PID2019-104253RB-C22, Ministry of Science and Innovation, Spain. Both started in June 2020 and completed in November 2024, and were conducted ethically.

Institutional Review Board Statement: This study was conducted in accordance with the guidelines of the Declaration of Helsinki. It was approved by the Ethics Committee of the University of Barcelona (10.13039/5011000011033, 22 December 2020), the Ethics Committee of the Rovira i Virgili University (CEIPSA-2020-PR-0002, 26 March 2021), and the Fundació Jordi Gol Ethics Committee (23/079-P, 18 December 2023). Additionally, the study was approved and authorized by the Northern Malaga Integrated Healthcare Area (CEIPSA-2020-PR-0002, 1 October 2022) and Clínica Guadalupe (CEIPSA-2020-PR-0002, 17 January 2023).

Informed Consent Statement: Informed written consent was obtained from all subjects involved in the study.

Data Availability Statement: The original contributions presented in this study are included in the article. Further inquiries can be directed to the corresponding authors.

Acknowledgments: The Eating Matters project would not have been possible without the selfless collaboration of all participants and the staff at the Health Centres Centro de Atención Primaria Florida Sud de L'Hospitalet de Llobregat and Clínica Guadalupe de Esplugues de Llobregat (Barcelona, Catalonia); Centro de Atención Primaria de Sant Salvador and Centro de Atención Primaria de El Morell (Tarragona, Catalonia); and Centro de Salud de Antequera and Centro de Salud de Archidona (Málaga, Andalusia).

Conflicts of Interest: The authors declare no conflicts of interest.

References

1. Sanchez-Garcia, E.; Cruz-Jentoft, A.J.; Ravasco, P.; Suominen, M.; Pitkälä, P.K. Nutritional care in older adults: Are we dc everything? An expert opinion review. *Curr. Med. Res. Opin.* **2024**, *40*, 1563–1576. [CrossRef] [PubMed]
2. Esperanza de Vida a Diferentes Edades. Available online: https://www.ine.es/ss/Satellite?L=es_ES&c=INESeccion_C&cid=1 944484459&p=1254735110672&pagename=ProductosYServicios/PYSLayout&param1=PYSDetalleFichaIndicador&param 259937499084 (accessed on 20 October 2024).
3. Gronich, N.; Saliba, W.; Schwartz, J.B. Prevalence and proportion by age and sex of chronic health conditions in a large health system. *PLoS ONE* **2024**, *19*, e0308031. [CrossRef] [PubMed] [PubMed Central]
4. Garcia, C.A.B.; Meira, K.C.; Souza, A.H.; Oliveira, A.L.G.; Guimarães, N.S. Obesity and associated factors in Brazilian ad Systematic review and meta-analysis of representative studies. *Int. J. Environ. Res. Public Health* **2024**, *21*, 1022. [Cross [PubMed] [PubMed Central]
5. Barbosa, B.B.; Baltar, V.T.; Horta, R.L.; Lobato, J.C.P.; Vieira, L.J.E.S.; Gallo, C.O.; Carioca, A.A.F. Cobertura do Sistema Vigilância Alimentar e Nutricional (SISVAN), estado nutricional de idosos e sua relação com desigualdades sociais no Br 2008–2019: Estudo ecológico de série temporal. *Epidemiol. Serv. Saude* **2022**, *32*. [CrossRef]
6. Wood, B.; Robinson, E.; Baker, P.; Paraje, G.; Mialon, M.; van Tulleken, C.; Sacks, G. What is the purpose of ultra-processed fo An exploratory analysis of the financialisation of ultra-processed food corporations and implications for public health. C *Health* **2023**, *19*, 85. [CrossRef] [PubMed] [PubMed Central]
7. Baker, P.; Machado, P.; Santos, T.; Sievert, K.; Backholer, K.; Hadjikakou, M.; Russell, C.; Huse, O.; Bell, C.; Scrinis, G.; e Ultra-processed foods and the nutrition transition: Global, regional and national trends, food systems transformations political economy drivers. *Obes. Rev.* **2020**, *21*, e13126. [CrossRef] [PubMed]
8. Godos, J.; Giampieri, F.; Al-Qahtani, W.H.; Scazzina, F.; Bonaccio, M.; Grosso, G. Ultra-Processed Food Consumption and Rela with Diet Quality and Mediterranean Diet in Southern Italy. *Int. J. Environ. Res. Public Health* **2022**, *19*, 11360. [CrossRef] [PubM [PubMed Central]
9. Monteiro, C.A.; Cannon, G.; Lawrence, M.; Costa Louzada, M.L.; Pereira Machado, P. Ultra-processed foods, diet quality, health using the NOVA classification system. *Public Health Nutr.* **2019**, *22*, 1764–1772.
10. Mendonça, R.D.; Pimenta, A.M.; Gea, A.; de la Fuente-Arrillaga, C.; Martinez-Gonzalez, M.A.; Lopes, A.C.; Bes-Rastrollo Ultraprocessed food consumption and risk of overweight and obesity: The University of Navarra Follow-Up (SUN) cohort st *Am. J. Clin. Nutr.* **2016**, *104*, 1433–1440. [CrossRef]
11. Chen, X.; Zhang, Z.; Yang, H.; Qiu, P.; Wang, H.; Wang, F.; Zhao, Q. Consumption of ultra-processed foods and health outcor A systematic review of epidemiological studies. *Nutr. J.* **2021**, *20*, 44. [CrossRef]
12. Srour, B.; Touvier, M.; Allès, B.; Mancini, F.R.; Bottigliengo, D.; Julia, C.; Hercberg, S.; Galan, P. Association between u processed food consumption and risk of mortality among middle-aged adults in France. *JAMA Intern. Med.* **2020**, *180*, 283– [CrossRef]
13. Larrea-Killinger, C.; Juzwiak, C.; Muñoz, A. "Nadie sabe lo que comemos": Confianza y desconfianza en los entornos alimenta en mujeres mayores de 65 años en España. *Anu. Antropol.* **2024**, *49*, 1–24. [CrossRef]
14. Larrea-Killinger, C.; Muñoz, A.; Echeverría, R.; Larrea, O.; Gracia-Arnaiz, M. Trust and distrust in food among non-depend elderly people in Spain. Study on socio-cultural representations through the analysis of cultural domains. *Appetite* **2** *197*, 107306. [CrossRef] [PubMed]
15. Company-Morales, M.; Casadó-Marín, L.; Muñoz, A.; Fontalba-Navas, A. Breaking the Silence on Food Risks for Elderly Pec Living Alone. *Nutrients* **2024**, *16*, 2655. [CrossRef] [PubMed] [PubMed Central]
16. Larrea-Killinger, C.; Muñoz, A.; Echeverría, R.; Gracia-Arnaiz, M. Comer importa. Desafíos alimentarios en sociedades envejecen. In *Itinerarios, Entornos y Consumo Alimentario en Personas Mayores: Etnografía Comparada en las Comunidades Autónoma Andalucía, Cataluña y Comunidad Valenciana*; Gracia-Arnaiz, M., Larrea-Killinger, C., Eds.; Tirant lo Blanch: Valencia, Spain, 2
17. FAO; IFAD; UNICEF; WFP; WHO. *The State of Food Security and Nutrition in the World 2023: Urbanization, Agrifood Syst Transformation and Healthy Diets Across the Rural–Urban Continuum*; FAO: Rome, Italy, 2023. Available online: https://www.w int/publications/m/item/the-state-of-food-security-and-nutrition-in-the-world-2023 (accessed on 15 September 2024).

Norte Navarro, A.I.; Ortiz Moncada, R. Calidad de la dieta española según el índice de alimentación saludable. *Nutr. Hosp.* **2011**, *26*, 330–336. [PubMed]
Sandri, E.; Cantín Larumbe, E.; Cerdá Olmedo, G. The Influence of Socio-Economic Factors on Diet and Active Lifestyle in the Spanish Female Population. *Nutrients* **2023**, *15*, 3319. [CrossRef] [PubMed] [PubMed Central]
Amo-Saus, E.; Pardo-García, I.; Martínez-Valero, A.P.; Escribano-Sotos, F. Health in Spanish older people: Dietary habits, lifestyles and related socioeconomic factors. *Prev. Med. Rep.* **2025**, *51*, 102995. [CrossRef] [PubMed] [PubMed Central]
Cederholm, T.; Barazzoni, R.; Austin, P.; Ballmer, P.; Biolo, G.; Bischoff, S.C.; Compher, C.; Correia, I.; Higashiguchi, T.; Holst, M.; et al. ESPEN guidelines on definitions and terminology of clinical nutrition. *Clin. Nutr.* **2017**, *36*, 49–64. [CrossRef] [PubMed]
Fox, J. Rcmdr: R Commander. R Package Version 2.9-0. 2024. Available online: https://CRAN.R-project.org/package=Rcmdr (accessed on 11 May 2025).
Kouiti, M.; Ortega-Rico, C.; Arrebola, J.P.; Gracia-Arnaiz, M.; Larrea-Killinger, C. Demographic and Socioeconomic Factors Associated to Fruits and Vegetables Consumption in Elderly Europeans: A Systematic Review. *Int. J. Environ. Res. Public Health* **2023**, *20*, 3442. [CrossRef] [PubMed] [PubMed Central]
Colleluori, G.; Villareal, D.T. Aging, obesity, sarcopenia and the effect of diet and exercise intervention. *Exp. Gerontol.* **2021**, *155*, 111561. [CrossRef]
Boucham, M.; Salhi, A.; El Hajji, N.; Gbenonsi, G.Y.; Belyamani, L.; Khalis, M. Factors associated with frailty in older people: An umbrella review. *BMC Geriatr.* **2024**, *24*, 737. [CrossRef] [PubMed] [PubMed Central]
Battista, F.; Bettini, S.; Verde, L.; Busetto, L.; Barrea, L.; Muscogiuri, G. Diet and physical exercise in elderly people with obesity: The state of the art. *Eur. J. Intern. Med.* **2024**, *130*, 9–18. [CrossRef] [PubMed]
Rezaei, M.; Ghadamgahi, F.; Jayedi, A.; Arzhang, P.; Yekaninejad, M.S.; Azadbakht, L. The association between food insecurity and obesity, a body shape index and body roundness index among US adults. *Sci. Rep.* **2024**, *14*, 23631. [CrossRef]
van de Geest, J.D.S.; Meijer, P.; Remmelzwaal, S.; Lakerveld, J. Moderators and mediators of the association between the obesogenicity of neighbourhoods and weight status in Dutch adults. *Health Place* **2024**, *90*, 103364. [CrossRef] [PubMed]
Papalini, S. Stress-induced overeating behaviors explained from a (transitory) relief-learning perspective. *Physiol Behav.* **2024**, *287*, 114707. [CrossRef] [PubMed]
Fernandez, D.M.; Larson, J.L.; Zikmund-Fisher, B.J. Associations between health literacy and preventive health behaviors among older adults: Findings from the health and retirement study. *BMC Public Health* **2016**, *16*, 596. [CrossRef] [PubMed] [PubMed Central]
Wieczorek, M.; Meier, C.; Kliegel, M.; Maurer, J. Relationship Between Health Literacy and Unhealthy Lifestyle Behaviours in Older Adults Living in Switzerland: Does Social Connectedness Matter? *Int. J. Public Health* **2023**, *68*, 1606210. [CrossRef] [PubMed] [PubMed Central]
Delerue Matos, A.; Barbosa, F.; Cunha, C.; Voss, G.; Correia, F. Social isolation, physical inactivity and inadequate diet among European middle-aged and older adults. *BMC Public Health* **2021**, *21*, 924. [CrossRef] [PubMed] [PubMed Central]

nutrients

MDPI

Article

Prolonged Water-Only Fasting Followed by a Whole-Plant-Food Diet Is a Potential Long-Term Management Strategy for Hypertension and Obesity

Evelyn Zeiler [1], Sahmla Gabriel [1], Mackson Ncube [1], Natasha Thompson [1], Daniel Newmire [2], Eugene L. Scharf Alan C. Goldhamer [4] and Toshia R. Myers [1,*]

[1] TrueNorth Health Foundation, Santa Rosa, CA 95404, USA; drevezeiler@gmail.com (E.Z.); macksonncube@gmail.com (M.N.)
[2] School of Health Promotion and Kinesiology, Texas Women's University, Denton, TX 76204, USA
[3] Department of Neurology, Mayo Clinic, Rochester, MN 55905, USA
[4] TrueNorth Health Center, Santa Rosa, CA 95404, USA; dracg@truenorthhealth.com
* Correspondence: drmyers@truenorthhealth.org

Abstract: Objective: This single-arm, pre–post interventional trial (clinicaltrials.gov, NCT04515095) investigates the safety, feasibility, and potential effectiveness of prolonged water-only fasting followed by a whole-plant-food diet in the long-term management of hypertension and other cardiometabolic disorders. **Methods:** Safety was assessed based on adverse events (AEs) that were recorded according to Common Terminology Criteria for Adverse Events (CTCAE) v5.0. Feasibility was assessed based on retention rate, ability to complete minimal fast length, and intervention acceptability. Twenty-nine participants with stage 1 and 2 hypertension and without type 2 diabetes were enrolled from a residential fasting center. **Results:** Study retention was 100% at the end of the refeed and 93% at the six-week follow-up visit. Median (range) fasting and refeeding duration were 11 (7–40) and 5 (3–17) days, respectively, and 90% of participants were able to complete at least 7 days of fasting. The majority of AEs were mild (grade 1) and transient and there were no higher-grade or serious AEs. At the end of the intervention, median systolic/diastolic blood pressure had normalized to below 130/80 mmHg, body weight reduced by >5%, and anti-hypertensive medication was completely discontinued. These results were sustained for at least six weeks and potentially up to one year. **Conclusions:** Our data suggest that the intervention may be a feasible, well-tolerated, low-risk option for lowering and managing high blood pressure, excess body weight, and other cardiometabolic disorders in people with stage 1 and 2 hypertension.

Keywords: hypertension; prolonged water-only fasting; prolonged fasting; adverse events; whole-plant-food diet; anti-hypertensive medication use; obesity

1. Introduction

More than half of US adults have hypertension (HTN), a primary modifiable risk factor for developing cardiovascular disease (CVD), kidney disease, and other conditions, with associated healthcare costs estimated at USD 131 billion annually [1–5]. Current treatment guidelines recommend diet and lifestyle modifications for all people with high blood pressure (BP) and the use of anti-hypertensive medications when systolic blood pressure (SBP) and/or diastolic blood pressure (DBP) reaches ≥140/90 mmHg (Stage 2 HTN) or in high-risk patients when SBP and/or DBP reaches ≥130/80 mmHg (Stage 1 HTN) [5]. However, up to 60% of medicated patients with HTN continue to have uncontrolled high BP, potentially due to modest BP reductions, high rates of adverse side effects, and low adherence rates associated with anti-hypertensive medications [6,7]. Additionally, lowering high BP with anti-hypertensive medications significantly reduces risk only in patients already at high risk for CVD [8]. Diet and lifestyle modifications may lower high BP, reduce associated CVD risks, and decrease rates of polypharmacy, but these interventions also suffer from low adherence rates [9–11]. Thus, there is a need for innovative treatment options to prevent and reverse high blood pressure, ideally with an overall improvement in cardiovascular health.

Medically supervised, prolonged water-only fasting followed by an exclusively whole-plant-food diet free of added salt, oil, and sugar (SOS-free diet) has a very low risk of causing severe or serious adverse events and effectively lowers borderline and high blood pressure [12–14]. The intervention may support adherence to diet and lifestyle modifications and also correlates with sustained improvements in biomarkers of CVD risk [15,16]. To further evaluate the potential of this intervention as a treatment for HTN, we conducted a single-arm pre–post interventional trial with long-term follow-up. The primary aim was to assess the safety and feasibility of the intervention in adults with stage 1 and stage 2 HTN and without type 2 diabetes. We systematically collected and reported adverse events and treatment deviations, along with study retention rates, participants' ability to complete the minimum fasting duration, and self-reported acceptability of the intervention. Additionally, we measured the immediate, sustained, and long-term effects of the intervention on blood pressure and other cardiometabolic risk factors.

2. Materials and Methods

2.1. Ethical Approval

This study was approved by the TrueNorth Health Foundation Institutional Review Board (TNHF2020-1HTN and TNHF2021-1HTNFU) and registered at clinicaltrials.gov (NCT04515095). The research was conducted in accordance with the approved protocol and complied with the standards of the Declaration of Helsinki. All participants provided written informed consent before data collection began.

2.2. Participant Enrollment and Study Protocol

This study was a single-arm pre–post intervention trial that recruited patients with stage 1 and 2 HTN who were undergoing an elective, medically supervised, water-only fast of at least seven days at a residential fasting center between August 2020 and September 2021. Thirty participants were enrolled, of which one was ineligible due to pre-existing hyponatremia that contraindicates fasting (Figure 1). Consenting participants of any sex, aged 30–75 years, with uncontrolled (SBP $\geq$ 130 mmHg and/or DBP $\geq$ 80 mmHg) or medication-controlled HTN, fasting glucose < 126 mg/dL and/or hemoglobin A1c < 7%, and prior approval by a non-research physician to water-only fast for at least seven consecutive days followed by a refeeding period of at least half the fasting length were eligible for inclusion. Exclusion criteria included SBP > 180 and/or DBP > 120 mmHg at the time of enrollment, active malignancy, active kidney disease, active inflammatory disorder (including classic autoimmune connective tissue disorders, multiple sclerosis, inflammatory bowel disorders), stroke or heart attack within the last 90 days, and the inability to discontinue medications and/or supplements. Study dates overlapped with NCT04514146, conducted at the same fasting center, and 18/29 participants were co-enrolled in that study [15].

During the treatment period, onsite study visits occurred daily and at baseline (BL), end-of-fast (EOF), and end-of-refeed (EOR). Two additional study visits occurred either onsite or remotely: an expected visit that occurred 6 weeks after departure from the fasting center (6wFU) and one unexpected visit that occurred 12 months after the 6wFU visit (12mFU). During daily visits, symptoms and vital signs were assessed, and adverse events (AEs) were recorded. Additionally, demographics, medical diagnoses, medication use, total body weight (BW), blood pressure (BP), abdominal circumference (AC), and blood and urine samples were collected at BL, EOF, EOR, weekly from BL to EOR, 6wFU, and 12mFU visits (see supplemental methods 1.1 and 1.2 for data collection details). Web-based versions of three questionnaires were administered: the SOS-Free Diet Screener [15] at BL, 6wFU, and 12mFU visits; the Treatment Adherence/Acceptability Scale (TAAS) [17] questionnaire at EOF and 6wFU visits; and the Food Acceptability Questionnaire (FAQ) [18] at BL, EOR,

6wFU, and 12mFU visits. Data collection and survey distribution were performed using the web-based software Research Electronic Data Capture (REDCap) [19]. Missing data are described in Figure 1 and the legend of respective tables.

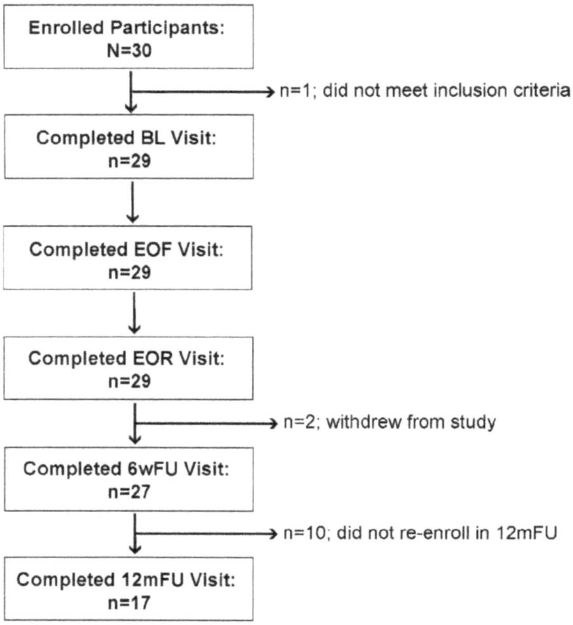

Figure 1. Enrollment and participation flow diagram. See "Participant Enrollment and Study Protocol" in the "Materials and Methods" section and "Participant Characteristics" in the "Results" section for details on eligibility and data collection. N, number of participants; BL, baseline; EOF, end-of-fast; EOR, end-of-refeed; 6wFU, six-week follow-up; 12mFU, 12-month follow-up. At EOF visit, 2/29 participants began refeeding before the blood draw and were excluded from serology and urinalysis. At the 6wFU visit, 2 out of 27 provided incomplete data: one provided all data except for anthropometric measurements, and one provided only blood pressure data.

2.3. Medically Supervised Water-Only Fasting Protocol

The prefeeding, fasting, and refeeding protocol took place at a residential fasting center. The protocol was previously described in detail [14]. Participants were approved to water-only fast by medical doctors not affiliated with this study after a thorough examination, which included detailed patient history, comprehensive physical exam, basic neurological and psychological status, complete blood count (CBC), comprehensive metabolic panel (CMP), urinalysis, and additional tests as clinically indicated, in order to rule out contraindications to fasting. Medication use while water-only fasting is contraindicated, and ability to safely discontinue medication use was a requirement for enrollment in this study. Participants received 24 h medical supervision during the entire treatment (i.e., prefeeding, water-only fasting, and refeeding). Vital signs were examined by medical personnel twice per day, and labs were ordered once per week or as requested by the attending physician.

2.3.1. Prefeeding

A prefeeding period began at least two days prior to the water-only fast, during which participants eliminated all recreational drugs (e.g., coffee, alcohol, nicotine, etc.) and specific foods (i.e., grains, legumes, dairy, meat, seafood, added sugar, oils, and salt, and all processed foods) and ate only the provided raw/steamed fruits and vegetables. During this time, participants were weaned off anti-hypertensive and other medications as determined appropriate by the attending physician based on clinical protocol and according to the individual participant's medical needs.

2.3.2. Fasting

Participants remained onsite during the entire fasting period, were encouraged to engage in a small amount of low-intensity physical activity (i.e., slow walking and light stretching), and did not operate heavy machinery (e.g., automobiles). During the water-only fast, participants drank a minimum of 1.2 L/day of steam-distilled water. If medically indicated (e.g., due to blood electrolyte imbalance, hypoglycemia, or gastroesophageal reflux disease) or desired by the participant, vegetable broth (VB; 80 kcal per day) was consumed. VB has such an insignificant number of calories that it does not prevent ketosis or reverse ketosis once it is initiated and is assumed to be equivalent to water. The fast continued for the predetermined amount of time or was modified according to the individual patient's needs. In cases of more severe adverse events or discomfort, the fast was temporarily or indefinitely broken with fruit and vegetable juice (500–600 kcal per day) or potato/zucchini blend (900 kcal per day).

2.3.3. Refeeding

The refeeding diet was administered in five phases: (1) fruit and vegetable juice; (2) raw fruits/vegetables; (3) raw/steamed vegetables and fruits; (4) raw/steamed fruits and vegetables, grains, and nuts or avocado; (5) unrestricted whole-plant foods free of added salt, oil, and sugar. Each of the five refeeding phases lasted 1 day for every 7–10 days of water-only fasting, for a period of time lasting at least one-half of the total fast length (e.g., 10 days of fasting would correspond to 5 days of refeeding with 1 day on each of the five phases). If medically indicated (e.g., due to food intolerance), the refeeding protocol was modified [14]. Before leaving the center, participants received basic nutrition education and were instructed to continue the exclusively whole-plant-food, SCS-free diet for at least the next six weeks. There were no further instructions after the 6wFU visit.

2.4. Adverse Events Recording and Analysis

While prefeeding, fasting, and refeeding, AEs were identified in daily interviews conducted by trained clinical research personnel, daily physical (i.e., daily vital signs) examinations, weekly blood analysis (i.e., CBC and CMP), and weekly urinalysis. AEs were recorded by date and according to Common Terminology Criteria for Adverse Events (CTCAE) [20] based on symptom categorization and severity (grade 1, mild; grade 2, moderate; grade 3, severe; grade 4, life-threatening; grade 5, death). The CTCAE describes AE terms according to the Medical Dictionary for Regulatory Activities (MedDRA) as lowest-level terms (LLT) that are grouped into a system organ class (SOC). For terms not specifically listed in the CTCAE and listed under the MedDRA SOC as 'other', new terms were added and graded according to the CTCAE guideline that described the AE as best as possible. All AEs were reported regardless of attribution. Pre-existing conditions were considered an AE if reoccurring or increasing in severity at any time during the intervention. The same AE may have occurred multiple times for the same participant and was counted as a new event if it decreased or increased in grade or had previously resolved but subsequently returned. AE outcomes (i.e., resolved, persisted, unknown) were determined as follows: the outcome was considered "resolved" if the symptom cleared completely or the severity of the event decreased (e.g., G2 decreased to G1). The outcome was considered "persisted" if the AE did not resolve at EOR or 6wFU visit. The outcome was considered "unknown" if the interview or specific analysis was not repeated (only AEs determined by CMP and CBC were monitored at 6wFU) or if the participant failed to report back at the 6wFU visit. The total number of AEs for all participants during the entire intervention was counted and presented based on SOC, LLT, grade, and outcome. Additionally, the top 10% of total AEs experienced by participants were presented based on LLT, grade, and treatment phase (i.e., prefeeding, fasting, and refeeding). AEs were further categorized as the highest-grade adverse event (HGAE) during the entirety of each participant's intervention.

2.5. Daily Vital Signs

Daily vital signs, including body weight (BW), BP, peripheral oxygen saturation (SpO_2), and body temperature (BT), were collected onsite by trained clinical research staff every morning from BL through EOR. Baseline values were calculated from day 2 daily vitals data. Participants were asked to rest in a seated position with their arms elevated to heart level on a table or pillow for five minutes prior to having their BP (Welch Allyn-Connex ProBP 3400, Hill-Rom Holding Inc., Chicago, IL, USA), BT (Welch Allyn Sure Temp plus 690, Hill-Rom Holding Inc., Chicago, IL, USA), peripheral oxygen saturation (SpO_2, Zacurate 500DL, Zacurate, Stafford, TX, USA), and pulse rate and rhythm (manually for 15 s or 1 min) measured. BW was self-reported using a floor scale (WW26, Conair LLC, Stamford, CT, USA). Participants were also observed and asked about hours of sleep, energy level, urination characteristics (dysuria, difficulty, changes), nausea, presyncope (i.e., near fainting), quantity of water intake, bowel movements (frequency, characteristics), and any other symptoms for the previous 24 h as well as about any unresolved complaints.

2.6. Questionnaires

2.6.1. SOS-Free Dietary Screener

Adherence to the recommended SOS-Free Diet was assessed with a 27-question screener as previously described [15]. The SOS-Free Dietary Screener was administered online at BL, 6wFU, and 12mFU visits. A non-adherence score was calculated based on the consumption of inclusionary and exclusionary foods over the previous 30 days. The minimum non-adherence score is zero (i.e., 100% adherent), and the maximum non-adherence score is 82.5 (i.e., 0% adherent).

2.6.2. Treatment Acceptability Adherence Scale

Acceptability of the treatment was assessed using the Treatment Acceptability/Adherence Scale (TAAS) [17]. The TAAS was administered online at EOF and 6wFU visits. The TAAS contains 10 questions with response options ranging from 1 (disagree strongly) to 4 (neither agree nor disagree) to 7 (agree strongly). Negatively worded questions (#3–5, #7–8, #10) were reverse scored, and total scores were obtained by summing all answers. Scoring ranged from 70 to 10, with higher scores indicating greater treatment acceptability. Individual questions are shown in Figure S1.

2.6.3. Food Acceptability Questionnaire

Acceptability of foods permitted on the SOS-Free Diet was assessed using the Food Acceptability Questionnaire [18]. The FAQ was administered online at BL, EOR, 6wFU, and 12mFU visits. The questionnaire contains 10 questions with response options ranging from 1 (not at all) to 7 (extremely). Negatively worded questions (#4 and #8) were reverse scored, and total scores were obtained by summing all answers. Scoring ranged from 70 to 10, with higher scores indicating greater acceptability of permissible foods. Individual questions are shown in Figure S2.

2.7. Statistical Analysis

Data cleaning and statistical analysis were conducted using R, with descriptive statistics reported as medians and interquartile ranges (IQR) [21]. The statistical analysis aimed to estimate within-group changes between visits (e.g., BL, EOF, EOR, 6wFU, and 12mFU). The analysis employed random intercept generalized linear mixed-effects models, with clinical parameters as dependent variables and participant ID as the grouping variable. Age and sex served as fixed effect control variables in all models; baseline HTN status was also included for binary outcome models.

Continuous outcomes were analyzed using lmerTest version 3.1.3 [22], while binary and count outcomes used lme4 version 1.1.32 [23]. Binary data were modeled using a binomial family parameter with a logit link, and count data used a Poisson family parameter with a log link. Regression coefficients and 95% confidence intervals (CI) were extracted using broom.mixed version 0.2.9.4 [24]. Missing data were addressed through complete case analysis, where case is defined as a visit within participant. Model diagnostics employed the modelDiagnostics function from multilevelTools version 0.0.1 [25], with model assumption violations addressed by comparing lmerTest results to Robust Scoring Equations estimator (RSE) results from robustlmm version 3.2.0 [26,27] using the Satterthwaite approximation from sjPlot version 2.8.14 [28]. RSE results were preferred when they differed substantially from the lmerTest analysis. The RSE method was not available for binary or count outcomes.

After data collection was complete, a post-hoc simulation-based power analysis [29] was conducted. This analysis used hypothetical population effect sizes and standard deviations [30] derived from the SBP and BMI models in Table 4 of Gabriel et al. [15] The goal was to estimate the sample size required to achieve 80% statistical power at an alpha level of 0.05 for parameter estimates assessing within-group changes from BL to 6wFU visits. For SBP, the power analysis indicated that 80% power could be attained with 32 participants. Adjusting the simulation to increase the magnitude of effect sizes associated with the visits by 10% resulted in achieving 80% power with a reduced sample size of 27 participants. For the exploratory secondary endpoint BMI, the analysis demonstrated that 80% statistical power could be reached with 27 participants.

The rates of change in clinical parameters were estimated using linear mixed-effect models [31] implemented with nlme version 3.1.160 [32]. Models included the clinical parameter as the dependent variable, day of study phase as a fixed effect, and participant ID as the random intercept. A random slope for day of study phase was included when supported by lower Akaike Information Criterion and Bayesian Information Criterion values. Separate models were fitted for prefeeding, fasting, and refeeding. For the body weight analysis, the fasting phase was divided into early (days 1–5) and late periods with phase, day of study phase, and their interaction included as fixed effects. Model assumptions were verified using residual and quantile-quantile plots. RSEs [26] with Satterthwaite approximation [28] were applied when necessary.

3. Results

3.1. Participant Characteristics

Baseline characteristics of participants (N = 29) are presented in Table 1. All participants had a diagnosis of stage 1 or 2 HTN, and 15 (52%) were taking anti-hypertensive medications. The most common pre-existing comorbidities were obesity (n = 15; 52%) and mixed and unspecified hyperlipidemia (n = 12; 41%) (Tables 1 and S1).

Table 1. Select baseline characteristics.

Total Participants, N	29
Total Medicated ^ Participants, n (%)	15 (52)
Female, n (%)	19 (66)
Median (IQR) Age, y	62 (58, 67)
SBP < 130 AND DBP < 80 mmHg, n (%)	5 † (17)
SBP ≥ 130 AND ≤ 139 mmHg AND/OR DBP ≥ 80 AND ≤ 89 mmHg, n (%)	12 * (41)
SBP ≥ 140 AND/OR DBP ≥ 90 mmHg, n (%)	12 ≠ (41)
Normal Weight BMI, n (%)	4 (14)
Overweight BMI, n (%)	10 (34)
Obese BMI, n (%)	15 (52)

N, the total number of participants; n, a subset of 29 participants; %, percentage; IQR, interquartile range; y, years; SBP, systolic blood pressure; DBP, diastolic blood pressure: Stage 1 HTN = 130–139/80–89 mmHg, Stage 2 HTN = ≥140/90 mmHg; BMI, body mass index: normal weight, 18.5–<25 kg/m^2; overweight, 25–<29 kg/m^2; obese ≥30 kg/m^2. ^ Medicated with anti-hypertensive medications; † 4 of 5 participants were taking anti-hypertensive medications. * 5 of 12 participants were taking anti-hypertensive medications. ≠ 6 of 12 participants were taking anti-hypertensive medications.

3.2. Treatment and Visit Characteristics

This study was conducted onsite at a residential fasting center, and participants' adherence to the fasting and refeeding protocol was monitored by trained medical personnel as part of standard practice. All 29 participants completed BL, EOF, and EOR visits. Of the 29 participants, 26 (90%) completed at least seven consecutive days of fasting (see full description of treatment deviations in Section 3.4). The median (range) prefeeding, water-only fasting, and refeeding duration was 2 (1–4), 11 (7–40), and 5 (3–17) days, respectively.

Participants had daily access to nutrition and health education, were instructed to continue eating an SOS-free diet while offsite between EOR and 6wFU visits, and did not receive further dietary instruction thereafter. Of the 29 participants, 27 (93%) attended the 6wFU visit, which occurred at a median (range) of 45 (40–58) days after the EOR visit (Figure 1). Of the 27 participants, 17 (63%) attended the unanticipated 12mFU visit, which occurred at a median (range) of 364 (358, 383) days after the 6wFU visit. Of these 17 participants, 5 voluntarily visited the fasting center for additional interventions between 6wFU and 12mFU visits. Of these, 2 participants visited the fasting center one time and 3 participants visited two times, with a median (range) fasting and refeeding length of 10 (8, 13) and 6 (4, 9) days, respectively.

Participants' adherence to an SOS-free diet during the follow-up periods was assessed using a previously described dietary screener with scores ranging from 0 (100% adherent) to 82 (0% adherent) [15]. Responses to individual questions are in Table S2. The mean (SD) score was 12 (10), 6 (3), and 6 (4) at BL, 6wFU, and 12mFU, respectively. Participants reported increased fruit and vegetable consumption and decreased consumption of animal products, added salt, and added oil.

3.3. Adverse Events Identified During Prefeeding, Fasting, and Refeeding

Daily interviews and physical examinations, as well as weekly hematology, serology, urinalyses, and additional testing as indicated, were used to identify AEs from BL through EOR visits. AEs were classified into categories and grades using CTCAE v.5.0 [20]. We identified 453 AEs, of which 381 (84%) were mild Grade 1 (G1), 64 (14%) were moderate Grade 2 (G2), and 8 (2%) were severe Grade 3 (G3) events (Table 2). There were no Grade 4 (life-threatening), Grade 5 (death), or serious AEs. There were 11 (2%), 350 (77%), and 92 (20%) AEs during prefeeding, fasting, and refeeding, respectively (Table 2). G1, G2, and G3 were the highest-grade AE (HGAE) experienced by 7% (2/29), 69% (20/29), and 24% (7/29) of participants, respectively.

Table 2. Total adverse events by grade and treatment phase.

	N (%)			
AE Grade	**Prefeeding**	**Fasting**	**Refeeding**	**All Phases**
1	9	289	83	381 (84)
2	2	54	8	64 (14)
3	0	7	1	8 (2)
4	0	0	0	0
5	0	0	0	0
Total	11 (2)	350 (77)	92 (20)	453 (100)

N (%), number and percentage of total adverse events; AE, adverse event; Grade 1, mild; Grade 2, moderate; Grade 3, severe; Grade 4, life-threatening; Grade 5, death. There were no Grade 4 or 5 events.

A detailed account of adverse event type, severity, prevalence, and outcomes can be found in Supplemental Tables S3 and S4. The most commonly occurring AEs (i.e., experienced by >10% of participants) by treatment stage are shown in Table S3. Overall, the five most common events were mild-to-moderate fatigue, mild decrease in blood bicarbonate, mild decrease in BUN/creatinine, mild-to-moderate high blood pressure, and mild-to-moderate nausea. During fasting, the three most common events were fatigue, hypertension, and decreased blood bicarbonate. There were 15 AE classifications that only occurred during fasting (Table S3), including presyncope and various mild changes in blood chemistry and/or blood count identified by CMP and CBC analysis (Tables S5–S8). During refeeding, fatigue was the most common event, and diarrhea occurred only during refeeding (Table S3). As expected, four-fifths of hyperglycemia events occurred during refeeding. The other hyperglycemic event was identified at the EOF visit and may be due to an unreported protocol deviation.

Total AEs, associated system organ class, and event outcome are shown in Table S4. The most frequently occurring G1 events were fatigue (n = 60/381), dizziness (n = 23/381), decreased blood bicarbonate (n = 22/381), decreased BUN/creatinine ratio (n = 18/381), nausea (n = 13/381), and decreased chloride (n = 13/381) and did not require intervention. Of the 381 G1 events, 33 were unresolved at EOR or 6wFU visits, and the outcome of 19/381 G1 events was unknown due to either unrepeated tests (9/19) or participant dropout (10/19). The most frequently occurring G2 events were fatigue (n = 19/64), hypertension (16/64), and presyncope (n = 10/64). All of the G2 events were resolved while onsite (n = 63/64) or before the 6wFU visit (n = 1/64). Of the eight G3 events, seven were hypertensive events, and one was a low neutrophil count. All G3 hypertensive events resolved before the EOR visit, but it is unknown if the low neutrophil count resolved due to participant dropout at the 6wFU visit.

We also assessed median changes in the clinical and laboratory markers used to assess AEs at each study visit. The median (IQR) for CBC variables remained within the normal range throughout this study (Table S5), but several values significantly changed, and some changes were considered to be AEs. For example, there was a statistically significant increase in red blood cells at the EOF visit, and there were six G1 AEs due to increased red blood cells that did not require intervention (Tables S4 and S6). There were also several CMP values with statistically significant changes (e.g., decreased sodium at the EOF visit that resulted in 5 G1 hyponatremia events that did not require intervention, Tables S4 and S8). However, the only abnormal median (IQR) values included low BUN [6 (4, 8) mg/dL] for participants >60 years old at the EOR visit, low BUN/creatinine ratio at EOF [8 (7, 11) mg/dL] and EOR [7 (6, 9) mg/dL] visits for the entire population, and decreased carbon dioxide [17 (15, 20) mmol/L] at the EOF visit (Tables S7 and S8). Median values increased to the normal range for carbon dioxide at the EOR visit and for BUN and BUN/creatinine ratio at the 6wFU visit.

Urinalysis confirmed that during fasting, the concentration of ketones increased while pH decreased, and both values reverted to baseline upon refeeding when glucose metabolism resumed (Table S9). At EOF, median urine volume (mL) decreased along with a slight increase in median (IQR) urine specific gravity (USG) to 1.008 (1.006, 1.010), which is well below the value (1.020) indicating dehydration (Table S10). Although the standard USG data do not suggest that clinically significant dehydration occurred during fasting, dipstick analysis indicates that at EOF, four participants had USG > 1.020, suggesting mild dehydration (Table S9). Median sodium (mmol/24 h) excretion also decreased to slightly below the reference range at EOF and EOR but normalized by the 6wFU (Table S10). Median potassium (mmol/24 h) excretion was slightly elevated at baseline but decreased to low-normal at EOF, and was also normalized by the 6wFU. Pulse significant increase from BL to EOF visits (β (95% CI): 7.66 beats/min (3.10 to 12.21)), corresponding to an estimated rate of change of 0.55 beats/min per day, respectively, during fasting, but the changes were not clinically significant (Tables 3, 4 and S11). There were no clinically meaningful changes observed for BT and SpO2 (Tables 3, 4 and S11). These results indicate that fasting causes various temporary minor changes that are likely necessary to maintain homeostasis during the fasted state.

Table 3. Vital signs by visit.

	Median (IQR)		
	BL	**EOF**	**EOR**
BW, kg	86.6 (80.1, 97.6)	79.1 (72.4, 87.8)	81.4 (73.8, 88.7)
SBP, mmHg <120	135 (123, 150)	125 (120, 131)	114 (108, 123)
DBP, mmHg <80	81 (76, 88)	84 (80, 85)	78 (74, 82)
BT, °C 36.1–37.2	36.7 (36.5, 36.9)	36.6 (36.5, 36.7)	36.7 (36.6, 36.9)
Pulse, min^{-1} 60–100	66 (60, 70)	73 (68, 83)	69 (64, 80)
SpO_2, % 95–100	98 (97, 99)	98 (97, 99)	98 (98, 98)

Normal reference ranges are listed below each variable. At BL, EOF, and EOR, there were 29 participants. IQR, interquartile range; BL, baseline; EOF, end-of-fast; EOR, end-of-refeed; BW, body weight; DBP, diastolic blood pressure; mmHg, millimeter mercury; kg; BT, body temperature; °C, degrees Celsius; min^{-1}, per minute; SpO_2, saturation of peripheral oxygen; %, percent.

Table 4. Significance of differences for vital signs.

	Estimates (95% CI) *p*-Value		
	EOF-BL	**EOR-BL**	**EOR-EOF**
Weight, kg ‡	−7.76 * (−8.85, −6.66) <0.001	−6.59 * (−7.69, −5.49) <0.001	1.17 * (0.07, 2.26) 0.038
SBP, mmHg	−9.34 * (−15.80, −2.89) 0.006	−18.93 * (−25.39, −12.48) <0.001	−9.59 * (−16.04, −3.13) 0.005
DBP, mmHg	0.71 (−2.76, 4.17) 0.693	−4.33 * (−7.79, −0.87) 0.017	−5.03 * (−8.50, −1.57) 0.006
BT, °C	−0.06 (−0.18, 0.06) 0.313	0.03 (−0.08, 0.15) 0.589	0.09 (−0.02, 0.21) 0.122
Pulse, min^{-1}	7.66 * (3.10, 12.21) 0.002	5.00 * (0.45, 9.55) 0.036	−2.66 (−7.21, 1.90) 0.258
SpO_2, % ‡	0.07 (−0.56, 0.71) 0.820	0.27 (−0.36, 0.89) 0.408	0.19 (−0.43, 0.82) 0.550

CI, confidence interval; BL, baseline; EOF, end-of-fast; EOR, end-of-refeed; BW, body weight; SBP, systolic blood pressure; DBP, diastolic blood pressure; mmHg, millimeter mercury; kg, kilogram; BT, body temperature; °C, degrees Celsius; min^{-1}, per minute; SpO_2, saturation of peripheral oxygen; %, percent. * Zero lies outside the 95% CI, so the finding is considered significant. ‡ Used robust mixed effects model on complete cases. Weight, SBP, and DBP models included 6wFU and 12mFU time points as described for Table S14 [15].

3.4. Deviations in Water-Only Fasting Intervention

As described in Section 3.2, 3/29 (10%) participants did not complete at least seven consecutive days of fasting. One fasted entirely on vegetable broth due to pre-existing cardiac arrhythmia. Of the other two participants, one temporarily interrupted the fast with a steamed potato/zucchini blend due to a G2 gastroesophageal reflux event, and one modified the fast with vegetable and fruit juice due to G2 hypoglycemia. Of the 26 participants, 17 completed at least seven consecutive days of fasting solely on water and 9 supplemented distilled water with vegetable broth (80 kcal/day) without interrupting ketosis. Six of those nine participants consumed vegetable broth while fasting because of a treatment-emergent AE, including G2 presyncope (n = 3), G1 gastroesophageal reflux (n = 1), G1 hypokalemia (n = 1), and G1 dry mouth (n = 1). The remaining 3 consumed vegetable broth for non-medical reasons. Additionally, of the 26 participants, 2 completed at least seven consecutive fasting days and had their fast prematurely terminated after day seven due to an AE, which included 1 participant with a G2 nausea event and 1 with concurrent G1 hypokalemia and G1 electrocardiogram QT-corrected prolonged events.

3.5. Changes in BW, Anti-Hypertensive Medication Use, and BP

BW and BP were also collected during daily vital signs monitoring throughout fasting and refeeding. At baseline (i.e., day 2 of daily rounding), 52%, 34%, and 14% had obesity, overweight, and normal weight, respectively (Table 1). At the EOR visit, 38%, 31%, 28%, and 3% had obesity, overweight, normal weight, and underweight, respectively (Table S12). Baseline median (IQR) BW had a clinically meaningful reduction from 87.0 (80.0, 96.3) kg at BL to 79.1 (72.4, 87.8) kg and 81.4 (73.8, 88.7) kg at EOF and EOR visits, respectively (Table 3); after controlling for age and sex, the average changes from BL to EOF (β (95% CI): −7.76 kg (−8.85 to −6.66)) and from BL to EOR visits (β (95% CI): −6.59 kg (−7.69 to −5.49)) were statistically significant (Table 4). This corresponded to an average BW loss of −0.54 kg/day ($p < 0.0001$) while fasting, with higher rates of loss early in fasting and an average gain of 0.23 kg/day ($p < 0.0001$) while refeeding (Table S11). The one person who was underweight at the EOF visit recovered to normal weight by the 6wFU (Table S12). Median weight loss was also maintained at 6wFU and 12mFU visits (Tables S13 and S14).

The population recruited for this study had a current diagnosis of stage 1 or 2 hypertension. At the BL visit, 15/29 (52%) participants were taking nineteen anti-hypertensive medications; 11/15 were taking one, and 4/15 were taking two medications (Table S15). Only 4/15 (27%) had achieved a medication-controlled SBP/DBP of <130/80 mmHg (Table 1). During the prefeeding period, all participants were tapered completely off anti-hypertensive medications by a trained physician according to their individual medical needs and remained off medications while at the residential fasting center. Participants' medication use after leaving the fasting center was determined independently by their primary care physician. As such, no participants were taking any anti-hypertensive medications at EOF or EOR visits. Overall, baseline median (IQR) SBP/DBP had clinically meaningful changes from 135 (123, 150)/81 (7, 88) at BL to 125 (120, 131)/84 (80, 85) and 114 (108, 123)/78 (74, 82) mmHg at EOF and EOR visits, respectively (Table 3, Figure 2A,B). The estimated changes in SBP/DBP from BL to EOF and in SBP from BL to EOF were found to be statistically significant after controlling for age and sex (Table 4). The reductions in BP were sustained at the 6wFU and 12mFU visits. The estimated loss (95% CI) in SBP/DBP from the BL visit was −10.24/−4.65 (−16.04/−7.71, −4.46/−1.57) and −8.80/−8.83 (−15.47/−12.35, −2.15/−1.57) mmHg at 6wFU and 12mFU visits, respectively (Tables S13 and S14).Of the 15 medicated participants, 14 were taking anti-hypertensive medications at the BL visit and returned for the 6wFU visit; of them, only 1/14 was taking one anti-hypertensive medication at a reduced dose (Table S15). Of the 17 participants, 7 attended the 12mFU visit and were taking anti-hypertensive medications; 5 were remedicated, and 2 were newly medicated (Table S15). Figure 2C–F shows the SBP/DBP distribution of medicated and unmedicated participants at each study visit.

As previously described for a subset (n = 18) of this population [15], median values and estimated changes in these and other select cardiometabolic markers are also presented in Tables S13 and S14. At BL, only median total cholesterol, LDL, and FLI were outside of the normal limits. Median (IQR) total cholesterol normalized during refeeding to 4.71 (4.12, 5.52) mmol/L and was sustained at 6wFU and 12mFU visits. Median LDL remained slightly elevated throughout this study, and median triglycerides increased slightly out of normal limits at the EOR visit but normalized again at the 6wFU visit. Median insulin remained within normal limits throughout this study; however, the statistical model estimated a significant decrease from BL to EOF visit, a significant increase from BL to EOR visit and a return to BL by the 6wFU visit. Median (IQR) FLI was abnormally high at the BL visit (ST13) and mixed effects modeling provided evidence for a statistically significantly decrease from BL levels at 6wFU and 12mFU visits (ST14). These results suggest that the intervention effectively reduces high BP and BW, and may be an effective long-term management strategy for treating HTN, obesity, and other cardiometabolic disorders.

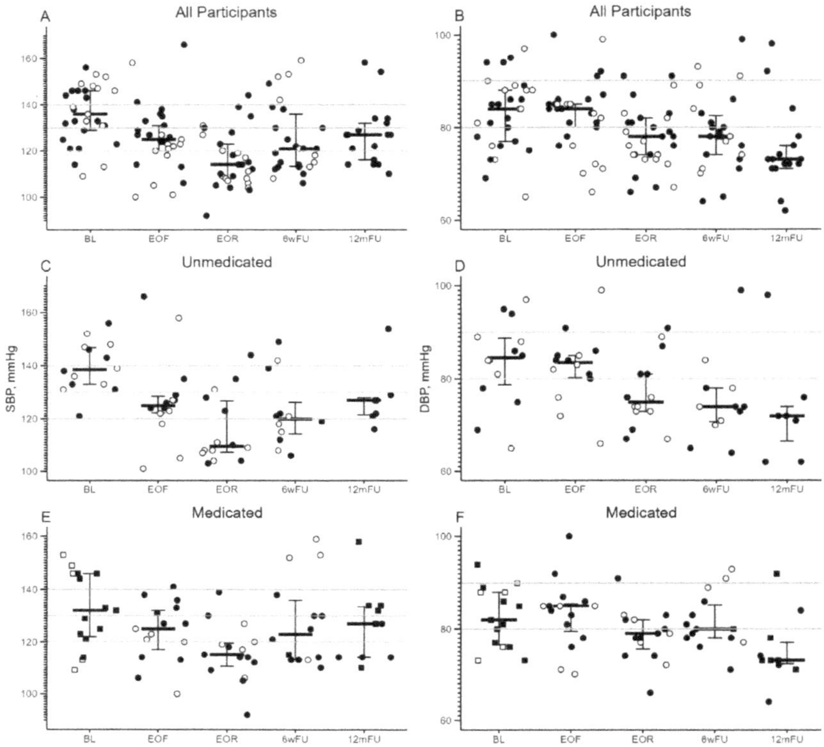

Figure 2. SBP (**A**,**C**,**E**) and DBP (**B**,**D**,**F**) by visit of all participants (**A**,**B**) and by baseline medication status (unmedicated (**C**,**D**,) and medicated (**E**,**F**)). Graphs include individual values as well as first (lower) and third (upper) quartiles and the median value. Circles and squares in panels (**C**–**F**) represent unmedicated and medicated SBP/DBP, respectively. Participants who attended the 6wFU visit (n = 27) and 12mFU visit (n = 17) are depicted as unfilled (open) and filled (black) symbols, respectively. Horizontal gray lines represent severity of HTN: SBP 120–129 mmHg, elevated blood pressure; SBP/DBP $\geq$ 130/80 mmHg, Stage 1 HTN; SBP/DBP $\geq$ 140/90 mmHg, Stage 2 HTN. A total of 3/29 and 12/29 participants did not provide data at 6wFU and 12mFU visits, respectively. SBP, systolic blood pressure; DBP, diastolic blood pressure; mmHg, millimeter mercury; BL, baseline; EOF, end-of-fast; EOR, end-of-refeed; 6wFU, six-week follow-up; 12mFU, 12-month follow-up; HTN, hypertension.

3.6. Water-Only Fasting and SOS-Free Diet Refeeding Treatment Acceptability

Participant acceptability of the entire fasting and refeeding intervention (BL to EOR) was assessed using the Treatment Acceptability/Adherence Screener (TAAS), with scores ranging from 10 (no acceptability/adherence) to 70 (full acceptability/adherence). Responses to individual TAAS questions are shown in Figure S1. Median (IQR) scores were 67 (63, 70) and 66 (60, 69) at EOF and 6wFU visits, respectively, suggesting a high degree of treatment acceptability.

Participant acceptability of foods permitted on an SOS-free diet was assessed using the Food Acceptability Questionnaire (FAQ), with scores ranging from 10 (no acceptability) to 70 (full acceptability). Responses to individual FAQ questions are shown in Figure S2. Median (IQR) scores were 47 (44, 52), 49 (45, 58), 48 (42, 55), and 45 (32, 70) at BL, EOR, 6wFU, and 12mFU visits, respectively. Together with the high study retention rate, these results suggest that participants found the medically supervised fasting and refeeding intervention to be highly acceptable.

4. Discussion

Here we present data that medically supervised, prolonged water-only fasting and whole-plant-food refeeding is well-tolerated, feasible, and potentially an effective treatment in people with multiple metabolic disorders. Importantly, the fasting and refeeding intervention was conducted at a residential fasting center using a protocol in which participants are thoroughly prescreened for potentially serious contraindications, have access to medical care 24 h per day, and are individually examined twice daily to identify potentially serious complications and, if necessary, modify the intervention accordingly. Using this protocol, more than 90% of participants in this study were able to complete at least seven consecutive days of fasting, and study attrition through the six-week follow-up visit was less than 10%. Participants also reported that the in-patient intervention was highly acceptable and preferable to conventional treatment with anti-hypertensive medications.

The most commonly identified AEs included transient mild (G1) or moderate (G2) fatigue, nausea, presyncope, dizziness, headache, and insomnia, which is in agreement with previously reported retrospective data from a larger mixed normotensive and hypertensive population using the same fasting protocol [14]. This study also utilized hematology and serology to thoroughly screen for AEs and identified some commonly occurring AEs not reported in our previous study. For example, 72% of participants experienced mild (G1) decreased blood bicarbonate while fasting, potentially due to the overproduction of ketoacids [33]. Symptoms of decreased blood bicarbonate include fatigue and nausea, which could potentially explain, at least in part, the high rates of fatigue and nausea commonly reported while fasting.

Seven of the eight severe (G3) events identified in this study were HTN and occurred during fasting, which is unsurprising given that this population had uncontrolled HTN and/or were weaned off anti-hypertensive medications before starting to fast. All of these HTN events were resolved while the participants were refeeding. Notably, fasting does not increase blood pressure in normotensive individuals [14,34]. The other G3 event was a low neutrophil count during refeeding that progressed from a G1 event during prefeeding. At the EOR visit, the participant's WBC count had also decreased to a G1 event. Overall, we observed a trend of significantly decreased WBC count at EOR, but the median value did not decrease below the lower normal level, and abnormal values were not associated with any negative clinical outcomes. Previous research suggests that prolonged fasting induces stem cell regeneration and leads to a transient reduction in WBC count such that the body discards old WBCs before the immune system is replenished with new ones [35]. We do not know the relevance of this or other changes in CBC or CMP, but the results are in line with previous reports and warrant a more thorough analysis beyond the scope of this manuscript [36]. There were no other G3, life-threatening (G4), death (G5), or serious adverse events identified in this study. These data indicate that medically supervised fasting and refeeding are well-tolerated and low-risk in people with stage 1 and 2 HTN.

Similar to previous reports, we observed clinically meaningful and significant reductions in median SBP, DBP, BW, BMI, AC, and FLI [12,13,15,37,38] that correlated with the intervention and were sustained at the 6wFU [15]. Remarkably, median unmedicated blood pressure was normotensive by the EOR visit. At the 6wFU visit, only one participant had resumed anti-hypertensive medication use, and unmedicated median SBP/DBP was below 130/80 mmHg. Furthermore, the 17 participants who returned for the unanticipated 12mFU visit sustained a median BP below 130/80 mmHg and maintained median BW loss of >5%, suggesting the intervention is in alignment with clinical guidelines and may support long-term outcomes necessary to reduce CVD risk. The role of diet in maintaining outcomes after fasting remains elusive, but these participants were only moderately adherent to the recommended diet, suggesting that even with imperfect dietary adherence, outcomes achieved during fasting are durable. The long-term BW loss data are especially encouraging given the long-held belief that weight lost through fasting is quickly regained [39].

The mechanism by which fasting reduces blood pressure is not fully understood. One hypothesis is that dehydration during fasting results in hypovolemia, or reduced blood volume, that reduces blood pressure. Indeed, our data suggest that at least some participants were mildly dehydrated during fasting. Although this might explain the observed drop in blood pressure during fasting, it is noteworthy that these values began to revert to baseline during refeeding and had normalized by the 6wFU visit, whereas the reduction in blood pressure persisted.

This study has several limitations that should be addressed in future research. A major limitation is the potential for selection bias since the small number of participants were recruited from existing patients at a single fasting center and the majority of enrolled participants were post-menopausal women. As such, the results from this "self-selected" population may not be representative of the general hypertensive population. This study also lacks a diet control group and/or usual care comparison, and this study was not powered to assess changes in blood pressure or other cardiometabolic markers. Therefore, it is inconclusive what long-term results are attributable to diet alone and how the intervention compares to standard interventions (e.g., combination therapy anti-hypertensive medications). Furthermore, only 59% of participants re-enrolled for the 12-month follow-up visit. Future studies should aim to enroll and randomize a sufficient number of participants from a more general hypertensive population, include appropriate control populations, control for potential confounders such as prior diet and activity levels, and have additional planned study visits. Another important methodological limitation is that BP data are based on single rather than 24 h ambulatory BP measurements [40]. The effect of these methodological limitations on study outcomes is unknown, but these results are comparable to other reports in different populations [12,13,37].

5. Conclusions

Hypertension is the most common chronic disease worldwide, and when uncontrolled, it is a risk factor for developing cardiovascular and other diseases. Standard medical care typically includes anti-hypertensive medications that only minimally lower overall health risk, may be associated with serious side effects, have low adherence rates, and have a high lifetime cost [4,8,41,42]. Our results suggest that this in-patient, medically supervised, prolonged water-only fasting and SOS-free diet refeeding protocol may be a well-tolerated, low-risk alternative for long-term management of high blood pressure and obesity. These findings are in support of additional research to include a more diverse population, optimize treatment length and frequency, determine the effects of diet and other lifestyle modifications on sustained outcomes, and compare this intervention to standard treatment.

Supplementary Materials: The following supporting information can be downloaded at: https://www.mdpi.com/article/10.3390/nu16223959/s1. Supplemental Methods: Method S1. Demographics, Medical Diagnoses, Medication Use, and Anthropometric Measurements; Method S2. Biospecimen Collection. Supplemental Tables: Table S1. Baseline ICD-10 Diagnosis and Code by Sex; Table S2. SOS-Free Diet Screener Serving Quantity Reported by Category at BL, 6wFU, and 12mFU; Table S3. Adverse Events Occurring in $\geq$10% of Participants by Treatment Stage and Grade; Table S4. Total Adverse Events by Classification, Grade, and Outcome; Table S5. CBC by Visit; Table S6. Significance of Differences for CBC; Table S7. CMP by Visit; Table S8. Significance of Differences for CMP; Table S9. 24 h Dipstick Urinalysis by Visit; Table S10. 24 h Standard Urinalysis by Event; Table S11. Daily Rate of Change for Body Weight, Blood Pressure, and Vital Signs; Table S12. Weight Class by Visit; Table S13. Cardiometabolic Biomarkers by Visit; Table S14. Significance of Differences for Cardiometabolic Markers; Table S15. Anti-Hypertensive Medication Use at BL, 6wFU, and 12mFU; Supplemental Figures: Figure S1. Percentage of participants responding to individual TAAS questions; Figure S2. Percentage of participants responding to individual FAQ questions. References [43–45] are cited in supplementary file.

Author Contributions: Conceptualization, E.L.S., A.C.G. and T.R.M.; data curation, E.Z., D.N. and M.N.; formal analysis, E.Z. and M.N.; funding acquisition, A.C.G.; investigation, E.Z., S.G. and N.T.; methodology, M.N., A.C.G. and T.R.M.; project administration, T.R.M.; supervision, T.R.M.; visualization, E.Z. and M.N.; writing—original draft, E.Z. and T.R.M.; writing—review and editing, E.Z., S.G., M.N., N.T., D.N., E.L.S., A.C.G. and T.R.M. All authors have read and agreed to the published version of the manuscript.

Funding: This research received no external funding.

Institutional Review Board Statement: This study was conducted according to the guidelines of the Declaration of Helsinki and approved by the Institutional Review Board of the TrueNorth Health Foundation (TNHF2020-1HTN, 16 August 2020 and TNHF2021-1HTNFU, 28 October 2021).

Informed Consent Statement: Informed consent was obtained from all subjects involved in this study.

Data Availability Statement: The minimal dataset, excluding AE data, are publicly available at https://doi.org/10.5061/dryad.9cnp5hqt8. The AE data presented in this study are available on request from the corresponding author. The AE data are not publicly available due to privacy reasons.

Acknowledgments: We would like to thank the study volunteers and dedicated staff at the TrueNorth Health Center.

Conflicts of Interest: A.C.G. is the owner of the TrueNorth Health Center and President of the Board of Directors of the TrueNorth Health Foundation. All other authors declare no conflicts of interest.

erences

Ostchega, Y.; Fryar, C.D.; Nwankwo, T.; Nguyen, D.T. Hypertension Prevalence Among Adults Aged 18 and Over: United States, 2017–2018. In *NCHS Data Brief*; National Center for Health Statistics: Hyattsville, MD, USA, 2020; pp. 1–8.

Oliveros, E.; Patel, H.; Kyung, S.; Fugar, S.; Goldberg, A.; Madan, N.; Williams, K.A. Hypertension in older adults: Assessment, management, and challenges. *Clin. Cardiol.* **2020**, *43*, 99–107. [CrossRef] [PubMed]

Franklin, S.S.; Larson, M.G.; Khan, S.A.; Wong, N.D.; Leip, E.P.; Kannel, W.B.; Levy, D. Does the relation of blood pressure to coronary heart disease risk change with aging? The Framingham Heart Study. *Circulation* **2001**, *103*, 1245–1249. [CrossRef]

Kirkland, E.B.; Heincelman, M.; Bishu, K.G.; Schumann, S.O.; Schreiner, A.; Axon, R.N.; Mauldin, P.D.; Moran, W.P. Trends in Healthcare Expenditures Among US Adults with Hypertension: National Estimates, 2003–2014. *J. Am. Hear. Assoc.* **2018**, *7*, e008731. [CrossRef]

Whelton, P.K.; Carey, R.M.; Aronow, W.S.; Casey, D.E., Jr.; Collins, K.J.; Himmelfarb, C.D.; DePalma, S.M.; Gidding, S.; Jamerson, K.A.; Jones, D.W.; et al. 2017 ACC/AHA/AAPA/ABC/ACPM/AGS/APhA/ASH/ASPC/NMA/PCNA Guideline for the Prevention, Detection, Evaluation, and Management of High Blood Pressure in Adults A Report of the American College of Cardiology/American Heart Association Task Force on Clinical Practice Guidelines. *J. Am. Coll. Cardiol.* **2018**, *71*, e127–e248. [PubMed]

Chobufo, M.D.; Gayam, V.; Soluny, J.; Rahman, E.U.; Enoru, S.; Foryoung, J.B.; Agbor, V.N.; Dufresne, A.; Nfor, T. Prevalence and control rates of hypertension in the USA: 2017–2018. *Int. J. Cardiol. Hypertens.* **2020**, *6*, 100044. [CrossRef]

Albasri, A.; Hattle, M.; Koshiaris, C.; Dunnigan, A.; Paxton, B.; Fox, S.E.; Smith, M.; Archer, L.; Levis, B.; Payne, R.A.; et al. investigators, Association between antihypertensive treatment and adverse events: Systematic review and meta-analysis. *BMJ* **2021**, *372*, n189. [CrossRef]

Ho, C.L.B.; Breslin, M.; Doust, J.; Reid, C.M.; Nelson, M.R. Effectiveness of blood pressure-lowering drug treatment by levels of absolute risk: Post hoc analysis of the Australian National Blood Pressure Study. *BMJ Open* **2018**, *8*, e017723. [CrossRef] [PubMed]

Virani, S.S.; Alonso, A.; Aparicio, H.J.; Benjamin, E.J.; Bittencourt, M.S.; Callaway, C.W.; Carson, A.P.: Chamberlain, A.M.; Cheng, S.; Delling, F.N.; et al. Heart Disease and Stroke Statistics-2021 Update: A Report from the American Heart Association. *Circulation* **2021**, *143*, e254–e743.

Artinian, N.T.; Fletcher, G.F.; Mozaffarian, D.; Kris-Etherton, P.; Van Horn, L.; Lichtenstein, A.H.; Kumanyika, S.; Kraus, W.E.; Fleg, J.L.; Redeker, N.S.; et al. American Heart Association Prevention Committee of the Council on Cardiovascular, Interventions to promote physical activity and dietary lifestyle changes for cardiovascular risk factor reduction in adults: A scientific statement from the American Heart Association. *Circulation* **2010**, *122*, 406–441.

Dhakal, A.; Takma, K.C.; Neupane, M. Adherence to lifestyle modifications and its associated factors in hypertensive patients. *J. Clin. Nurs.* **2022**, *31*, 2181–2188. [CrossRef]

Goldhamer, A.; Lisle, D.; Parpia, B.; Anderson, S.V.; Campbell, T.C. Medically supervised water-only fasting in the treatment of hypertension. *J. Manip. Physiol. Ther.* **2001**, *24*, 335–339. [CrossRef] [PubMed]

Goldhamer, A.C.; Lisle, D.J.; Sultana, P.; Anderson, S.V.; Parpia, B.; Hughes, B.; Campbell, T.C. Medically supervised water-only fasting in the treatment of borderline hypertension. *J. Altern. Complement. Med.* **2002**, *8*, 643–650. [CrossRef]

Finnell, J.S.; Saul, B.C.; Goldhamer, A.C.; Myers, T.R. Is fasting safe? A chart review of adverse events during medically supervised, water-only fasting. *BMC Complement. Altern. Med.* **2018**, *18*, 67. [CrossRef] [PubMed]

15. Gabriel, S.; Ncube, M.; Zeiler, E.; Thompson, N.; Karlsen, M.C.; Goldman, D.M.; Glavas, Z.; Beauchesne, A.; Scharf, Goldhamer, A.C.; et al. A Six-Week Follow-Up Study on the Sustained Effects of Prolonged Water-Only Fasting and Refeed on Markers of Cardiometabolic Risk. *Nutrients* **2022**, *14*, 4313. [CrossRef] [PubMed]
16. Myers, T.R.; Saul, B.; Karlsen, M.; Beauchesne, A.; Glavas, Z.; Ncube, M.; Bradley, R.; Goldhamer, A.C. Potential Effect Prolonged Water-Only Fasting Followed by a Whole-Plant-Food Diet on Salty and Sweet Taste Sensitivity and Perceived Inten Food Liking, and Dietary Intake. *Cureus* **2022**, *14*, e24689. [CrossRef] [PubMed]
17. Milosevic, I.; Levy, H.C.; Alcolado, G.M.; Radomsky, A.S. The Treatment Acceptability/Adherence Scale: Moving Beyond Assessment of Treatment Effectiveness. *Cogn. Behav. Ther.* **2015**, *44*, 456–469. [CrossRef]
18. Fruge, A.D.; Smith, K.S.; Riviere, A.J.; Demark-Wahnefried, W.; Arthur, A.E.; Murrah, W.M.; Morrow, C.D.; Arnold, R Braxton-Lloyd, K. Primary Outcomes of a Randomized Controlled Crossover Trial to Explore the Effects of a High Chlorop Dietary Intervention to Reduce Colon Cancer Risk in Adults: The Meat and Three Greens (M3G) Feasibility Trial. *Nutrients* **2** *11*, 2349. [CrossRef]
19. Harris, P.A.; Taylor, R.; Thielke, R.; Payne, J.; Gonzalez, N.; Conde, J.G. Research electronic data capture (REDCap)—A metad driven methodology and workflow process for providing translational research informatics support. *J. Biomed. Inform.* **2** *42*, 377–381. [CrossRef]
20. NIH. Common Terminology Criteria for Adverse Events (CTCAE). Available online: https://ctep.cancer.gov/protocoldevelopm electronic_applications/ctc.htm (accessed on 21 October 2024).
21. Team, R.C. *R: A Language and Environment for Statistical Computing*; R Foundation for Statistical Computing: Vienna, Austria, 2
22. Kuznetsova, A.; Brockhoff, P.B.; Christensen, R.H.B. lmerTest Package: Tests in Linear Mixed Effects Models. *J. Stat. Softw.* **2** *82*, 1–26. [CrossRef]
23. Bates, D.; Mächler, M.; Bolker, B.; Walker, S. Fitting Linear Mixed-Effects Models Using lme4. *J. Stat. Softw.* **2015**, *67*, 1- [CrossRef]
24. Bolker, B.; Robinson, D.; Menne, D.; Gabry, J.; Buerkner, P.; Hua, C.; Petry, W.; Wiley, J.; Kennedy, P.; Szöcs, E.; et al. broom.mi Tidying Methods for Mixed Models. 2024. Available online: https://github.com/bbolker/broom.mixed (accessed on 21 October 2(
25. Wiley, J.F. *multilevelTools: Multilevel and Mixed Effects Model Diagnostics and Effect Sizes*; R Foundation for Statistical Comput Vienna, Austria, 2020.
26. Koller, M. robustlmm: An R Package for Robust Estimation of Linear Mixed-Effects Models. *J. Stat. Softw.* **2016**, *75*, 1- [CrossRef]
27. Koller, M.; Stahel, W.A. Robust Estimation of General Linear Mixed Effects Models. In *Robust and Multivariate Statistical Meth* Springer: Berlin/Heidelberg, Germany, 2023.
28. Lüdecke, D.; Bartel, A.; Schwemmer, C.; Powell, C.; Djalovski, A.; Titz, J. *sjPlot: Data Visualization for Statistics in Social Scienc Package Version 2.8.15*; R Foundation for Statistical Computing: Vienna, Austria, 2023.
29. Brookes, S.T.; Whitely, E.; Egger, M.; Smith, G.D.; Mulheran, P.A.; Peters, T.J. Subgroup analyses in randomized trials: Ri of subgroup-specific analyses; power and sample size for the interaction test. *J. Clin. Epidemiol.* **2004**, *57*, 229–236. [Cross [PubMed]
30. O'Keefe, D.J. Brief Report: Post Hoc Power, Observed Power, A Priori Power, Retrospective Power, Prospective Power, Achie Power: Sorting Out Appropriate Uses of Statistical Power Analyses. *Commun. Methods Meas.* **2010**, *1*, 291–299. [CrossRef]
31. Bolger, N.L.; Philippe, J. *Intensive Longitudinal Methods: An Introduction to Diary and Experience Sampling Research*; Guilford P New York, NY, USA, 2013.
32. Pinheiro, J.; Bates, D.; DebRoy, S.; Sarkar, D.; Heisterkamp, S.; Willigen, B.V.; Ranke, J.; Team, R.C. *nlme: Linear and Nonli Mixed Effects Models, Version 3.1-166*; R Foundation for Statistical Computing: Vienna, Austria, 2023.
33. Kraut, J.A.; Madias, N.E. Metabolic acidosis: Pathophysiology, diagnosis and management. *Nat. Rev. Nephrol.* **2010**, *6*, 274– [CrossRef] [PubMed]
34. Dai, Z.; Zhang, H.; Wu, F.; Chen, Y.; Yang, C.; Wang, H.; Sui, X.; Guo, Y.; Xin, B.; Guo, Z.; et al. Effects of 10-Day Complete Fas on Physiological Homeostasis, Nutrition and Health Markers in Male Adults. *Nutrients* **2022**, *14*, 3860. [CrossRef]
35. Cheng, C.W.; Adams, G.B.; Perin, L.; Wei, M.; Zhou, X.; Lam, B.S.; Da Sacco, S.; Mirisola, M.; Quinn, D.I.; Dorff, T.B.; e Prolonged fasting reduces IGF-1/PKA to promote hematopoietic-stem-cell-based regeneration and reverse immunosuppress *Cell Stem Cell* **2014**, *14*, 810–823. [CrossRef]
36. Ogłodek, E.; Pilis, W. Is Water-Only Fasting Safe? *Glob. Adv. Integr. Med. Health* **2021**, *10*, 21649561211031178. [CrossRef]
37. Maifeld, A.; Bartolomaeus, H.; Lober, U.; Avery, E.G.; Steckhan, N.; Marko, L.; Wilck, N.; Hamad, I.; Susnjar, U.; Mahler, A.; e Fasting alters the gut microbiome reducing blood pressure and body weight in metabolic syndrome patients. *Nat. Commun.* **2** *12*, 1970. [CrossRef]
38. Laurens, C.; Grundler, F.; Damiot, A.; Chery, I.; Le Maho, A.L.; Zahariev, A.; Le Maho, Y.; Bergouignan, A.; Gauquelin-Koch Simon, C.; et al. Is muscle and protein loss relevant in long-term fasting in healthy men? A prospective trial on physiolog adaptations. *J. Cachexia Sarcopenia Muscle* **2021**, *12*, 1690–1703. [CrossRef]
39. Fanti, M.; Mishra, A.; Longo, V.D.; Brandhorst, S. Time-Restricted Eating, Intermittent Fasting, and Fasting-Mimicking Diet Weight Loss. *Curr. Obes. Rep.* **2021**, *10*, 70–80. [CrossRef]
40. Pena-Hernandez, C.; Nugent, K.; Tuncel, M. Twenty-Four-Hour Ambulatory Blood Pressure Monitoring. *J. Prim. Care Commu Health* **2020**, *11*, 2150132720940519. [CrossRef] [PubMed]

Kaiser, E.A.; Lotze, U.; Schäfer, H.H. Increasing complexity: Which drug class to choose for treatment of hypertension in the elderly? *Clin. Interv. Aging* **2014**, *2014*, 459–475.
Gebreyohannes, E.A.; Bhagavathula, A.S.; Abebe, T.B.; Tefera, Y.G.; Abegaz, T.M. Adverse effects and non-adherence to antihypertensive medications in University of Gondar Comprehensive Specialized Hospital. *Clin. Hypertens.* **2019**, *25*, 1. [CrossRef] [PubMed]
LabCorp. Blood Specimens: Chemistry and Hematology. Available online: https://www.labcorp.com/test-menu/resources (accessed on 21 October 2024).
ICD10 Data. Available online: https://icd.who.int/browse10/2019/en (accessed on 21 October 2024).
Weir, C.B.; Jan, A. *BMI Classification Percentile and Cut Off Points*; StatPearls: Treasure Island, FL, USA, 2023.

nutrients

MDPI

Article

Usefulness of Body Fat and Visceral Fat Determined by Bioimpedanciometry versus Body Mass Index and Waist Circumference in Predicting Elevated Values of Different Risk Scales for Non-Alcoholic Fatty Liver Disease

María Gordito Soler [1], Ángel Arturo López-González [2,3,*], Daniela Vallejos [2,3], Emilio Martínez-Almoyna Rifá [2], María Teófila Vicente-Herrero [2] and José Ignacio Ramírez-Manent [2,4,5,6]

1 Pharmaceutical, 41013 Seville, Seville, Spain; mgorditosoler@hotmail.com
2 Investigation Group ADEMA SALUD, University Institute for Research in Health Sciences (IUNICS), 07010 Palma, Balearic Islands, Spain; d.vallejos@eua.edu.es (D.V.); emilio@mompra.com (E.M.-A.R.); correoteo@gmail.com (M.T.V.-H.); joseignacio.ramirez@ibsalut.es (J.I.R.-M.)
3 Faculty of Dentistry, University School ADEMA, 07010 Palma, Balearic Islands, Spain
4 Institut d'Investigació Sanitària de les Illes Balears (IDISBA), Balearic Islands Health Research Institute Foundation, 07010 Palma, Balearic Islands, Spain
5 Balearic Islands Health Service, 07010 Palma, Balearic Islands, Spain
6 Faculty of Medicine, University of the Balearic Islands, 07010 Palma, Balearic Islands, Spain
* Correspondence: angarturo@gmail.com; Tel.: +34-687548105

Abstract: Background: Obesity constitutes a public health problem worldwide and causes non-alcoholic fatty liver disease (MALFD), the leading cause of liver disease in developed countries, which progresses to liver cirrhosis and liver cancer. MAFLD is associated with obesity and can be evaluated by validated formulas to assess MAFLD risk using different parameters such as the body mass index (BMI) and waist circumference (WC). However, these parameters do not accurately measure body fat. As MAFLD is strongly associated with obesity, we hypothesize that measuring body and visceral fat by electrical bioimpedance is an efficient method to predict the risk of MAFLD. The objective of our work was to demonstrate that electrical bioimpedance is a more efficient method than the BMI or WC to predict an elevated risk of MAFLD. Methods: A cross-sectional, descriptive study involving 8590 Spanish workers in the Balearic Islands was carried out. The study's sample of employees was drawn from those who underwent occupational medicine examinations between January 2019 and December 2020. Five MAFLD risk scales were determined for evaluating very high levels of body fat and visceral fat. The determination of body and visceral fat was performed using bioimpedanciometry. Student's *t*-test was employed to ascertain the mean and standard deviation of quantitative data. The chi-square test was used to find prevalences for qualitative variables, while ROC curves were used to define the cut-off points for body and visceral fat. The calculations included the area under the curve (AUC), the cut-off points along with their Youden index, sensitivity, and specificity. Correlation and concordance between the various scales were determined using Pearson's correlation index and Cohen's kappa, respectively. Results: As both total body fat and visceral fat increase, the risk of MAFLD increases with a statistically significant result ($p < 0.001$), presenting a higher risk in men. The areas under the curve (AUC) of the five scales that assess overweight and obesity to determine the occurrence of high values of the different MAFLD risk scales were very high, most of them exceeding 0.9. These AUC values were higher for visceral and body fat than for the BMI or waist circumference. FLD-high presented the best results in men and women with the AUC at around 0.97, both for visceral fat and total body fat, with a high Youden index in all cases (women body fat = 0.830, visceral fat = 0.892; men body fat = 0.780, visceral fat = 0.881). Conclusions: In our study, all the overweight and obesity scales show a very good association with the scales assessing the risk of MAFLD. These values are higher for visceral and body fat than for waist circumference and the BMI. Both visceral fat and body fat are better associated than the BMI and waist circumference with MAFLD risk scales.

Keywords: non-alcoholic fatty liver disease; visceral fat; body fat; obesity; waist circumference; body mass index

1. Introduction

Obesity is a metabolic disorder in which there is an accumulation of excessive fat in the body, which is harmful to health. Nowadays, it is considered a public health problem in both developed and developing countries and is recognized as a 21st century pandemic [1]. The impact of obesity on health is very high, both because of the pathology it presents in itself and because it is a risk factor for multiple diseases. Currently, it is a cause of greater mortality in developed countries than low weight in developing countries [2].

Among the pathologies that obesity promotes are heart disease and stroke [3], diabetes and insulin resistance [4], different types of cancer [3], musculoskeletal disorders [3], and different liver diseases such as non-alcoholic fatty liver disease (MAFLD), non-alcoholic steatohepatitis (MASH), liver cirrhosis, and hepatocellular carcinoma [5,6].

Fatty liver and obesity are closely related. This relationship is due to poor metabolic health that facilitates the development of what can be called fatty liver disease associated with metabolic dysfunction (MAFLD) [7]. MAFLD is currently defined as a chronic liver disease with >5% fat deposition in liver cells in the absence of excessive alcohol intake and other secondary causes [8]. This increase in fat in the liver is responsible for increased insulin resistance, which plays an essential role in the development of MAFLD. The adipocyte behaves like an endocrine organ and produces various cytokines, which include tumor necrosis factor (TNF-α), angiotensinogen, free fatty acids that are mainly responsible for lipotoxicity, and leptin. The latter increases in obese individuals—who produce resistance to it—exert a pro-inflammatory action and the development of MAFLD, and may well play an important role in the progression to liver fibrosis, which, in patients with MAFLD, constitutes the most important risk factor for developing liver cirrhosis and liver cancer [9].

About 20 years ago, MAFLD was strongly associated with obesity, type 2 diabetes mellitus (T2DM), metabolic syndrome (MS), and dyslipidemia [10]. Nowadays, a second type of MAFLD would be related to infectious diseases such as Hepatitis C and HIV or drugs [11]. However, the majority of MAFLD occurs in developed and developing countries due to an unhealthy lifestyle, with an intake of foods rich in carbohydrates and saturated fats (Fast Food), along with a lack of physical exercise, causing obesity [12].

Today, linked to obesity, MAFLD is the leading cause of chronic liver disease in developed countries, with a global prevalence of around 30%, which reaches 90% of patients with morbid obesity [13].

The gold standard for diagnosing any liver pathology is a biopsy; however, it is an aggressive, expensive, painful, and not risk-free test [14].

Liver ultrasound is a non-invasive method and well tolerated by the patient. However, the interpretation of hepatic steatosis is operator-dependent, requires training time for the technician [15], and the classification of steatosis is established subjectively at three levels: mild, moderate, and severe. Further, an experienced sonographer can only detect hepatic steatosis when the fat content in the liver is at least between 2.5 and 20% [16], so approximately 5% of patients with initial steatosis would not be diagnosed [17].

Transient elastography (LSM) is also useful for the diagnosis of MAFLD. However, although its usefulness has been demonstrated in cases of advanced fibrosis in MAFLD, with a sensitivity in these cases of 97% in patients with a BMI < 30 kg/m^2, it is not useful in incipient or poorly developed cases [18]. It is an operator-dependent technique requiring training time; subcutaneous fat reduces the propagation of ultrasound, thereby affecting the measurements made in people with obesity; and it has the cost of the ultrasound machine [19].

As MAFLD is closely associated with obesity, different formulas have been validated to evaluate the risk of MAFLD. They use different parameters that evaluate obesity, such as the body mass index (BMI) and waist circumference (WC). However, although widely used, these parameters do not accurately measure body fat. The BMI is obtained by dividing weight (in kg) by height (in meters) squared. This formula has several limitations: firstly, it does not provide any information on how body fat is distributed; secondly, when establishing a relationship between height and weight, the BMI is not able to differentiate between muscle, bone, or adipose tissue, so individuals with large muscle mass will obtain a high BMI without having excess adipose tissue [20].

Visceral fat in adults is associated with insulin resistance [21], which plays a prominent role in the development of MAFLD. WC is a valid parameter for indirect measurement of visceral adipose tissue [22]; however, we consider that there are valid economic methods to assess both total body fat and visceral fat. These systems include bioelectrical impedance (BIA), which measures the electrical resistance of the different components of the body by applying a constant low intensity alternating current to them. It is a simple, fast, harmless, low-cost, and affordable technique in medical consultations. This technique is valid for studying body composition in healthy, normal weight individuals and in the study of overweight and moderate obesity. However, it does not seem to have the same usefulness in the study of morbid obesity [23].

It is important to highlight the fact that liver fibrosis can be prevented, reversed, or stabilized if the cause that triggers it is eliminated [24]; and if this is insufficient, immunosuppressive, anti-inflammatory, or antiviral drugs may be considered. New antifibrotic drugs, such as angiotensin inhibitors, are not yet available [25].

As previously mentioned, the most common cause of MAFLD today is unhealthy lifestyle habits, which facilitate the deposition of fat in the liver and are frequently associated with obesity. Modifying lifestyle habits to prevent MAFLD is the basis of preventive and restorative treatment for MAFLD [26]. Therefore, the detection of MAFLD in its early stages is of vital importance for establishing appropriate measures and preventing its evolution to liver fibrosis, liver cirrhosis, and hepatocellular carcinoma.

As MAFLD is strongly associated with obesity, we hypothesize that measuring body and visceral fat by electrical bioimpedance is an efficient method to predict the risk of MAFLD.

The objective of our work was to demonstrate that electrical bioimpedance is a more efficient method than the BMI or WC to predict an elevated risk of MAFLD.

2. Material and Methods

2.1. Participants

A cross-sectional, descriptive study including 8590 Spanish workers in the Balearic Islands was carried out. The study's sample of employees was drawn from those who underwent occupational medicine exams between January 2019 and December 2020.

Inclusion criteria:

- Individuals in the 18–69 age range;
- Consent to take part in the research;
- Giving permission for the data to be used for epidemiological research;
- Being employed by one of the participating companies in the research and not being temporarily disabled at the time of the study;
- A flowchart of the study participants is presented in Figure 1.

2.2. Determination of Variables

Following process standardization to prevent interobserver bias, occupational health professionals from the participating firms conducted all measurements, whether anthropometric (height, weight, and waist circumference), analytical, or clinical:

- Variables such as age, sex, performing regular physical exercise, physical exercise days per week, and smoking were collected;
- Anthropometric and clinical determinations: weight, height, waist and hip circumference, and both systolic and diastolic blood pressure;

– Analytical determinations: fasting blood glucose, lipid profile, and hepatic enzymes.

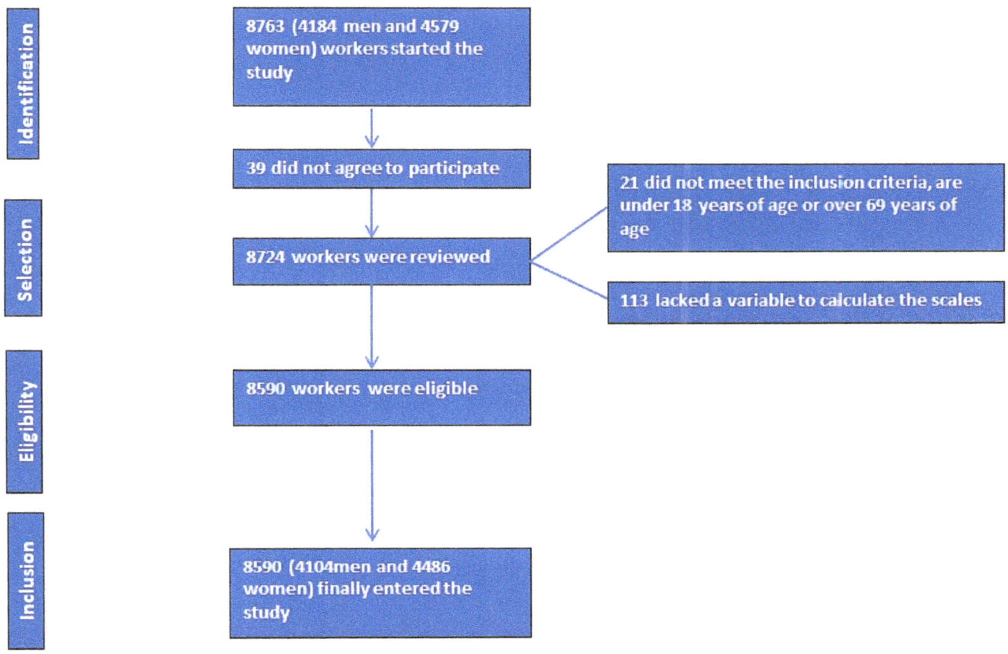

Figure 1. PRISMA flowchart of participants in the study.

2.2.1. Anthropometric Determinations

Measurements of height (in cm) and weight (in kg) were taken using a SECA 700 scale. The measurements were carried out following the ISAK's international standards for anthropometric assessment [27].

With the subject standing, feet together, and abdomen relaxed, waist circumference was measured using a tape measure parallel to the floor at the midpoint between the last palpable rib and the iliac crest [28].

Body and visceral fat determination was performed by bioimpedanciometry using a Tanita DC 430MA model. High values of body and visceral fat are considered to be those shown by the bioimpedance scale (from 10 for visceral fat and variable according to age for body fat).

2.2.2. Clinical Determinations

Blood pressure was measured after 10 min of rest, with the subject seated and without crossed legs, using an OMRON-M3 model blood pressure monitor. Three measurements were made at one-minute intervals, and the average of the three was calculated.

2.2.3. Analytical Determinations

The blood sample was taken after a minimum of 12 h of fasting and was then processed in 48 to 72 h. The measurement of triglycerides, total cholesterol, and blood sugar was performed automatically by enzymatic procedures. The dextran sulfate-$MgCl_2$ precipitation technique was employed for HDL-cholesterol.

By using the Friedewald formula, which is only reliable when triglycerides do not exceed 400, LDL-cholesterol can be calculated indirectly. The unit of measurement for all analytical parameters is mg/dL.

$$\text{LDL} = \text{Total cholesterol total} - \text{HDL-c} - \text{triglycerides}/5$$

2.2.4. Risk Scales

The non-alcoholic fatty liver disease and liver fibrosis risk scales listed below were applied:

- FLI (fatty liver index) [29] FLI = (e0.953 × loge (triglycerides) + 0.139 × BMI + 0.718 × loge (ggt) + 0.053 × waist circumference − 15.745)/(1 + e0.953 × loge (triglycerides) + 0.139 × BMI + 0.718 × loge (ggt) + 0.053 × waist circumference − 15.745) × 100. High risk is defined as beginning at 60.
- Hepatic steatosis index (HSI) [29] HSI = 8 × ALT/AST + BMI + 2 (if type 2 diabetes yes) + 2 (if female). Thirty-six is regarded as high risk.
- Zhejian University index (ZJU) [29] ZJU index = BMI + FBG + TG + 3 × ALT/AST +2 (if female). Fasting blood glucose (FBG) was in mmol/L; WC was in cm, triglycerides (TG).
- A high-risk situation is defined as 38.
- Fatty Liver Disease Index (FLD) [30] FLD= BMI + TG + 3 × (ALT/AST) + 2 × Hyperglycemia (presence= 1; absence = 0)
- High risk is defined as beginning at 37.
- Lipid accumulation product (LAP) [31]. Men: (waist (cm) − 65) × (triglycerides (mMol)).
  Women: (waist (cm) − 58) × (triglycerides (mMol)).
  High risk is considered starting from 42.7.

Anyone who had smoked at least one cigarette in the previous month (or its equivalent in other forms of consumption) or who had given up smoking less than a year before was considered a smoker.

The Spanish Society of Epidemiology's recommendation, based on the 2011 National Classification of Occupations, was used to determine socioeconomic class. Class I comprises managers, directors, and university professionals; Class II includes intermediate vocations and self-employed individuals; and Class III includes manual workers [32].

2.3. *Statistical Analysis*

Student's *t*-test was employed to ascertain the mean and standard deviation of quantitative data. The chi-square test was used to find prevalences for qualitative variables. ROC curves were used to define the cut-off points for cardiac ages as moderate and high. The calculations included the area under the curve (AUC), the cut-off points along with their Youden index, sensitivity, and specificity. The correlation and concordance between the various scales were determined using Pearson's correlation index and Cohen's kappa, respectively. Statistical analysis was performed using SPSS 29.0, with $p < 0.05$ as the recognized threshold for statistical significance.

3. Results

The anthropometric and clinical details of the study participants are displayed in Table 1. The analyses comprised a total of 8590 workers (4104 men, 47.8%, and 4486 women, 52.2%). The average age of the sample was marginally higher than 41, with the bulk of participants in the 30- to 49-year-old age range. Labourers were primarily from social class I. In both genders, just over 15% smoked. Of the men and women, 25.9% and 35.1%, respectively, did not exercise regularly.

Table 2 displays the average body and visceral fat values for both sexes based on the results of the various MAFLD risk scales.

Table 1. Characteristics of study participants.

	Men n = 4104	Women n = 4486	p-Value
	Mean (SD)	**Mean (SD)**	
Age (years)	41.6 (10.6)	41.5 (10.5)	0.492
Height (cm)	175.8 (7.2)	162.5 (6.1)	<0.001 *
Weight (kg)	81.2 (14.8)	63.9 (13.6)	<0.001 *
Waist circumference (cm)	89.8 (12.5)	77.0 (12.0)	<0.001 *
Hip circumference (cm)	101.8 (8.7)	99.6 (10.9)	<0.001 *
Systolic blood pressure (mmHg)	128.6 (13.3)	117.2 (14.1)	<0.001 *
Diastolic blood pressure (mmHg)	79.9 (10.2)	74.9 (9.9)	<0.001 *
Glycemia (mg/dL)	93.4 (17.8)	88.9 (12.6)	<0.001 *
Total cholesterol (mg/dL)	191.8 (36.0)	189.0 (34.8)	<0.001 *
HDL-cholesterol (mg/dL)	49.2 (11.3)	59.5 (12.8)	<0.001 *
LDL-cholesterol (mg/dL)	124.0 (54.6)	113.8 (30.7)	<0.001 *
Triglycerides (mg/dL)	107.8 (69.4)	81.5 (46.3)	<0.001 *
GGT (UI)	31.5 (30.0)	18.5 (15.9)	<0.001 *
AST (UI)	24.4 (17.3)	18.2 (7.7)	<0.001 *
ALT (UI)	29.3 (34.9)	17.3 (13.4)	<0.001 *
	%	%	p-value
18–29 years	15.5	16.8	0.005 *
30–39 years	27.8	25.1	
40–49 years	32.7	34.4	
50–59 years	19.0	19.7	
60–69 years	5.0	4.0	
Social class I	57.1	50.8	<0.001 *
Social class II	20.2	23.8	
Social class III	22.7	25.4	
Non-smokers	84.5	84.2	0.348
Smokers	15.5	15.8	
GGT high	18.6	12.3	<0.001 *
AST high	17.8	11.3	<0.001 *
ALT high	19.5	12.5	<0.001 *
Non physical activity	25.9	35.1	<0.001*
Physical activity 1–3 days/week	27.0	26.5	
Physical activity over 3 days/week	47.1	38.4	

(*) Statistical significance HDL High density lipoprotein. LDL Low density lipoprotein. GGT Gamma-glutamyl transpeptidase. AST Aspartate Aminotransferase. ALT Alanine Aminotransferase UI International unit. SD Standard deviation. (upper normal limits: GGT > 55 men and > 38 women. AST > 33 in both and ALT > 40 men and >35 women).

The mean body fat values were consistently higher in women and rose as the risk of MAFLD increased. Visceral fat and the MAFLD risk scales showed a similar link but with greater values in men in this instance.

Alongside the rise in the various scales measuring the risk of non-alcoholic fatty liver disease (MAFLD), there was a corresponding rise in the prevalence of extremely high body fat values. This prevalence was typically greater in women. Similar trends were revealed in the prevalence of high visceral fat levels, with men showing the highest prevalence in this instance. Table 3 contains all of the data.

Table 2. Mean body fat and visceral fat values according to NAFLD risk scale values.

Body Fat	Men			Women		
	n	Mean (SD)	*p*-Value	*n*	Mean (SD)	*p*-Value
low FLI	2114	14.7 (5.3)	<0.001 *	3646	26.6 (6.1)	<0.001 *
moderate FLI	930	21.4 (5.0)		478	37.3 (3.8)	
high FLI	1060	27.8 (6.2)		362	42.2 (5.3)	
low HSI	625	11.5 (4.4)	<0.001 *	1320	22.2 (4.8)	<0.001 *
moderate HSI	1015	16.5 (5.0)		1891	28.1 (4.9)	
high HSI	1751	25.5 (6.5)		1275	37.4 (5.7)	
low ZJU	879	11.7 (4.3)	<0.001 *	1589	22.1 (4.6)	<0.001 *
moderate ZJU	1867	17.9 (5.0)		1798	29.4 (4.4)	
high ZJU	1358	27.0 (6.1)		1099	38.4 (5.1)	
low FLD	1293	12.9 (4.7)	<0.001 *	2695	24.4 (5.1)	<0.001 *
moderate FLD	2215	20.4 (5.3)		1477	34.3 (4.3)	
high FLD	596	31.0 (5.7)		314	43.5 (4.8)	
normal LAP	3120	17.7 (6.9)	<0.001 *	3978	27.8 (6.9)	<0.001 *
high LAP	984	27.0 (6.5)		508	40.3 (6.1)	
Visceral Fat	*n*	**Mean (SD)**	*p*-Value	*n*	**Mean (SD)**	
low FLI	2114	4.8 (2.8)	<0.001 *	3646	3.6 (2.2)	<0.001 *
moderate FLI	930	8.6 (2.9)		478	7.9 (1.8)	
high FLI	1060	13.3 (4.3)		362	10.9 (3.2)	
low HSI	625	3.1 (2.0)	<0.001 *	1320	2.3 (1.3)	<0.001 *
moderate HSI	1015	5.9 (2.9)		1891	4.0 (1.9)	
high HSI	1751	11.4 (4.5)		1275	8.1 (3.3)	
low ZJU	879	3.2 (2.0)	<0.001 *	1589	2.2 (1.3)	<0.001 *
moderate ZJU	1867	6.6 (2.8)		1798	4.4 (1.8)	
high ZJU	1358	12.6 (4.3)		1099	8.6 (3.2)	
low FLD	1293	3.9 (2.4)	<0.001 *	2695	2.9 (1.6)	<0.001 *
moderate FLD	2215	8.1 (3.2)		1477	6.4 (2.3)	
high FLD	596	15.4 (4.2)		314	11.6 (3.0)	
normal LAP	3120	6.4 (3.8)	<0.001 *	3978	4.1 (2.6)	<0.001 *
high LAP	984	12.5 (4.5)		508	9.7 (3.4)	

(*) Statistical significance. FLI Fatty liver index, HSI Hepatic steatosis index, ZJU Zhejian University index, FLD Fatty liver disease index, LAP Lipid accumulation product. SD standard deviation.

The areas under the curve (AUC) of the five scales that assess overweight and obesity to determine the occurrence of high values of the different MAFLD risk scales were very high, most of them exceeding 0.9. These AUC values were higher for visceral and body fat than for the BMI or waist circumference. In all cases, these AUCs were higher in women. See Figures 2 and 3 and Table 4.

Table 5 presents the cut-off points for all the overweight and obesity scales (with their sensitivity, specificity, and Youden index) to determine elevated values of the different MAFLD risk scales. As already seen for the AUC, the highest Youden index values were found for visceral and body fat, and these values were also higher in women.

Tables 6a,b and 7a,b present the values of Pearson's correlation coefficients and Cohen's kappa indices for both the overweight and obesity scales and the MAFLD risk scales in both sexes. The degree of correlation in both sexes, although especially in women, was generally very high for both scales that assess overweightness and MAFLD.

The degree of concordance, determined with Cohen's kappa index, shows much lower values for the overweight-obesity scales and higher values for the MAFLD scales, especially FLI with FLD and ZJU and HSI with ZJU.

Table 3. Prevalence of very high body fat and visceral fat values according to MAFLD risk scales.

Very High Body Fat	**Men**			**Women**		
	n	%	*p*-**Value**	*n*	%	*p*-**Value**
low FLI	2114	0.3	<0.001 *	3646	0.8	<0.001 *
moderate FLI	930	8.6		478	27.6	
high FLI	1060	42.5		362	66.4	
low HSI	625	0	<0.001 *	1320	0	<0.001 *
moderate HSI	1015	0.4		1891	0.4	
high HSI	1751	30.3		1275	31.0	
low ZJU	879	0	<0.001 *	1589	0	<0.001 *
moderate ZJU	1867	1.2		1798	0.3	
high ZJU	1358	38.0		1099	36.2	
low FLD	1293	0	<0.001 *	2695	0	<0.001 *
moderate FLD	2215	4.6		1477	10.3	
high FLD	596	73.3		314	79.5	
normal LAP	3120	5.4	<0.001 *	3978	4.7	<0.001 *
high LAP	984	39.0		508	49.6	
High Visceral Fat	*n*	%	*p*-**Value**	*n*	%	*p*-**Value**
low FLI	2114	0	<0.001 *	3646	0.1	<0.001 *
moderate FLI	930	10.2		478	3.2	
high FLI	1060	54.1		362	28.9	
low HSI	625	0	<0.001 *	1320	0	<0.001 *
moderate HSI	1015	2.1		1891	1.7	
high HSI	1751	36.1		1275	9.0	
low ZJU	879	0	<0.001 *	1589	0	<0.001 *
moderate ZJU	1867	1.2		1798	1.1	
high ZJU	1358	47.6		1099	10.4	
low FLD	1293	0	<0.001 *	2695	0	<0.001 *
moderate FLD	2215	10.8		1477	3.3	
high FLD	596	72.0		314	34.8	
normal LAP	3120	6.7	<0.001 *	3978	0.4	<0.001 *
high LAP	984	45.1		508	20.9	

(*) Statistical significance. FLI Fatty liver index, HSI Hepatic steatosis index, ZJU Zhejian University index, FLD Fatty liver disease index, LAP Lipid accumulation product.

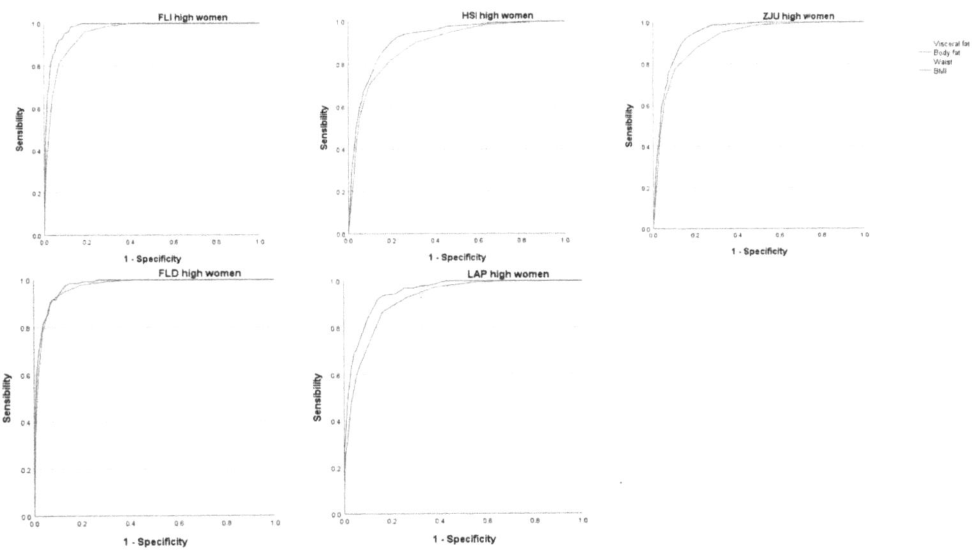

Figure 2. ROC curves in women. FLI Fatty liver index, HSI Hepatic steatosis index. ZJU Zhejian University index, FLD Fatty liver disease index, LAP Lipid accumulation product.

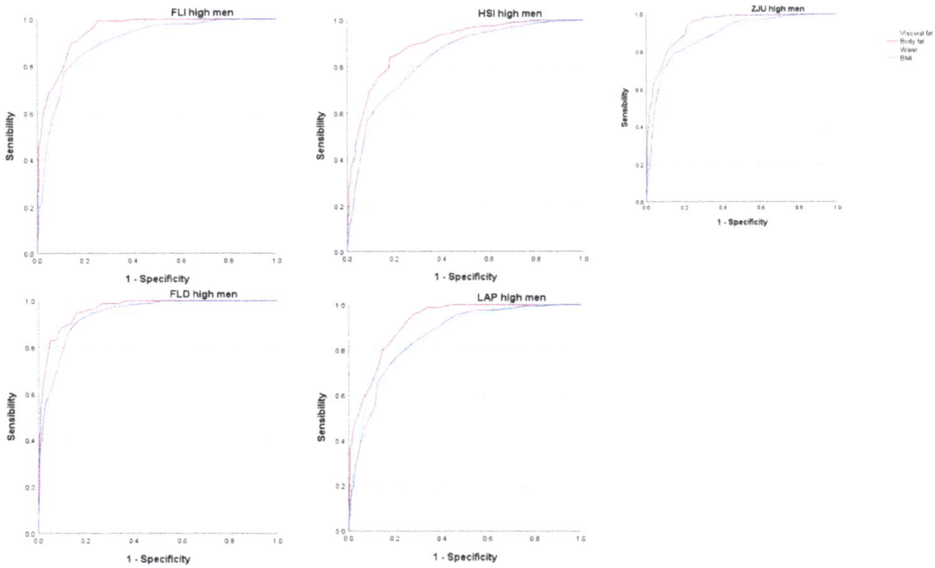

Figure 3. ROC curves in men. FLI Fatty liver index, HSI Hepatic steatosis index, ZJU Zhejian University index, FLD Fatty liver disease index, LAP Lipid accumulation product.

Table 4. Areas under the curve for body and visceral fat predict high values of MAFLD risk scales by sex.

n = 4486	BMI Women	Waist Women	Body Fat Women	Visceral Fat Women
high FLI	0.952 (0.944–0.960)	0.941 (0.931–0.951)	0.978 (0.974–0.982)	0.965 (0.959–0.972)
high HSI	0.887 (0.876–0.898)	0.900 (0.889–0.910)	0.917 (0.908–0.926)	0.941 (0.933–0.948)
high ZJU	0.914 (0.905–0.924)	0.924 (0.916–0.932)	0.943 (0.936–0.949)	0.964 (0.959–0.969)
high FLD	0.969 (0.962–0.976)	0.963 (0.956–0.971)	0.975 (0.969–0.980)	0.985 (0.981–0.989)
high LAP	0.920 (0.909–0.930)	0.912 (0.901–0.924)	0.950 (0.942–0.958)	0.919 (0.908–0.930)
***n* = 4104**	**BMI Men**	**Waist Men**	**Body Fat Men**	**Visceral Fat Men**
high FLI	0.880 (0.868–0.893)	0.899 (0.888–0.910)	0.936 (0.928–0.944)	0.948 (0.941–0.954)
high HSI	0.838 (0.826–0.851)	0.837 (0.824–0.849)	0.914 (0.905–0.922)	0.895 (0.885–0.905)
high ZJU	0.882 (0.870–0.894)	0.888 (0.877–0.899)	0.952 (0.945–0.958)	0.936 (0.929–0.944)
high FLD	0.937 (0.926–0.948)	0.938 (0.929–0.947)	0.975 (0.966–0.984)	0.963 (0.957–0.970)
high LAP	0.854 (0.841–0.867)	0.860 (0.847–0.872)	0.875 (0.863–0.887)	0.919 (0.911–0.927)

FLI Fatty liver index, HSI Hepatic steatosis index, ZJU Zhejian University index, FLD Fatty liver disease index, LAP Lipid accumulation product. BMI Body mass index.

Table 5. Body and visceral fat cut-off points for predicting high values of MAFLD risk scales by sex.

n = 4486	Body Fat Women	Visceral Fat Women	BMI Women	Waist Women
	Cut-Off-Sens-Specif-Youden	Cut-Off-Sens-Specif-Youden	Cut-Off-Sens-Specif-Youden	Cut-Off-Sens-Specif-Youde
high FLI	36.5–92.4–92.1–0.845	8.0–89.8–89.5–0.793	28.6–88.2–87.8–0.760	91.0–87.5–87.0–0.745
high HSI	32.8–85.6–84.2–0.698	6.0–89.0–89.0–0.780	25.8–81.7–80.6–0.623	80.0–86.9–86.2–0.731
high ZJU	33.3–88.6–87.1–0.757	6.0–91.8–91.4–0.832	26.6–84.5–82.7–0.672	82.0–91.8–91.4–0.832
high FLD	37.7–91.7–91.3–0.830	8.0–94.7–94.5–0.892	30.4–92.8–90.6–0.814	91.0–90.9–90.2–0.811
high LAP	34.4–87.9–87.6–0.755	6.0—85.4–85.4–0.708	27.1–89.8–81.2–0.710	86.0–83.3–82.4–0.657
***n* = 4104**	**Body Fat Men**	**Visceral Fat Men**	**BMI Men**	**Waist Men**
high FLI	23.1–86.6–86.5–0.731	10.0–86.0–85.5–0.715	27.8–80.9–80.8–0.617	95.0–84.2–81.8–0.660
high HSI	21.3–82.2–81.6–0.638	8.0–83.8–83.5–0.673	26.5–76.3–76.3–0.526	91.0–77.6–72.3–0.499
high ZJU	22.5–85.2–84.2–0.694	9.0–88.8–88.8–0.776	27.4–83.3–82.9–0.662	93.0–82.9–82.5–0.654
high FLD	25.0–89.0–89.0–0.780	11.0–94.2–93.9–0.881	29.9–89.1–86.3–0.754	98.5–89.0–86.2–0.752
high LAP	22.3–83.6–82.0–0.656	9.0–78.7–78.1–0.568	27.0–78.7–77.4–0.561	93.0–76.5–76.4–0.529

FLI Fatty liver index, HSI Hepatic steatosis index, ZJU Zhejian University index, FLD Fatty liver disease index, LAP Lipid accumulation product. BMI Body mass index sens Sensitivity. Specif Specificity.

Table 6. a. Pearson's correlation. b. Pearson's correlation.

(a)

Women	**Body fat**	**Visceral fat**	**BMI**	**Waist**
Body fat	1	0.864	0.875	0.834
Visceral fat		1	0.873	0.845
BMI			1	0.895
Waist				1
Men	**Body fat**	**Visceral fat**	**BMI**	**Waist**
Body fat	1	0.856	0.803	0.789
Visceral fat		1	0.853	0.842
BMI			1	0.893
Waist				1

(b)

Women	**FLI**	**HSI**	**ZJU**	**FLD**	**LAP**
FLI	1	0.865	0.905	0.905	0.853
HSI		1	0.972	0.976	0.678
ZJU			1	0.996	0.755
FLD				1	0.750
LAP					1
Men	**FLI**	**HSI**	**ZJU**	**FLD**	**LAP**
FLI	1	0.791	0.898	0.897	0.776
HSI		1	0.938	0.946	0.595
ZJU			1	0.991	0.736
FLD				1	0.728
LAP					1

BMI Body mass index, FLI Fatty liver index, HSI Hepatic steatosis index, ZJU Zhejian University index, FLD Fatty liver disease index, LAP Lipid accumulation product.

Table 7. a. Kappa Cohen indices. b. Kappa Cohen indices.

(a)

Women	**Body fat**	**Visceral fat**	**BMI**	**Waist**
Body fat	1	0.396	0.729	0.555
Visceral fat		1	0.343	0.710
BMI			1	0.632
Waist				1
Men	**Body fat**	**Visceral fat**	**BMI**	**Waist**
Body fat	1	0.680	0.698	0.629
Visceral fat		1	0.668	0.670
BMI			1	0.729
Waist				1

(b)

Women	**FLI**	**HSI**	**ZJU**	**FLD**	**LAP**
FLI	1	0.749	0.902	0.942	0.348
HSI		1	0.918	0.632	0.260
ZJU			1	0.684	0.301
FLD				1	0.267
LAP					1
Men	**FLI**	**HSI**	**ZJU**	**FLD**	**LAP**
FLI	1	0.746	0.855	0.806	0.480
HSI		1	0.857	0.608	0.355
ZJU			1	0.719	0.440
FLD				1	0.307
LAP					1

BMI Body mass index, FLI Fatty liver index, HSI Hepatic steatosis index, ZJU Zhejian University index, FLD Fatty liver disease index, LAP Lipid accumulation product.

4. Discussion

The ability of electrical bioimpedance to predict the high risk of MAFLD was evaluated in a sample of 8590 Spanish workers of both sexes: 4104 men and 4486 women. All of them belonged to the Autonomous Community of the Balearic Islands (Spain) and were between 18 and 69 years of age.

Regarding the characteristics of the population, it should be noted that they mostly belong to social class I, the majority of whom are between 30 and 49 years of age. The percentage of smokers is the same by sex, around 16%, and the group of women performs less physical exercise than the group of men. It is noteworthy that in our study population, the number of smokers is much lower than the data obtained in the European Health Survey in Spain in 2020, where the smoking population had a percentage of around 20% in women and 30% in men [33]. This could be influenced by the fact that all the participants in the sample come from the Balearic Islands, where the smoking habit is somewhat lower than the national average—approximately 17.2% according to the results of the INE (National Statistics Institute) of Spain in 2022 [34]—which is more in line with our results.

The objective of our study was to demonstrate that electrical bioimpedance is a more efficient method than the BMI or WC in the ability to predict a high risk of MAFLD. To do this, the amount of total body fat and visceral fat determined by electrical bioimpedance was compared against five validated formulas to calculate the risk of MAFLD, of which the BMI or WC are a part.

When we assessed the association between the average values of visceral fat and body fat with the five formulas (FLI, HSI, ZJU, FLD, LAP), we observed that as both total body fat and visceral fat increased, so did the risk of MAFLD, with a statistically significant result in all cases ($p < 0.001$ in all scales). These results coincide with a Spanish study carried out on 219,477 workers, where the relationship between several overweight and obesity scales (including the BMI and different estimators of body and visceral fat) and MAFLD risk scales was evaluated. Their results show that as overweight-obesity increases, the risk of MAFLD also increases in parallel in all the scales used [35]. Our results show that this increased risk is greater in the group of women than in the group of men. The association between increased body fat and MAFLD has already been defined in previous studies, in which an association of up to 80% is established between obesity and MAFLD [36].

When assessing the association between the risk of MAFLD and high body fat values, we found the same results. That is, there was a significant increase in the risk of MAFLD that was more pronounced in the group of women. However, when this association was assessed with high visceral fat values, the increased risk, in this case, was observed to be higher in the group of men. This is consistent with other studies that have found a greater association between visceral fat and the risk of MALFD in men [37]. In men, there is a greater predisposition to the accumulation of visceral fat, with more lipolytic capacity than subcutaneous fat and a greater supply of fatty acids to the liver, which may lead to MALFD [38].

In the analysis of the ROC curves, the AUC of the five scales used to assess overweight and obesity presented a very high value, with all of them showing a result between good and excellent. For women, for all five MAFLD risk scales used, the AUC was higher for both percent total body fat and visceral fat. Even when using the FLD high-risk scale, the AUC gave us a value greater than 0.97, which implies an excellent test result—as such a high result is obtained in very few tests. The same occurred when assessing the percentage of body fat with the FLI high-risk scale, in which the AUC also gave us a value greater than 0.97. Even so, it is worth noting that, for all the risk scales used, the AUC was greater than 0.90 for both the percentage of visceral fat and the percentage of body fat, which implies a very good test result.

In the case of men, the results were similar, although the AUC showed lower values than in women in practically all cases. Even so, we must highlight the highest AUC value when using the FLD high-risk scale for the percentage of total body fat, with a result greater than 0.97, which is excellent. On the other hand, the lowest AUC values were found for the

LAP high-risk scales when assessing total body fat, with an AUC of 0.875, and in the HSI high-risk scale when assessing visceral fat, with an AUC of 0.895.

These values, being the lowest AUC obtained, offer a good test result that is very close to very good. Notably, for both risk scales, the AUC presented lower values when related to the BMI or WC.

In the five MALFD risk scales used, the AUC was higher when total body fat or visceral fat was used than when the BMI or WC was used.

The risk of MALFD for all scales was observed to increase more in men than in women as visceral fat increased. In the case of the ROC curves, the AUC for the percentage of visceral fat was higher in women. This tells us that although visceral fat is associated with a higher risk of MALFD in men, the Youden index is higher for women. That is to say, the performance of this test is greater or, in other words, has a greater sensitivity-specificity relationship. It can be seen how it oscillates from the lowest value with a Youden index of 0.708 for high LAP (sensitivity 85.4-specificity 85.4) to the highest value obtained with a high FLD, with a Youden index of 0.892 (sensitivity 94.7-specificity 94.5).

In the Pearson correlation coefficient, a linear correlation can be observed between body fat and visceral fat through the BMI and WC. This strength of correlation is very high, in all cases greater than 0.7 for both sexes, although it shows slightly higher figures in women.

Since MAFLD was not evaluated directly but rather indirectly through MAFLD risk formulas, the Pearson correlation coefficient between the different formulas was also performed to check the validity between them when determining said risk. In all the formulas used, a correlation between high and very high can be seen, with the highest value between ZJU and FLD of 0.996 in women and 0.991 in men, which implies a very high and almost total correlation. The lowest correlation was obtained between HSI and LAP, with a value of 0.678 in women and 0.595 in men. Even so, the results were greater than 0.5 in both cases, which expresses a high or strong correlation.

Likewise, in order to gauge the degree of agreement, Cohen's Kappa index was evaluated. In the case of comparing the different scales to assess obesity, the greatest degree of agreement was found to have occurred between the BMI and total body fat, and between waist circumference and visceral fat, with good agreement, especially in the group of women. The good agreement between waist circumference and visceral fat confirms that waist circumference is a good indirect measure of the amount of visceral adipose tissue [39].

Regarding Cohen's Kappa index between the different MAFLD risk formulas, a very good agreement was found between almost all of them except for what corresponds to the LAP. The latter presented values between insignificant and low in both men and women. This could be because the BMI is used in the other four formulas, whereas waist circumference is used in the LAP.

5. Strengths and Limitations

Among the strengths of the study, it is worth highlighting the large sample size, almost 9000 persons, and the fact that the determination of body and visceral fat was performed with objective and validated methods, such as bioimpedance measurement.

The main limitation of the study is that MAFLD was not determined by objective methods but by using risk scales, even though these are validated.

6. Conclusions

In our study, all the overweight and obesity scales show a very good association with the scales assessing the risk of MAFLD. Nonetheless, these values are higher for visceral and body fat than for waist circumference and the BMI.

Both visceral fat and body fat are better associated than the BMI and waist circumference with MAFLD risk scales.

The use of bioimpedanciometry in primary care and occupational medicine consultations can be very useful in predicting the risk of MAFLD.

Author Contributions: Conceptualization: Á.A.L.-G. and J.I.R.-M.; Data collection and analysis: M.G.S. and D.V. Data curation: M.G.S. Methodology: E.M.-A.R. and D.V. Validation: M.T.V.-H.; Formal analysis: Á.A.L.-G.; Investigation: M.G.S.; Draft: M.G.S., Á.A.L.-G., M.T.V.-H. and E.M.-A.R.; Revision: J.I.R.-M. and Á.A.L.-G. All authors have read and agreed to the published version of the manuscript.

Funding: This research received no external funding.

Institutional Review Board Statement: The research team is committed to always adhering to the ethical guidelines for health sciences research that have been established on a national and international level (the Declaration of Helsinki), with particular consideration paid to participant anonymity and data confidentiality. The Ethics and Research Committee of the Balearic Islands (CEI-IB) was consulted in order to acquire approval (IB 4383/20), which was accomplished using indicator IB 4383/20. The study was voluntary, meaning that after being fully informed about its purpose, participants gave their written and verbal consent to take part in it. In order to do this, they were provided with an information sheet outlining the purpose of the study and an informed consent form. The codes used to identify the data collected for the study make it impossible for anybody other than the project coordinator to link the data to the participants. There will be no publication of the participants' identities in any study report. No information that could be used to identify them will be shared by the investigators. The research team guarantees that all participants in this study may exercise their rights of access, rectification, cancellation, and opposition of the data collected. In any event, the team pledges to strictly adhere to Organic Law 3/2018, of December 5, on the protection of personal data and guarantee of digital rights.

Informed Consent Statement: Informed consent was obtained from all subjects involved in this study.

Data Availability Statement: Study data are stored in a database that complies with all security measures at the ADEMA-Escuela Universitaria. The Data Protection Delegate is Ángel Arturo López González.

Conflicts of Interest: The authors declare no conflicts of interest.

References

1. Puljiz, Z.; Kumric, M.; Vrdoljak, J.; Martinovic, D.; Kurir, T.T.; Krnic, M.O.; Urlic, H.; Puljiz, Z.; Zucko, J.; Dumanic, P.; et al. Obe Gut Microbiota, and Metabolome: From Pathophysiology to Nutritional Interventions. *Nutrients* **2023**, *15*, 2236. [CrossR [PubMed]
2. Hancková, M.; Betáková, T. Pandemics of the 21st Century: The Risk Factor for Obese People. *Viruses* **2021**, *14*, 25. [CrossR [PubMed]
3. Wei, S.; Nguyen, T.T.; Zhang, Y.; Ryu, D.; Gariani, K. Sarcopenic obesity: Epidemiology, pathophysiology, cardiovascular dise mortality, and management. *Front. Endocrinol.* **2023**, *14*, 1185221. [CrossRef]
4. Suárez, R.; Chapela, S.P.; Álvarez-Córdova, L.; Bautista-Valarezo, E.; Sarmiento-Andrade, Y.; Verde, L.; Frias-Toral, E.; Sarno Epigenetics in Obesity and Diabetes Mellitus: New Insights. *Nutrients* **2023**, *15*, 811. [CrossRef] [PubMed]
5. Koperska, A.; Wesołek, A.; Moszak, M.; Szulińska, M. Berberine in Non-Alcoholic Fatty Liver Disease—A Review. *Nutrients* **2** *14*, 3459. [CrossRef] [PubMed]
6. Ramírez Manent, J.I.; Gordito Soler, M.; Perelló Viola, N.; Montero Muñoz, N.; Altisench Jané, B. Anthropometric parame related to high-risk values of different scales of nonalcoholic fatty liver disease and liver fibrosis in 146.318 spanish adults. *A J. Health Sci.* **2022**, *37*, 73–82.
7. Eslam, M.; Sanyal, A.J.; George, J.; International Consensus Panel. MAFLD: A Consensus-Driven Proposed Nomenclature Metabolic Associated Fatty Liver Disease. *Gastroenterology* **2020**, *158*, 1999–2014.e1. [CrossRef] [PubMed]
8. Chalasani, N.; Younossi, Z.; LaVine, J.E.; Charlton, M.; Cusi, K.; Rinella, M.; Harrison, S.A.; Brunt, E.M.; Sanyal, A.J. The diagnc and management of nonalcoholic fatty liver disease: Practice guidance from the American Association for the Study of Li Diseases. *Hepatology* **2018**, *67*, 328–357. [CrossRef]
9. Stojsavljević, S.; Gomerčić Palčić, M.; Virović Jukić, L.; Smirčić Duvnjak, L.; Duvnjak, M. Adipokines and proinflammat cytokines, the key mediators in the pathogenesis of nonalcoholic fatty liver disease. *World J. Gastroenterol.* **2014**, *20*, 18070–18 [CrossRef]
10. Cortez-Pinto, H.; Camilo, M.E.; Baptista, A.; De Oliveira, A.G.; De Moura, M.C. Non-alcoholic fatty liver: Another feature of metabolic syndrome? *Clin. Nutr.* **1999**, *18*, 353–358. [CrossRef] [PubMed]
11. Eslam, M.; Newsome, P.N.; Sarin, S.K.; Anstee, Q.M.; Targher, G.; Romero-Gomez, M.; Zelber-Sagi, S.; Wong, V.W.-S.; Dufc J.-F.; Schattenberg, J.M.; et al. A new definition for metabolic dysfunction-associated fatty liver disease: An international exp consensus statement. *J. Hepatol.* **2020**, *73*, 202–209. [CrossRef]

Nonguierma, E.; Lesco, E.; Olak, R.; Welch, H.; Alam, N.Z.; Bonyadi, J.; Hopkins, L. Improving Obesogenic Dietary Behaviors among Adolescents: A Systematic Review of Randomized Controlled Trials. *Nutrients* **2022**, *14*, 4592. [CrossRef]
Younossi, Z.M.; Golabi, P.; Paik, J.M.; Henry, A.; Van Dongen, C.; Henry, L. The global epidemiology of nonalcoholic fatty liver disease (NAFLD) and nonalcoholic steatohepatitis (NASH): A systematic review. *Hepatology* **2023**, *77*, 1335–1347. [CrossRef] [PubMed]
Liu, C.-F.; Chien, L.-W. Predictive Role of Neutrophil-Percentage-to-Albumin Ratio (NPAR) in Nonalcoholic Fatty Liver Disease and Advanced Liver Fibrosis in Nondiabetic US Adults: Evidence from NHANES 2017–2018. *Nutrients* **2023**, *15*, 1892. [CrossRef]
Ballestri, S.; Nascimbeni, F.; Lugari, S.; Lonardo, A.; Francica, G. A critical appraisal of the use of ultrasound in hepatic steatosis. *Expert. Rev. Gastroenterol. Hepatol.* **2019**, *13*, 667–681. [CrossRef]
Bril, F.; Ortiz-Lopez, C.; Lomonaco, R.; Orsak, B.; Freckleton, M.; Chintapalli, K.; Hardies, J.; Lai, S.; Solano, F.; Tio, F.; et al. Clinical value of liver ultrasound for the diagnosis of nonalcoholic fatty liver disease in overweight and obese patients. *Liver Int.* **2015**, *35*, 2139–2146. [CrossRef]
Paige, J.S.; Bernstein, G.S.; Heba, E.; Costa, E.A.C.; Fereirra, M.; Wolfson, T.; Gamst, A.C.; Valasek, M.A.; Lin, G.Y.; Han, A.; et al. A Pilot Comparative Study of Quantitative Ultrasound, Conventional Ultrasound, and MRI for Predicting Histology-Determined Steatosis Grade in Adult Nonalcoholic Fatty Liver Disease. *Am. J. Roentgenol.* **2017**, *208*, W168–W177. [CrossRef]
Wong, V.W.-S.; Vergniol, J.; Wong, G.L.-H.; Foucher, J.; Chan, H.L.-Y.; Le Bail, B.; Choi, P.C.-L.; Kowo, M.; Chan, A.W.-H.; Merrouche, W.; et al. Diagnosis of fibrosis and cirrhosis using liver stiffness measurement in nonalcoholic fatty liver disease. *Hepatology* **2009**, *51*, 454–462. [CrossRef] [PubMed]
Sigrist, R.M.S.; Liau, J.; Kaffas, A.E.; Chammas, M.C.; Willmann, J.K. Ultrasound Elastography: Review of Techniques and Clinical Applications. *Theranostics* **2017**, *7*, 1303–1329. [CrossRef]
Bray, G.A. Beyond BMI. *Nutrients* **2023**, *15*, 2254. [CrossRef] [PubMed] [PubMed Central]
McLaughlin, T.; Lamendola, C.; Liu, A.; Abbasi, F. Preferential Fat Deposition in Subcutaneous Versus Visceral Depots Is Associated with Insulin Sensitivity. *J. Clin. Endocrinol. Metab.* **2011**, *96*, E1756–E1760. [CrossRef] [PubMed]
Ross, R.; Neeland, I.J.; Yamashita, S.; Shai, I.; Seidell, J.; Magni, P.; Santos, R.D.; Arsenault, B.; Cuevas, A.; Hu, F.B.; et al. Waist circumference as a vital sign in clinical practice: A Consensus Statement from the IAS and ICCR Working Group on Visceral Obesity. *Nat. Rev. Endocrinol.* **2020**, *16*, 177–189. [CrossRef] [PubMed]
Gómez-Ambrosi, J.; González-Crespo, I.; Catalán, V.; Rodríguez, A.; Moncada, R.; Valentí, V.; Romero, S.; Ramírez, B.; Silva, C.; Gil, M.J.; et al. Clinical usefulness of abdominal bioimpedance (ViScan) in the determination of visceral fat and its application in the diagnosis and management of obesity and its comorbidities. *Clin. Nutr.* **2017**, *37*, 580–589. [CrossRef] [PubMed]
Pouwels, S.; Sakran, N.; Graham, Y.; Leal, A.; Pintar, T.; Yang, W.; Kassir, R.; Singhal, R.; Mahawar, K.; Ramnarain, D. Non-alcoholic fatty liver disease (NAFLD): A review of pathophysiology, clinical management and effects of weight loss. *BMC Endocr. Disord.* **2022**, *22*, 63. [CrossRef] [PubMed]
Cusi, K.; Isaacs, S.; Barb, D.; Basu, R.; Caprio, S.; Garvey, W.T.; Kashyap, S.; Mechanick, J.I.; Mouzaki, M.; Nadolsky, K.; et al. American Association of Clinical Endocrinology Clinical Practice Guideline for the Diagnosis and Management of Nonalcoholic Fatty Liver Disease in Primary Care and Endocrinology Clinical Settings: Co-Sponsored by the American Association for the Study of Liver Diseases (AASLD). *Endocr. Pract.* **2022**, *28*, 528–562. [PubMed]
Lee, K.-C.; Wu, P.-S.; Lin, H.-C. Pathogenesis and treatment of non-alcoholic steatohepatitis and its fibrosis. *Clin. Mol. Hepatol.* **2023**, *29*, 77–98. [CrossRef]
Stewart, A.; Marfell-Jones, M.; Olds, T.; Ridder, H. *International Standards for Anthropometric Assessment*; International Society for the Advancement of Kinanthropometry–ISAK: Lower Hutt, New Zealand, 2011.
Fang, H.; Berg, E.; Cheng, X.; Shen, W. How to best assess abdominal obesity. *Curr. Opin. Clin. Nutr. Metab. Care* **2018**, *21*, 360–365. [CrossRef]
Mohebbi, V.; Aramayo, A.; Morales, J. Determination of scales related to cardiovascular risk and fatty liver in 5.370 Spanish farmers. *Acad. J. Health Sci.* **2021**, *36*, 26–33.
Fuyan, S.; Jing, L.; Wenjun, C.; Zhijun, T.; Weijing, M.; Suzhen, W.; Yongyong, X. Fatty liver disease index: A simple screening tool to facilitate diagnosis of nonalcoholic fatty liver disease in the Chinese population. *Dig. Dis. Sci.* **2013**, *58*, 3326–3334. [CrossRef]
Kahn, H.S. The "lipid accumulation product" performs better than the body mass index for recognizing cardiovascular risk: A population-based comparison. *BMC Cardiovasc. Disord.* **2005**, *5*, 26, Erratum in: *BMC Cardiovasc. Disord.* **2006**, *6*, 5. [CrossRef]
Domingo-Salvany, A.; Bacigalupe, A.; Carrasco, J.M.; Espelt, A.; Ferrando, J.; Borrell, C.; del Grupo de Determinantes Sociales de Sociedad Española de Epidemiología. Propuestas de clase social neoweberiana y neomarxista a partir de la Clasificación Nacional de Ocupaciones 2011 [Proposals for social class classification based on the Spanish National Classification of Occupations 2011 using neo-Weberian and neo-Marxist approaches]. *Gac Sanit.* **2013**, *27*, 263–272. (In Spanish)
Determinantes de Salud (Consumo de Tabaco, Exposición Pasiva al Humo de Tabaco, Alcohol, Problemas Medioambientales en la Vivienda). Available online: https://www.ine.es/ss/Satellite?L=es_ES&c=INESeccion_C&cid=1259926698156&p=1254735110672&pagename=ProductosYServicios/PYSLayout (accessed on 11 May 2024).
INEbase/Indicadores de Calidad de Vida. Available online: https://www.ine.es/jaxi/Datos.htm?path=/t00/ICV/dim3/10/&file=33201.px (accessed on 11 May 2024).

35. Martínez-Almoyna Rifá, E.; Tomás-Gil, P.; Coll Villalonga, J.L.L.; Ramírez-Manent, J.I.; Martí-Lliteras, P.; López-González, Relationship between nonalcoholic fatty liver disease and liver fibrosis risk scales with overweight and obesity scales in 219, spanish workers. *Acad. J. Health Sci.* **2023**, *38*, 92–100.
36. Lazarus, J.V.; Mark, H.E.; Villota-Rivas, M.; Palayew, A.; Carrieri, P.; Colombo, M.; Ekstedt, M.; Esmat, G.; George, J.; Marche G. The global NAFLD policy review and preparedness index: Are countries ready to address this silent public health challeng *Hepatol.* **2022**, *76*, 771–780. [CrossRef] [PubMed]
37. Baek, J.; Jung, S.J.; Shim, J.-S.; Jeon, Y.W.; Seo, E.; Kim, H.C. Comparison of Computed Tomography-based Abdominal Adipo Indexes as Predictors of Non-alcoholic Fatty Liver Disease Among Middle-aged Korean Men and Women. *J. Prev. Med. Pu Health* **2020**, *53*, 256–265. [CrossRef] [PubMed]
38. Della Torre, S. Non-alcoholic Fatty Liver Disease as a Canonical Example of Metabolic Inflammatory-Based Liver Disease Show a Sex-Specific Prevalence: Relevance of Estrogen Signaling. *Front. Endocrinol.* **2020**, *11*, 572490. [CrossRef]
39. Pouliot, M.-C.; Després, J.-P.; Lemieux, S.; Moorjani, S.; Bouchard, C.; Tremblay, A.; Nadeau, A.; Lupien, P.J. Waist circumfere and abdominal sagittal diameter: Best simple anthropometric indexes of abdominal visceral adipose tissue accumulation related cardiovascular risk in men and women. *Am. J. Cardiol.* **1994**, *73*, 460–468. [CrossRef]

nutrients

MDPI

icle

besity Is Associated with Fatty Liver and Fat Changes in the idneys in Humans as Assessed by MRI

dar Raphael [1,2,3], Eyal Klang [2,3], Eli Konen [2,3], Yael Inbar [2,3], Avshalom Leibowitz [3,4], Yael Frenkel-Nir [3,5], a Apter [2,3,†] and Ehud Grossman [6,*,†]

1 Arrow Projects for Medical Research Education, The Chaim Sheba Medical Center, Tel Hashomer 5266202, Israel; aharonith@gmail.com
2 Department of Imaging, The Chaim Sheba Medical Center, Tel Hashomer 5266202, Israel; eyalkla@hotmail.com (E.K.); eli.konen@sheba.health.gov.il (E.K.); yael.inbar@sheba.health.gov.il (Y.I.); saraapter@gmail.com (S.A.)
3 Faculty of Medicine, Tel Aviv University, Tel Aviv 5266202, Israel; avshalom.leibowitz@sheba.health.gov.il (A.L.); yael.frenkelnir@sheba.health.gov.il (Y.F.-N.)
4 Internal Medicine D the Chaim Sheba Medical Center, Tel Hashomer 5266202, Israel
5 Medical Management Department, The Chaim Sheba Medical Center, Tel Hashomer 5266202, Israel
6 Adelson Medical School, Ariel University, Ariel 4077625, Israel
* Correspondence: pres@ariel.ac.il; Tel.: +972-39066153
† These authors contributed equally to this manuscript.

Abstract: Background: Obesity is associated with metabolic syndrome and fat accumulation in various organs such as the liver and the kidneys. Our goal was to assess, using magnetic resonance imaging (MRI) Dual-Echo phase sequencing, the association between liver and kidney fat deposition and their relation to obesity. Methods: We analyzed MRI scans of individuals who were referred to the Chaim Sheba Medical Center between December 2017 and May 2020 to perform a study for any indication. For each individual, we retrieved from the computerized charts data on sex, and age, weight, height, body mass index (BMI), systolic and diastolic blood pressure (BP), and comorbidities (diabetes mellitus, hypertension, dyslipidemia). Results: We screened MRI studies of 399 subjects with a median age of 51 years, 52.4% of whom were women, and a median BMI 24.6 kg/m^2. We diagnosed 18% of the participants with fatty liver and 18.6% with fat accumulation in the kidneys (fatty kidneys). Out of the 67 patients with fatty livers, 23 (34.3%) also had fatty kidneys, whereas among the 315 patients without fatty livers, only 48 patients (15.2%) had fatty kidneys ($p < 0.01$). In comparison to the patients who did not have a fatty liver or fatty kidneys ($n = 267$), those who had both ($n = 23$) were more obese, had higher systolic BP, and were more likely to have diabetes mellitus. In comparison to the patients without a fatty liver, those with fatty livers had an adjusted odds ratio of 2.91 (97.5% CI; 1.61–5.25) to have fatty kidneys. In total, 19.6% of the individuals were obese (BMI $\geq$ 30), and 26.1% had overweight (25 < BMI < 30). The obese and overweight individuals were older and more likely to have diabetes mellitus and hypertension and had higher rates of fatty livers and fatty kidneys. Fat deposition in both the liver and the kidneys was observed in 15.9% of the obese patients, in 8.3% of the overweight patients, and in none of those with normal weight. Obesity was the only risk factor for fatty kidneys and fatty livers, with an adjusted OR of 6.3 (97.5% CI 2.1–18.6). Conclusions: Obesity is a major risk factor for developing a fatty liver and fatty kidneys. Individuals with a fatty liver are more likely to have fatty kidneys. MRI is an accurate modality for diagnosing fatty kidneys. Reviewing MRI scans of any indication should include assessment of fat fractions in the kidneys in addition to that of the liver.

Keywords: obesity; fatty liver; fatty kidneys; MRI

1. Introduction

Obesity has grown to epidemic proportions, with over 4 million people dying each year because of being overweight or obese, according to the global burden of disease [1].

By 2030, nearly one in two adults will have obesity, and it is projected that nearly one in four adults will have severe obesity [2].

Obesity can lead to type 2 diabetes (T2D), hypertension, and dyslipidemia and is associated with metabolic syndrome (MS), which is a combination of abdominal obesity, elevated blood pressure, high triglyceride and low HDL cholesterol levels, and high fasting glucose levels [3,4]. Using a rat model, we showed that a high-fructose diet (HFD) could cause MS and fatty liver disease [5,6]. MS is a known risk factor for developing non-alcoholic fatty liver disease (NAFLD) [7]. Studies have shown that individuals with MS are at a higher risk of developing NAFLD than those without MS [8]. The exact mechanism by which MS leads to NAFLD is not fully understood; it is believed, however, that insulin resistance plays a key role. Insulin resistance can lead to increased production of free fatty acids and triglycerides, which can accumulate in the liver and cause fatty liver disease. In a recent study, we showed that a HFD could also cause fat accumulation in the kidneys [9]. Obesity can also increase the risk of developing fatty kidneys, as it is associated with insulin resistance, inflammation, and oxidative stress, which can all contribute to the development of fatty kidneys [10]. Additionally, high blood pressure, high triglyceride levels, and high blood glucose levels, all of which are components of MS, can contribute to the development of fatty kidney disease [4]. This can lead to inflammation and scarring of the kidney tissue, which can result in reduced kidney function and, in severe cases, renal failure. Fatty liver and fatty kidney disease are two distinct conditions, although they share a common underlying mechanism: the accumulation of excess fat in the respective organs. Magnetic Resonance Imaging (MRI) is an accurate method for assessing and monitoring lipid content in the liver [11,12]. This technique can be utilized to assess kidney parenchyma lipid content. The aim of the present study was two-fold. First, we sought to use a new MRI methodology (dual-echo phase sequencing) to assess the rates of fatty kidney and fatty liver disease in a large group of subjects and evaluate the association between these distinct conditions. The second aim was to evaluate the association between obesity and fatty liver and fatty kidney disease.

2. Methods

2.1. Study Population

We reviewed 695 MRI abdominal scans that were performed for any indication at the Sheba Medical Center between December 2017 and May 2020. In most cases, the indications for MRI scan were an evaluation of suspected malignancy or follow-up after the removal of an abdominal or gynecological tumor. We excluded MRI scans that were performed on pregnant women (81) or children younger than 16 (110), were of bad quality (18), and/or had no dual-echo phase scans (87). We therefore included in this study 399 MRI scans. (Figure 1). For each subject, we retrieved from computerized charts data on sex, age, weight, height, body mass index (BMI), systolic and diastolic blood pressure (BP), comorbidities (diabetes mellitus, hypertension, dyslipidemia), and renal function tests. Dyslipidemia was defined when an individual either used lipid-lowering agents or had the diagnostic ICD-9 code of dyslipidemia in his chart. We were blind with respect to each patient's metabolic status and whether they had a known affliction with NAFLD for each scan.

2.2. MRI Assessment

We assessed the fat fractions of the liver and kidneys using MRI dual-echo phase sequencing, a method that is based on the relative chemical shift between water and the methylene peak of fat. Volumetric liver fat can be detected by determining the relative signal loss between in-phase (IP) and opposed-phase (OP) images. This method is one of the imaging methods accepted for identifying and characterizing liver fat fractions [12]. We employed the fat signal fraction formula, i.e., $\eta = \frac{IP-OP}{2IP}$, to evaluate fat accumulation in the kidneys [13]. We measured each kidney at three points (defined on the coronal images): the upper, middle, and lower poles. We then chose the maximal value to calculate the kidney fat fraction. As described by Krievina G. et al. [14], we found higher rates of fat accumulation in the left kidney, and therefore we focused on the left kidney for each case. An illustration of the evaluation of fat in the liver and the kidneys is presented in Figure 2.

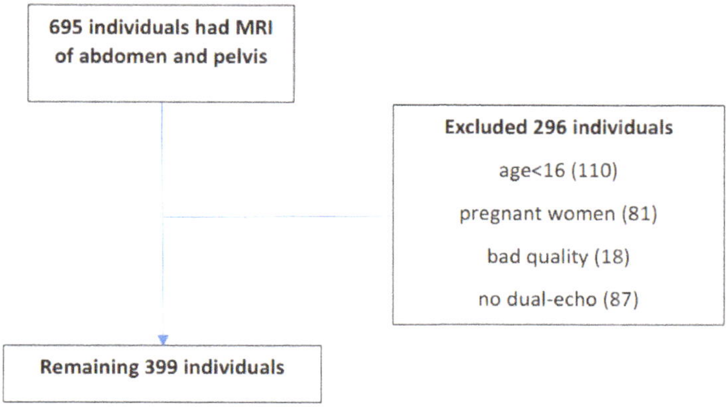

Figure 1. Study population flow chart.

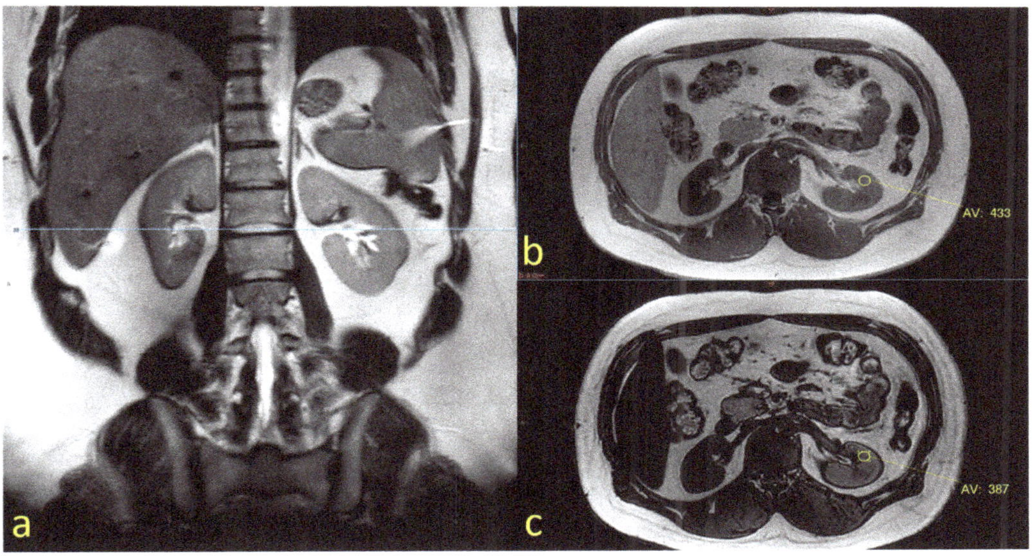

Figure 2. Assessment of renal fat using dual-phase MRI sequences: Measurements were performed on three levels of the kidney as defined on control T2Wis: upper pole, renal hilum (**a**), and lower pole. In-phase (IP) (TR 127.85, TE 2.30) (**b**) and opposed phase (OP) (TR 127.85, TE 1.15) (**c**) images of (**a**) 28 Y male. Assessment of the fat fraction was performed using the following equation: $\eta = \frac{IP-OP}{2IP}$ (Ref. [13]).

Fatty liver was defined as liver steatosis grade 1 and above that correlated with 5% or more of the fat fraction. This definition is based on histologic studies on liver steatosis [12]. Since a fatty kidney is not clearly defined in the literature and since there is no research on the correlation between MRI findings and histologic structure in this regard, we decided to set a threshold of a fat fraction of 4% to define a fatty kidney.

2.3. Statistical Analysis

The significance level was set at $p < 0.05$ for all analyses. Continuous variables were expressed as medians and interquartile ranges (IQRs), while categorical variables were presented as percentages.

We compared the rates of cases of fatty livers to the rates of cases with fat changes in the kidney. Using the chi-squared test, we analyzed the association between the presence of fatty liver and fatty kidneys. We also divided the patients into 3 groups according to BMI: normal weight (BMI $\leq$ 25 kg/m^2), overweight 25 < BMI < 30 kg/m^2), and obese (BMI $\geq$ 30 kg/m^2). We calculated the rates of fatty liver and kidneys in the different groups.

We then assessed the associations between these clinical variables and the presence of fatty liver, fatty kidneys, and both. Continuous variables were compared using the non-parametric Mann–Whitney U test for paired comparisons, while categorical variables were analyzed using the chi-squared test.

To further investigate the associations, we performed adjusted odds ratio (aOR) analyses using logistic regression models. First, we calculated the aOR for fatty kidneys as the target, using age, sex, diabetes, hypertension, dyslipidemia, and fatty liver as independent variables. Next, we calculated the aOR for subjects with both fatty kidney and fatty liver disease, using age, sex, diabetes, dyslipidemia, and BMI $\geq$ 30 as independent variables.

3. Results

3.1. Subjects' Characteristics

We screened the MRIs of 399 subjects whose mean age was 51 $\pm$ 19 (median 51) years, consisting of 52.4% women and exhibiting a mean BMI of 25.8 $\pm$ 5.6 (median 24.6) kg/m^2. Hypertension was identified in 86 subjects (21.6%). Diabetes mellitus and dyslipidemia were identified in less than 10% of the subjects (Table 1).

Table 1. Basic characteristics of the study cohort arranged by fatty liver group.

	Total (n = 399)	Fatty Liver (n = 72)	Non-Fatty Liver (n = 327)	p
Female sex, n, (%)	209 (52.4)	34 (47.2)	175 (53.5)	0.33
Age, y, median (IQR)	51 (35–67)	56 (44–67)	49 (33–67)	0.141
Weight, kg, median (IQR) *	72 (60–85)	88 (74–102)	68.5 (58–79)	<0.0001
Height, cm, median (IQR) *	168 (162–175)	167 (162–175)	168 (161–175)	0.800
BMI, kg/m^2, median (IQR) *	24.6 (21.8–29.3)	30.8 (27.4–34.1)	24.1 (21.3–27.3)	<0.0001
Systolic BP, mmHg, median # (IQR)	121 (110–140)	127 (115–142)	120 (109–138)	0.033
Diastolic BP, mmHg, median # (IQR)	73 (66–80)	77 (72–81)	73 (66–80)	0.017
Hypertension, n, (%)	86 (21.6)	22 (30.6)	64 (19.6)	0.040
Diabetes Mellitus, n, (%)	38 (9.5)	12 (16.7)	26 (8)	0.023
Dyslipidemia, n, (%)	24 (6)	9 (12.5)	15 (4.6)	0.011

Fatty liver—grade 1 and grade 2 steatosis. Non fatty liver—grade 0 steatosis. BMI = Body mass Index; BP = blood pressure. * Missing data for 79 subjects. # Missing data for 52 subjects.

3.2. The rates of Fatty Liver and Fatty Kidney Disease

Among the subjects we screened, 72 (18%) had fatty livers. The subjects with fatty liver disease were more obese and were more likely to have hypertension, diabetes mellitus, and dyslipidemia than those without a fatty liver (Table 1).

For the evaluation of fatty kidneys, we excluded 17 patients who had undergone a left nephrectomy. Out of 382 patients, 71 (18.6%) had fatty kidneys. Those with fatty kidneys were more obese and had higher systolic BP levels than those without fatty kidneys (Table 2). They also had higher creatinine and urea levels (0.89 vs. 0.76 and 35 vs. 30 for creatinine and urea, respectively, with $p < 0.05$ for both).

To analyze the association between fatty liver and fatty kidneys, we included 382 patients who had undergone an evaluation of both their liver and kidneys. Figure 3 depicts a case with a fatty liver and a fatty kidney. Out of the 67 patients with fatty livers, 23 (34.3%) also had fatty kidneys, whereas among the 315 patients without a fatty liver, only 48 patients (15.2%) had fatty kidneys. In comparison to patients who had neither a fatty liver nor fatty kidneys (n = 267), those who had both (n = 23) were more obese and had higher systolic BP and were more likely to have diabetes mellitus (Table 3).

Table 2. Basic characteristics of the study cohort according to fatty kidney group.

	Total (n = 382)	**Fatty Kidneys (n = 71)**	**Lack of Fatty Kidneys (n = 311)**	p
Female sex, n, (%)	203 (53.1)	31 (43.7)	172 (55.3)	0.076
Age, y, median (IQR)	50 (34–66)	56 (35–70)	49 (34–64)	0.076
Weight, kg, median (IQR) *	71 (60–84)	75 (65–88)	70 (58–83)	0.006
Height, cm, median (IQR) *	168 (160–175)	169 (162–174)	168 (160–175)	0.616
BMI, kg/m^2, median (IQR) *	24.6 (21.6–29.1)	27.2 (23.1–30.0)	24.4 (21.4–28.7)	0.013
ystolic BP, mmHg, median # (IQR)	120 (110–140)	126 (114–143)	120 (109–137)	0.032
astolic BP, mmHg, median # (IQR)	73 (66–80)	76 (66–80)	73 (66–80)	0.464
Hypertension, n, (%)	79 (20.7)	17 (23.9)	62 (19.9)	0.452
Diabetes Mellitus, n, (%)	35 (9.2)	8 (11.3)	27 (8.7)	0.496
Dyslipidemia, n, (%)	20 (5.2)	4 (5.6)	16 (5.1)	0.867

Fatty kidney was defined as ≥4% fatty change. A non-fatty kidney was defined as <4%. BMI = Body mass index; BP = blood pressure. * Missing data for 77 subjects. # Missing data for 52 subjects.

Table 3. Basic characteristics of the study cohort according to fatty kidney and fatty liver groups.

	Fatty Liver (n = 67)			**Non-Fatty Liver (n = 315)**		
	Fatty Kidney (n = 23, 34.33%)	**No Fatty Kidneys (n = 44, 65.67%)**	p	**Fatty Kidney (n = 48, 15.24%)**	**Non-Fatty Kidney (n = 267, 84.76%)**	p
Female sex, n, (%)	12 (52.2)	21 (47.7)	0.730	19 (39.6)	151 (56.6)	0.030
Age, y, median (IQR)	56 (45–70)	51 (40.5–61.75)	0.326	54.5 (34–70)	49 (33–65)	0.201
Veight, kg, median (IQR) *	90 (81–101)	85 (72–103)	0.211	72 (61–81)	68 (57–77)	0.182
leight, cm, median (IQR) *	165 (159–178)	168 (162–175)	0.790	170 (165–173)	168 (160–175)	0.375
MI, kg/m^2, median (IQR) *	32.0 (29.7–35.6)	29.8 (25.0–23.4)	0.059	24.3 (21.6–27.6)	24.0 (21.0–27.1)	0.394
Systolic BP, mmHg, median (IQR) #	133 (114–156)	120 (115–141)	0.115	125 (111–140)	120 (108–136)	0.104
Diastolic BP, mmHg, median (IQR) #	78 (74–82)	76 (70–80)	0.440	73 (66–78)	72 (65–80)	0.864
Hypertension, n, (%)	8 (34.8)	11 (25)	0.399	9 (18.8)	51 (19.1)	0.955
Diabetes Mellitus, n, (%)	5 (21.7)	5 (11.4)	0.258	3 (6.3)	22 (8.2)	0.639
Dyslipidemia, n, (%)	2 (8.7)	4 (9.1)	0.957	2 (4.2)	12 (4.5)	0.919

BMI = Body mass index; BP = blood pressure. * Missing data for 77 subjects. # Missing data for 52 subjects.

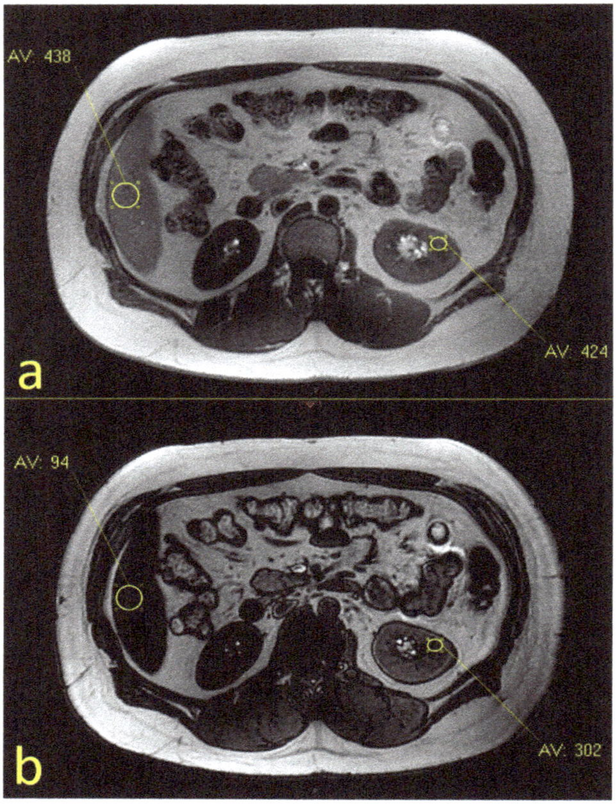

Figure 3. Assessment of renal and liver fat using dual-phase MRI sequences: (Same patient as in Figure 2): In-phase (**a**) (IP) (TR 127.85, TE 2.30) and opposed-phase (OP) (**b**) (TR 127.85, TE 1.15) axial images demonstrating fat fractions of 14% in the lower pole of the kidney and of 39% in the liver.

In comparison to the patients without a fatty liver, those with a fatty liver had an adjusted odds ratio of 2.91 (97.5% CI; 1.61–5.25) with respect to having fatty kidneys (Table 4).

Table 4. Adjusted odds ratio for fatty kidney.

Parameter	Odds Ratio	CI 2.5%	CI 97.5%	p-Value
Age	1.0	1.0	1.0	0.086
Sex	1.6	0.9	2.7	0.082
Diabetes Mellitus	1.0	0.4	2.5	0.987
Hypertension	0.9	0.4	1.8	0.688
Dyslipidemia	0.8	0.2	2.7	0.722
Fatty Liver	2.9	1.6	5.2	0.001

3.3. The Association between Body Mass Index and Fatty Liver and Fatty Kidneys

Height and weight data were available for 322 subjects. Most subjects had normal weights, and 19.6% were obese. In the normal-weight group, 18 subjects had a very low BMI (<18.5 kg/m^2). Inclusion or exclusion of the subgroup with a very low BMI did not affect the findings for the normal-weight group.

The overweight and obese patients were older and more likely to have diabetes mellitus and hypertension and had higher rates of fatty liver and fatty kidney disease (Table 5). Fatty deposition in both the liver and the kidneys was observed in 15.9% of the obese patients, 8.3% of the overweight patients, and none of those with normal weight (Table 5). Obesity was the only risk factor for fatty kidney and fatty liver disease, with an adjusted OR of 6.3 (97.5% CI 2.1–18.6) (Table 6).

Table 5. The rates of fatty liver and fatty kidney disease according to body mass index.

	Total (*n* = 322)	**BMI ≤ 25** (*n* = 175, 54.3%)	**25 < BMI < 30** (*n* = 84, 26.1%)	**BMI ≥ 30** (*n* = 63, 19.6%)	***p* Value**
Female sex, n, (%)	166 (51.6)	91 (52)	40 (47.6)	35 (55.6)	0.625
Age >50 y, n (%)	166 (51.6)	74 (42.3)	49 (58.3)	43 (68.3)	0.0006
Systolic BP > 130 mmHg, n (%)	116 (36.0)	44 (25.1)	33 (39.2)	39 (62.0)	<0.0001
Diastolic BP > 80 mmHg, n (%)	74 (23.0)	37 (21.1)	18 (21.4)	19 (30.2)	0.319
Hypertension, n, (%)	82 (25.5)	27 (15.4)	23 (27.4)	32 (50.8)	<0.0001
Diabetes Mellitus, n, (%)	37 (11.5)	13 (7.4)	7 (8.3)	17 (27)	<0.0001
Dyslipidemia, n, (%)	23 (7.1)	8 (4.6)	7 (8.3)	8 (12.7)	0.088
Fatty liver, n, (%)	57 (17.7)	7 (4)	18 (21.4)	32 (50.8)	<0.0001
Fatty kidney, n, (%)	56 (17.4)	22 (12.6)	22 (26.2)	12 (19)	0.007
Fatty liver and fatty kidney, n, (%)	17 (5.3)	0 (0)	7 (8.3)	10 (15.9)	<0.0001

BMI = body mass index; BP = blood pressure. Differences in baseline characteristics between the groups were tested using the chi-squared test.

Table 6. A: Adjusted OR for fatty kidneys. B: Adjusted OR for fatty kidneys + fatty liver.

		A		
Parameter	**Odds Ratio**	**CI 2.5%**	**CI 97.5%**	***p*-Value**
Age	1.0	1.0	1.0	0.086
Sex	1.6	0.9	2.7	0.082
Diabetes mellitus	1.0	0.4	2.5	0.987
Hypertension	0.9	0.4	1.8	0.688
Dyslipidemia	0.8	0.2	2.7	0.722
Fatty Liver	2.9	1.6	5.2	0.001
		B		
Parameter	**Odds Ratio**	**CI 2.5%**	**CI 97.5%**	***p*-Value**
Age	1.0	1.0	1.0	0.958
Sex	0.6	0.2	1.8	0.359
Diabetes mellitus	1.7	0.4	6.8	0.478
Hypertension	1.3	0.3	4.8	0.694
Dyslipidemia	0.5	0.1	4.9	0.545
BMI ≥ 30 kg/m^2	6.3	2.1	18.6	0.001

BMI = Body mass index.

4. Discussion

In this study, we used MRI to assess, in a large cohort, the fat content of the liver and kidneys and relate it to BMI.

We found a fatty liver in 18% of the individuals. This rate is slightly less than the current estimation of global prevalence, i.e., 25%, described in a meta-analysis by Younossi. Z et al. [15].

However, we used strict MRI criteria that may underestimate mild cases of fatty liver disease. MRI-proton density fat fraction is considered a reliable, non-invasive method for assessing liver steatosis and is commonly used in clinical practice [12]. The advantages of this method include its results close correlation with histopathological examination results and the convenience of the quantification of steatosis [12].

We found fatty kidneys in 18.6% of the individuals. Among 2923 participants of the Framingham Heart Study, Foster M.C. et al. [16] found fat deposits in the kidney in 30.1% of the participants, but they measured the fat deposition in the renal sinus by using CT scans and used sex-specific 90th percentiles of a healthy referent subsample to define fatty kidneys. We measured the fat deposition in the renal parenchyma by using MRI dual sequences, and we defined fatty kidneys as constituting cases in which a fate percentage of at least 4% was detected in the parenchyma of the kidneys.

The term "fatty kidney" was first coined in the literature in 1883 [17]. Since then, several studies have tried to assess lipid accumulation in the kidneys [18–20]. The true prevalence of fatty kidney disease is unknown because, until now, there was no precise modality for diagnosing fatty kidneys. In addition, various studies have measured fat deposition in different parts of the kidneys [21–25]. Most studies have measured fat deposition in the renal hilum, while some measured it in the pararenal space or the perirenal space, and some measured it in the renal parenchyma. In the present study, we measured fat deposition in the renal parenchyma. We used MRI dual sequences to estimate the fat content in the parenchyma of the kidneys. We defined a cut-off point of 4% fat content in the kidneys to diagnose fatty kidneys. We do not have results of a kidney biopsy that would allow us to show a correlation between our estimation and the actual fat accumulation in the kidneys of our patients. Thus, we cannot be certain that our cut-off point of a 4% fat content in the kidneys is sensitive enough. However, it is clear that we detected patients with abnormal fat accumulation in the kidneys. It is not clear whether we need a 4% fat content in the kidneys to define fatty kidneys or if we can define fatty kidneys with even less fat accumulation. The optimal method for the assessment of renal fat accumulation and the cut-off point for the definition of fatty kidneys remain to be determined.

Fatty kidney disease is associated with hypertension. In an analysis of individuals from the Framingham Heart Study, Foster et al. [16] showed that those with fatty kidneys had a higher odds ratio for hypertension (OR: 2.12; $p < 0.0001$), which persisted after adjusting for body mass index (OR: 1.49; $p < 0.0001$) or visceral adipose tissue (OR: 1.24; $p = 0.049$). In a study by Chughtai HL. et al., patients with a systolic BP > 160 mm Hg or a diastolic BP > 100 mm Hg had higher levels of renal sinus fat, quantified via MRI, than those with a BP less than 160/100 mm Hg [18]. In the present study, we also observed, in those with fatty kidneys, higher levels of systolic BP than in those without fatty kidneys. Fat deposition in the kidneys can increase renal interstitial pressure through the compression of renal veins and lymph vessels in the kidneys [18]. This leads to the activation of the renin angiotensin system and, in the presence of volume expansion, increased sodium reabsorption in the loop of Henle and decreased sodium excretion [20]. Activation of the renin angiotensin system and sodium and volume retention may explain the elevated BP associated with obesity and fatty kidneys [20]. Fatty kidney disease has also been linked to kidney injuries and an increased prevalence of chronic kidney disease. In the present study, we found decreased renal function in those with fatty kidneys. Several mechanisms, such as pro-inflammatory signals, oxidative stress, mitochondrial dysfunction, and dysregulation of serum leptin–adiponectin levels, may be responsible for such kidney injuries [10]. Several clinical trials have demonstrated associations between fatty kidneys and comorbidities including atherosclerosis, cardiovascular events, microalbuminuria, and vascular calcification [18,26,27].

We observed a combination of a fatty liver and fatty kidneys in 6% of the individuals.

The main risk factor for the combination of a fatty liver and fatty kidneys was obesity. We also showed that obese individuals with a fatty liver are at a high risk of having fatty kidneys. The association between obesity and fatty liver disease is well known [28]. However, the association between obesity and fatty kidneys is less known. This association was clearly observed in animal models of obesity. Data from animal studies suggest that obesity leads to kidney damage and hypertension through lipotoxicity, oxidative stress, inflammation, and fibrosis [29–31]. Obese mice fed a high-fat diet developed lipid accumulation in the glomeruli and proximal tubules. This lipid accumulation was associated with albuminuria, increased systolic BP and oxidative stress, and a larger glomerular tuft area and mesangial matrix [30]. It is not clear whether obesity itself leads to fatty kidneys or if food ingredients determine whether fat will accumulate in the kidneys. Unfortunately, we do not have data on the dietary content of our cohort. However, we have data from recent animal studies. We showed in a rat model that a high-fructose diet (HFD) can induce metabolic-like syndrome and increase triglyceride accumulation in the kidneys [9]. In this model, oil red staining revealed lipid droplet formation and increased adipophilin mRNA expression in the kidneys, supporting the formation of fatty kidneys. Unlike a HFD, a high-sucrose diet increased BP and caused mild worsening of insulin resistance in spontaneous hypertensive rats, but it did not cause metabolic syndrome [32]. These animal studies suggest that high-fat and high-fructose diets are important components in the development of fatty kidneys.

It is uncertain whether the hypertension and renal impairment associated with obesity are specifically present because of renal fat accumulation or are related to weight gain and adiposity. Through modeling structure and serial adjustment for BMI and visceral adipose tissue, Katharina Mueller-Peltzer et al. showed the independent role of renal fat accumulation in the pathogenesis of hypertension and chronic kidney disease [33].

The question remains whether weight reduction will reduce lipid accumulation in the liver and the kidney. Regarding the liver, two recent studies showed that weight reduction improved parameters of a fatty liver [34,35]. Regarding the kidneys, most dietary weight loss trials failed to show renal benefits. Small studies have shown that dietary weight loss improves albuminuria and attenuates the decline in renal function in patients with chronic kidney disease [36]. Bariatric surgery has yielded data showing that weight loss has a beneficial effect on the kidneys. Weight loss with bariatric surgery normalized hyperfiltration and reduced hypertension and albuminuria [37]. A recent review of bariatric surgery with up to 7 years of follow-up data showed an improvement of chronic kidney disease and less development of end-stage renal disease [38], which supports the concept that ectopic renal fat is worsened by obesity and improved with weight loss, as seen in the case of a fatty liver.

Fatty kidney disease is a common condition in obese individuals and is associated with a fatty liver and an increased risk of hypertension and chronic kidney disease. Fatty kidneys may be associated with BP regulation and chronic kidney disease in humans and provide additional insight into the pathophysiologic role of adiposity in renal dysfunction. Further research is necessary to evaluate the longitudinal associations of fatty kidneys with markers of renal function and metabolic risk factors.

Our study strengthens the association between obesity, a fatty liver, and fatty kidneys.

Our study has certain limitations. The cohort was composed of patients who underwent abdominal MRI for any indication and as such may not accurately represent the general population. While reviewing the scans, we did not take into account their indications. In addition, we had no data on their diets and the drug therapy they received, and therefore we cannot comment on the impact of diet and drug therapy on the development of a fatty liver and fatty kidneys.

Nevertheless, this study provides evidence that reviewing MRI scans of any indication should include measuring fat fractions in the kidneys in addition to the liver. Patients who have been found to have a fatty liver and fat changes in their kidneys should undergo further testing, such as being subjected to a urine protein test and kidney function and BP measurements. This will allow us to track down undiagnosed conditions such as hypertension, diabetes, and dyslipidemia, diseases whose early diagnosis can prevent morbidity.

While we do not yet see the value of ordering an imaging study just to make a diagnosis of fatty kidney disease, we do believe that radiologists reviewing abdominal MRI scans can specifically assess and report ectopic and increased renal fat. A renewed focus on the kidneys will help develop and refine radiologic diagnostic criteria for fatty kidney disease, much like what has been conducted for the liver.

5. Conclusions

Obesity is a major risk factor for fatty liver and fatty kidney disease. Individuals with a fatty liver are more likely to have fatty kidneys. MRI is an accurate modality for diagnosing fatty kidney disease. Reviewing MRI scans of any indication should include an assessment of the fat fraction in the kidneys in addition to that of the liver.

Author Contributions: H.R.—Data acquisition, data analysis, and preparation of the first draft. E.K. (Eyal Klang)—creation of software and data analysis. E.K. (Eli Konen)—Data analysis and interpretation of the data. Y.I.—Data analysis and interpretation of the data. A.L.—Study design and interpretation of the data. Y.F.-N.—Interpretation of the data and substantial revision of the manuscript. S.A.—Data analysis, interpretation of the data, and revision of the manuscript. E.G.—Study design, data analysis, interpretation of the data, and finalization of the manuscript. All authors have read and agreed to the published version of the manuscript.

Funding: This research received no external funding.

Institutional Review Board Statement: The study was approved by the Local Helsinki Committee (Approval date 21 March 2021, Approval code: SNC-8267-21).

Informed Consent Statement: Inform consent was not required.

Data Availability Statement: Data are not available.

Conflicts of Interest: The authors declare no conflicts of interest.

References

1. Collaborators GBDRF. Global burden of 87 risk factors in 204 countries and territories, 1990-2019: A systematic analysis for Global Burden of Disease Study 2019. *Lancet* **2020**, *396*, 1223–1249. [CrossRef] [PubMed]
2. Ward, Z.J.; Bleich, S.N.; Cradock, A.L.; Barrett, J.L.; Giles, C.M.; Flax, C.; Long, M.W.; Gortmaker, S.L. Projected U.S. State-Le Prevalence of Adult Obesity and Severe Obesity. *N. Engl. J. Med.* **2019**, *381*, 2440–2450. [CrossRef] [PubMed]
3. Engin, A. The Definition and Prevalence of Obesity and Metabolic Syndrome. *Adv. Exp. Med. Biol.* **2017**, *960*, 1–17.
4. Grundy, S.M.; Cleeman, J.I.; Daniels, S.R.; Donato, K.A.; Eckel, R.H.; Franklin, B.A.; Gordon, D.J.; Krauss, R.M.; Savage, Smith, S.C., Jr.; et al. Diagnosis and management of the metabolic syndrome: An American Heart Association/National He Lung, and Blood Institute Scientific Statement. *Circulation* **2005**, *112*, 2735–2752. [CrossRef] [PubMed]
5. Leibowitz, A.; Bier, A.; Gilboa, M.; Peleg, E.; Barshack, I.; Grossman, E. Saccharin Increases Fasting Blood Glucose but Not Li Insulin Resistance in Comparison to a High Fructose-Fed Rat Model. *Nutrients* **2018**, *10*, 341. [CrossRef] [PubMed]
6. Bier, A.; Khasbab, R.; Haberman, Y.; Braun, T.; Hadar, R.; Sosnovski, K.; Amir, A.; Leibowitz, A.; Grossman, E. Antibic Treatment Does Not Ameliorate the Metabolic Changes in Rats Presenting Dysbiosis After Consuming a High Fructose D *Nutrients* **2020**, *12*, 203. [CrossRef]
7. Hamaguchi, M.; Kojima, T.; Takeda, N.; Nakagawa, T.; Taniguchi, H.; Fujii, K.; Omatsu, T.; Nakajima, T.; Sarui, Shimazaki, M.; et al. The metabolic syndrome as a predictor of nonalcoholic fatty liver disease. *Ann. Intern. Med.* **20** *143*, 722–728. [CrossRef] [PubMed]
8. Mottillo, S.; Filion, K.B.; Genest, J.; Joseph, L.; Pilote, L.; Poirier, P.; Rinfret, S.; Schiffrin, E.L.; Eisenberg, M.J. The metabc syndrome and cardiovascular risk a systematic review and meta-analysis. *J. Am. Coll. Cardiol.* **2010**, *56*, 1113–1132. [CrossR [PubMed]
9. Bier, A.; Shapira, E.; Khasbab, R.; Sharabi, Y.; Grossman, E.; Leibowitz, A. High-Fructose Diet Increases Renal ChREBPb Expression, Leading to Intrarenal Fat Accumulation in a Rat Model with Metabolic Syndrome. *Biology* **2022**, *11*, 618. [CrossR [PubMed]
10. Tsuboi, N.; Okabayashi, Y.; Shimizu, A.; Yokoo, T. The Renal Pathology of Obesity. *Kidney Int. Rep.* **2017**, *2*, 251–260. [CrossR [PubMed]

Dzyubak, B.; Li, J.; Chen, J.; Mara, K.C.; Therneau, T.M.; Venkatesh, S.K.; Ehman, R.L.; Allen, A.M.; Yin, M. Automated Analysis of Multiparametric Magnetic Resonance Imaging/Magnetic Resonance Elastography Exams for Prediction of Nonalcoholic Steatohepatitis. *J. Magn. Reson. Imaging* **2021**, *54*, 122–131. [CrossRef] [PubMed]

Starekova, J.; Hernando, D.; Pickhardt, P.J.; Reeder, S.B. Quantification of Liver Fat Content with CT and MRI: State of the Art. *Radiology* **2021**, *301*, 250–262. [CrossRef] [PubMed]

Adams, L.A.; Waters, O.R.; Knuiman, M.W.; Elliott, R.R.; Olynyk, J.K. NAFLD as a risk factor for the development of diabetes and the metabolic syndrome: An eleven-year follow-up study. *Am. J. Gastroenterol.* **2009**, *104*, 861–867. [CrossRef] [PubMed]

Krievina, G.; Tretjakovs, P.; Skuja, I.; Silina, V.; Keisa, L.; Krievina, D.; Bahs, G. Ectopic Adipose Tissue Storage in the Left and the Right Renal Sinus is Asymmetric and Associated With Serum Kidney Injury Molecule-1 and Fibroblast Growth Factor-21 Levels Increase. *EBioMedicine* **2016**, *13*, 274–283. [CrossRef] [PubMed]

Younossi, Z.M.; Koenig, A.B.; Abdelatif, D.; Fazel, Y.; Henry, L.; Wymer, M. Global epidemiology of nonalcoholic fatty liver disease-Meta-analytic assessment of prevalence, incidence, and outcomes. *Hepatology* **2016**, *64*, 73–84 [CrossRef] [PubMed]

Foster, M.C.; Hwang, S.J.; Porter, S.A.; Massaro, J.M.; Hoffmann, U.; Fox, C.S. Fatty kidney, hypertension, and chronic kidney disease: The Framingham Heart Study. *Hypertension* **2011**, *58*, 784–790. [CrossRef] [PubMed]

Rickards, E. Remarks on the Fatty Transformation of the Kidney. *Br. Med. J.* **1883**, *2*, 2–3. [CrossRef] [PubMed]

Chughtai, H.L.; Morgan, T.M.; Rocco, M.; Stacey, B.; Brinkley, T.E.; Ding, J.; Nicklas, B.; Hamilton, C.; Hundley, W.G. Renal sinus fat and poor blood pressure control in middle-aged and elderly individuals at risk for cardiovascular events. *Hypertension* **2010**, *56*, 901–906. [CrossRef] [PubMed]

Mende, C.; Einhorn, D. Fatty kidney disease: The importance of ectopic fat deposition and the potential value of imaging. *J. Diabetes* **2022**, *14*, 73–78. [CrossRef] [PubMed]

Mende, C.W.; Einhorn, D. Fatty Kidney Disease: A New Renal and Endocrine Clinical Entity? Describing the Role of the Kidney in Obesity, Metabolic Syndrome, and Type 2 Diabetes. *Endocr. Pract.* **2019**, *25*, 854–858. [CrossRef] [PubMed]

Gjela, M.; Askeland, A.; Frokjaer, J.B.; Mellergaard, M.; Handberg, A. MRI-based quantification of renal fat in obese individuals using different image analysis approaches. *Abdom. Radiol.* **2022**, *47*, 3546–3553. [CrossRef] [PubMed]

Lin, L.; Dekkers, I.A.; Tao, Q.; Paiman, E.H.M.; Bizino, M.B.; Jazet, I.M.; Lamb, H.J. MR Assessed Changes of Renal Sinus Fat in Response to Glucose Regulation in West European and South Asian Patients With Type 2 Diabetes. *J. Magn. Reson. Imaging* **2024**, *37*, 483–490. [CrossRef] [PubMed]

Moritz, E.; Dadson, P.; Saukko, E.; Honka, M.J.; Koskensalo, K.; Seppala, K.; Pekkarinen, L.; Moriconi, D.; Helmio, M.; Salminen, P.; et al. Renal Sinus Fat Is Expanded in Patients with Obesity and/or Hypertension and Reduced by Bariatric Surgery Associated with Hypertension Remission. *Metabolites* **2022**, *12*, 617. [CrossRef] [PubMed]

Yildiz, A.B.; Vehbi, S.; Copur, S.; Gurses, B.; Siriopol, D.; Karakaya, B.A.D.; Hasbal, N.B.; Tekin, B.; Akyildiz, M.; van Raalte, D.H.; et al. Kidney and liver fat accumulation: From imaging to clinical consequences. *J. Nephrol.* **2024**, *37*, 483–490. [CrossRef] [PubMed]

Zelicha, H.; Schwarzfuchs, D.; Shelef, I.; Gepner, Y.; Tsaban, G.; Tene, L.; Yaskolka Meir, A.; Bilitzky, A.; Komy, O.; Cohen, N.; et al. Changes of renal sinus fat and renal parenchymal fat during an 18-month randomized weight loss trial. *Clin. Nutr.* **2018**, *37*, 1145–1153. [CrossRef] [PubMed]

Bassols, J.; Martinez-Calcerrada, J.M.; Prats-Puig, A.; Carreras-Badosa, G.; Xargay-Torrent, S.; Lizarraga-Mollinedo, E.; Feliu-Alsina, M.; Riera-Perez, E.; Osiniri, I.; de Zegher, F.; et al. Perirenal fat is related to carotid intima-media thickness in children. *Int. J. Obes.* **2018**, *42*, 641–647. [CrossRef] [PubMed]

Manno, C.; Campobasso, N.; Nardecchia, A.; Triggiani, V.; Zupo, R.; Gesualdo, L.; Silvestris, F.; De Pergola, G. Relationship of para- and perirenal fat and epicardial fat with metabolic parameters in overweight and obese subjects. *Eat Weight Disord.* **2019**, *24*, 67–72. [CrossRef] [PubMed]

Leone, A.; Bertoli, S.; Bedogni, G.; Vignati, L.; Pellizzari, M.; Battezzati, A. Association between Mediterranean Diet and Fatty Liver in Women with Overweight and Obesity. *Nutrients* **2022**, *14*, 3771. [CrossRef] [PubMed]

Bobulescu, I.A.; Dubree, M.; Zhang, J.; McLeroy, P.; Moe, O.W. Effect of renal lipid accumulation on proximal tubule Na^+/H^+ exchange and ammonium secretion. *Am. J. Physiol. Renal Physiol.* **2008**, *294*, F1315–F1322. [CrossRef] [PubMed]

Deji, N.; Kume, S.; Araki, S.; Soumura, M.; Sugimoto, T.; Isshiki, K.; Chin-Kanasaki, M.; Sakaguchi, M.; Koya, D.; Haneda, M.; et al. Structural and functional changes in the kidneys of high-fat diet-induced obese mice. *Am. J. Physiol. Renal Physiol.* **2009**, *296*, F118–F126. [CrossRef] [PubMed]

do Carmo, J.M.; Tallam, L.S.; Roberts, J.V.; Brandon, E.L.; Biglane, J.; da Silva, A.A.; Hall, J.E. Impact of obesity on renal structure and function in the presence and absence of hypertension: Evidence from melanocortin-4 receptor-deficient mice. *Am. J. Physiol. Regul. Integr. Comp. Physiol.* **2009**, *297*, R803–R812. [CrossRef] [PubMed]

Oron-Herman, M.; Kamari, Y.; Grossman, E.; Yeger, G.; Peleg, E.; Shabtay, Z.; Shamiss, A.; Sharabi, Y. Metabolic syndrome: Comparison of the two commonly used animal models. *Am. J. Hypertens.* **2008**, *21*, 1018–1022. [CrossRef] [PubMed]

Mueller-Peltzer, K.; von Kruchten, R.; Lorbeer, R.; Rospleszcz, S.; Schulz, H.; Peters, A.; Bamberg, F.; Schlett, C.L.; Mujaj, B. Adipose tissue is associated with kidney function parameters. *Sci. Rep.* **2023**, *13*, 9151. [CrossRef] [PubMed]

Aoko, O.; Maharaj, T.; Boland, F.; Cheriyan, D.; Ryan, J. Meta-analysis: Impact of intragastric balloon therapy on NAFLD-related parameters in patients with obesity. *Aliment. Pharmacol. Ther.* **2024**, *59*, 8–22. [CrossRef] [PubMed]

35. Nunes, B.C.M.; de Moura, D.T.H.; Kum, A.S.T.; de Oliveira, G.H.P.; Hirsch, B.S.; Ribeiro, I.B.; Gomes, I.L.C.; de Oliveira, C.P. Mahmood, S.; Bernardo, W.M.; et al. Impact of Endoscopic Sleeve Gastroplasty in Non-alcoholic Fatty Liver Disease: A System Review and Meta-analysis. *Obes. Surg.* **2023**, *33*, 2917–2926. [CrossRef] [PubMed]
36. Navaneethan, S.D.; Yehnert, H.; Moustarah, F.; Schreiber, M.J.; Schauer, P.R.; Beddhu, S. Weight loss interventions in chr kidney disease: A systematic review and meta-analysis. *Clin. J. Am. Soc. Nephrol.* **2009**, *4*, 1565–1574. [CrossRef] [PubMed]
37. Chang, A.R.; Chen, Y.; Still, C.; Wood, G.C.; Kirchner, H.L.; Lewis, M.; Kramer, H.; Hartle, J.E.; Carey, D.; Appel, L.J.; et al. Baria surgery is associated with improvement in kidney outcomes. *Kidney Int.* **2016**, *90*, 164–171. [CrossRef] [PubMed]
38. Friedman, A.N.; Wahed, A.S.; Wang, J.; Courcoulas, A.P.; Dakin, G.; Hinojosa, M.W.; Kimmel, P.L.; Mitchell, J.E.; Pomp, Pories, W.J.; et al. Effect of Bariatric Surgery on CKD Risk. *J. Am. Soc. Nephrol.* **2018**, *29*, 1289–1300. [CrossRef] [PubMed]

nutrients

MDPI

icle

on-Interventional Weight Changes Are Associated with lterations in Lipid Profiles and in the Triglyceride-to-HDL holesterol Ratio

ri Weinstein [1,2], Elad Maor [2,3], Alon Kaplan [1,2], Tammy Hod [2,4,5], Avshalom Leibowitz [1,2,6], Ehud Grossman [7] and di Shlomai [1,2,6,8,*]

1 Internal Medicine D, Sheba Medical Center, Ramat Gan 5262504, Israel; shiri.weinstein@sheb.health.gov.il (S.W.); alon.kaplan@sheba.health.gov.il (A.K.); avshalom.leibowitz@sheba.health.gov.il (A.L.)
2 Faculty of Medicine, Tel-Aviv University, Tel-Aviv 6997801, Israel; elad.maor@sheba.health.gov.il (E.M.); tamar.hod@sheba.health.gov.il (T.H.)
3 Leviev Heart Center, Sheba Medical Center, Ramat Gan 5262504, Israel
4 Renal Transplant Center, Sheba Medical Center, Ramat Gan 5262504, Israel
5 Nephrology Department, Sheba Medical Center, Ramat Gan 5262504, Israel
6 The Hypertension Unit, Sheba Medical Center, Ramat Gan 5262504, Israel
7 Adelson School of Medicine, Ariel University, Ariel 407000, Israel; ehud.grossman@ariel.ac.il
8 The Institute of Endocrinology, Diabetes and Metabolism, Sheba Medical Center, Ramat Gan 5262504, Israel
* Correspondence: gadi.shlomai@sheba.health.gov.il

Abstract: Background: Obesity is associated with dyslipidemia, and weight loss can improve obese patients' lipid profile. Here, we assessed whether non-interventional weight changes are associated with alterations in lipid profile, particularly the triglyceride (TG)-to-high-density lipoprotein cholesterol (HDL-C) ratio (TG/HDL-C). Methods: In this retrospective analysis of subjects referred to medical screening, body mass index (BMI), low-density lipoprotein cholesterol (LDL-C), TG, and HDL-C levels were measured annually. Patients were divided according to BMI changes between visits. The primary outcomes were the changes in LDL-C, TG, HDL-C, and the TG/HDL-C ratio between visits. Results: The final analysis included 18,828 subjects. During the year of follow-up, 9.3% of the study population lost more than 5% of their weight and 9.2% gained more than 5% of their weight. The effect of weight changes on TG and on the TG/HDL-C ratio was remarkable. Patients with greater BMI increases showed greater increases in their TG/HDL-C ratio, and conversely, a decreased BMI level had lower TG/HDL-C ratios. This is true even for moderate changes of more than 2.5% in BMI. Conclusions: Non-interventional weight changes, even modest ones, are associated with significant alterations in the lipid profile. Understanding that modest, non-interventional weight changes are associated with alterations in the TG/HDL-C ratio may aid in better risk stratification and primary prevention of CV morbidity and mortality.

Keywords: weight change; BMI change; lipids; triglyceride-to-HDL ratio

1. Introduction

Overweight and obesity are associated with an increased risk of cardiovascular (CV)-related morbidity such as hypertension (HTN), type 2 diabetes mellitus (DM), ischemic heart disease (IHD), chronic kidney disease (CKD), and dyslipidemia [1–5]. Dyslipidemia is an established risk factor for developing atherosclerosis and subsequent CV events [6–8], and interventional weight loss among overweight and obese patients improves their lipid profile [9–12]. High triglyceride (TG) levels are associated with other lipid abnormalities that predispose an individual to atherosclerosis development, including low levels of high-density lipoprotein cholesterol (HDL-C), high levels of low-density lipoprotein cholesterol (LDL-C), and atherogenic TG-rich lipoprotein remnants [13]. High TG is also associated with insulin resistance and DM, both of which are independent CV risk factors [14,15]. Insulin resistance induces the liver production and release of very low-density lipoprotein (VLDL) particles, which carry TGs in the bloodstream. Insulin resistance also decreases hepatic uptake of VLDL and LDL, resulting in increasing levels of these lipoproteins in the plasma and decreasing lipoprotein lipase activity, a major mediator of VLDL clearance [16]. While high TG levels are associated with insulin resistance and atherosclerosis [17–19], HDL-C promotes reverse cholesterol transport, removes excess cholesterol from arteries, and exerts anti-inflammatory and antioxidant properties [13]. In the past few years, the TG/HDL-C ratio has emerged as a surrogate marker for metabolic syndrome [20,21], increased CV risk [22–25], increased ischemic stroke risk [24,26], and CKD progression [27] and an independent predictor for all-cause mortality [28].

The effects of different dietary patterns on the lipid profile, particularly on the TG/HDL-C ratio, have been previously explored [29–35]. It has been reported that greater adherence to an unhealthy Western diet predicts an increased risk of abnormal blood lipids [31], that the atherogenic TG/HDL-C ratio is reduced significantly by the consumption of fresh fish [32], and that certain dietary patterns are associated with a low TG/HDL-C ratio and a lower risk for DM [30]. Furthermore, metabolic surgery in obese individuals has been shown to significantly reduce TG levels and the TG/HDL-C ratio [36,37]. However, previous studies, including recent reports, have suggested that reduced-calorie diets may result in clinically meaningful weight loss and improved glycemic control regardless of different compositions of fat, protein, and carbohydrates [38,39].

Most studies, to date, have focused on the association of various interventional weight-loss programs with specific lipid profile parameters. However, there is a paucity of data regarding the effects of non-interventional minor weight changes on the lipid profile and specifically the TG/HDL-C ratio. Most clinic patients do not participate in a structured weight loss program, yet their weight may change between clinic visits. We sought to explore the effects of any non-interventional weight changes on lipid profiles, regardless of the dietary restriction or particular nutritional habits. Specifically, we aimed to assess whether non-interventional weight changes are associated with alterations in LDL-C, HDL-C, TG, and particularly in the TG/HDL-C ratio. Our hypothesis was that even subtle weight changes may significantly affect patients' lipid profiles.

2. Materials and Methods

2.1. Study Population

All subjects enrolled were asymptomatic men and women examined annually at the Chaim Sheba Medical Center Institute for medical screening between the years 2000 and 2020. The annual examination includes filling out a standard questionnaire regarding demographic characteristics, a complete medical history, any unusual medical events that occurred since the previous visit, and lifestyle and health-related habits. Until 2016, the electronic medical records (EMR) system included a dietary questionnaire regarding any dietary restrictions or habits, such as low-calorie diet, low-fat diet, low-carbohydrate diet, or any combination of these diets. However, with the implementation of a new EMR system, self-reported dietary restrictions are no longer available and therefore not included in our data analysis. Data regarding the dietary habits of our cohort up to 2016 are illustrated in Supplementary Figure S1. Height and weight were measured while wearing light clothing without shoes and recorded at each encounter for all participants. Participants underwent a thorough physical examination. The body mass index (BMI) was calculated as weight in kg divided by the squared height in meters. No weight loss intervention program was applied and all weight changes were subject-driven and unguided by the investigators. Blood for lab tests, including LDL-C, HDL-C, and TG levels, was drawn by a trained nurse following at least eight hours of fasting.

2.2. Inclusion and Exclusion Criteria

The complete database included 21,111 individuals with two consecutive annual clinic visits. Individuals were excluded if height; weight; or TG, LDL-C, or HDL-C level records were missing; or if they had extreme BMI values (less than 15 kg/m^2 or more than 50 kg/m^2). After patient exclusion, the final study cohort comprised 18,828 participants. Data on diet restrictions (as self-reported) were collected from 14,104 subjects.

2.3. Definitions and Outcome

Participants were divided according to the percent change in BMI between the first and second visits: BMI reduction of more than 5% ("large reduction"), BMI reduction between 2.5% and 5% ("moderate reduction"), BMI reduction of <2.5% or elevation of <2.5% ("unchanged"), BMI elevation between 2.5% and 5% ("moderate increase"), and BMI elevation of more than 5% ("large increase").

The primary outcomes were changes in LDL-C, TG, HDL-C, and the TG/HDL-C ratio between visits.

2.4. Statistical Analysis

Trends in characteristics for categorical variables were assessed using chi-square tests. The logistic regression model was calculated to assess the relationship between the baseline characteristics of patients and increases of at least 10% in the TG/HDL-C ratio. Age, gender, initial BMI, BMI change, diagnosis of IHD, diagnosis of HTN, diagnosis of DM, and obesity (defined as BMI above 30 kg/m^2) were tested individually and in a multivariable logistic regression model as clinically and epidemiologically relevant variables. Subset analysis was performed for gender, initial BMI, and initial TG/HDL-C ratio. All analyses were performed using R software (R Development Core Team, version 4.1.0) [40]. A 2-sided p-value < 0.05 was used for statistical significance.

3. Results

The final analysis included 18,828 patients, of whom 72% were male. Baseline demographic and clinical characteristics according to pre-specified groups of BMI change are presented in Table 1. Gender proportions of roughly two-thirds male were generally consistent across the pre-specified groups (Table 1). The mean BMI for our cohort was approximately 28 kg/m^2 and was consistently in the overweight range across groups. Most patients in our study had a mean BMI in the overweight category (47%), followed by obesity (27%) and normal weight (26%) (Table 1). The frequency of hypertension was about 30% for the entire cohort without significant differences across groups, while mean SBP and DBP were in the range of stage 2 hypertension with a mean SBP of 126 mm Hg and a mean DBP of 79 mm Hg (Table 1). Rates of IHD and DM in our entire cohort were around 10% and were consistent across groups (Table 1).

The dietary habits of participants enrolled until the end of 2016 are illustrated in Figure S1. Of the participants, 63% indicated specific restrictions on their dietary habits. Of them, 21% self-reported adherence to a low-calorie diet, 13% to a low-fat diet, and 12% to a low-carbohydrate diet (Figure S1).

The mean baseline BMI was 26 kg/m^2 and there was no significant change in mean BMI between visits for the entire study population (Table 2). However, 20.8% of patients reduced their BMI by at least 2.5% and 23.6% increased their BMI by more than 2.5%, and 9.3% of the patients reduced their BMI by at least 5% and 9.2% of patients increased their BMI by at least 5% (Table 2). On the second visit, patients in the pre-specified "large reduction" group had a mean percent decrease of 3.8% and 11% in LDL-C and TG, respectively, and a 5.8% increase in HDL-C (Figure 1, Table 2). Patients in the pre-specified "large increase" group had a mean percent increase of 3.9% and 18% in LDL-C and TG, respectively, and a 0.41% decrease in HDL-C (Figure 1, Table 2). The TG/HDL-C ratio decreased by 13% and increased by 20% in the pre-specified "large reduction" and "large increase" groups, respectively.

Table 1. Baseline characteristics.

	Large Reduction (*N* = 1754)	Moderate Reduction (*N* = 2163)	Unchanged (*N* = 10,524)	Moderate Increase (*N* = 2664)	Large Increase (*N* = 1723)	Total (*N* = 18,828)	*p* Valu
Gender							<0.00
Males	1169 (67%)	1592 (74%)	7852 (75%)	1944 (73%)	1075 (62%)	13,632 (72%)	
Females	585 (33%)	571 (26%)	2672 (25%)	720 (27%)	648 (38%)	5196 (28%)	
Age (years)							<0.00
Mean (SD)	48.9 (±10.3)	50.4 (±10.7)	50.0 (±10.3)	49.2 (±10.4)	48.1 (±9.9)	49.7 (±10.4)	
1st visit BMI (kg/m^2)							<0.00
Mean (SD)	27.9 (±4.5)	26.4 (±3.6)	25.8 (±3.7)	25.6 (±3.8)	25.3 (±4.0)	26.0 (±3.8)	
BMI categories							<0.00
<18.5	5 (0%)	9 (0%)	109 (1%)	19 (1%)	30 (2%)	172 (1%)	
18.5–25	452 (26%)	788 (36%)	4547 (43%)	1308 (49%)	843 (49%)	7938 (42%)	
25–30	832 (47%)	1045 (48%)	4633 (44%)	1020 (38%)	653 (38%)	8183 (43%)	
>30	465 (27%)	321 (15%)	1235 (12%)	317 (12%)	197 (11%)	2535 (13%)	
IHD	200 (11%)	266 (12%)	1251 (12%)	285 (11%)	166 (10%)	2168 (12%)	0.033
SBP (mm Hg)							<0.00
Mean (SD)	125.9 (±18.4)	124.7 (±17.7)	124.2 (±17.3)	122.9 (±16.7)	121.4 (±16.6)	124.0 (±17.3)	
DBP (mm Hg)							<0.00
Mean (SD)	79.1 (±11.1)	78.1 (±10.4)	77.7 (±10.4)	77.3 (±10.2)	76.3 (±10.5)	77.7 (±10.5)	
HTN	501 (29%)	667 (31%)	3048 (29%)	725 (27%)	489 (28%)	5430 (29%)	0.093
DM	182 (10%)	220 (10%)	981 (9%)	256 (10%)	150 (9%)	1789 (10%)	0.356

Abbreviations: BMI, body mass index; IHD, ischemic heart disease; SBP, systolic blood pressure; DBP, diastolic blood pressure; HTN, hypertension; DM, diabetes mellitus.

Table 2. Body mass index and lipid levels.

	Large Reduction (*N* = 1754)	Moderate Reduction (*N* = 2163)	Unchanged (*N* = 10,524)	Moderate Increase (*N* = 2664)	Large Increase (*N* = 1723)	Total (*N* = 18,828)	*p* Valu
1st visit BMI (kg/m^2)							<0.001
Mean (SD)	27.9 (±4.5)	26.4 (±3.6)	25.8 (±3.7)	25.5 (±3.8)	25.3 (±4.0)	26.0 (±3.8)	
2nd visit BMI (kg/m^2)							<0.001
Mean (SD)	25.4 (±3.8)	25.4 (±3.5)	25.8 (±3.7)	26.5 (±3.9)	27.3 (±4.4)	25.9 (±3.8)	
%BMI change							<0.001
Mean (SD)	−8.6 (±4.2)	−3.6 (±0.7)	0.1 (±1.3)	3.6 (±0.7)	8.0 (±4.7)	0.1 (±4.5)	
1st visit LDL (mg/dL)							<0.001
Mean (SD)	123.5 (±30.0)	122.4 (±28.2)	121.5 (±28.2)	120.0 (±27.1)	120.4 (±29.4)	121.5 (±28.4)	
2nd visit LDL (mg/dL)							<0.001
Mean (SD)	116.5 (±28.8)	119.4 (±28.1)	121.3 (±28.0)	121.7 (±27.2)	122.8 (±29.1)	120.8 (±28.1)	
%LDL change							<0.001
Mean (SD)	−3.8 (±20.1)	−1.0 (±17.3)	1.3 (±17.4)	2.9 (±17.0)	3.9 (±18.6)	1.0 (±17.8)	
1st visit HDL (mg/dL)							<0.001
Mean (SD)	47.1 (±12.3)	47.3 (±12.0)	48.2 (±12.5)	48.3 (±12.0)	49.9 (±13.4)	48.2 (±12.4)	
2nd visit HDL (mg/dL)							0.004
Mean (SD)	49.3 (±12.6)	48.3 (±11.9)	48.7 (±12.3)	48.5 (±11.8)	49.6 (±13.0)	48.8 (±12.3)	
%HDL change							<0.001
Mean (SD)	5.8 (±15.4)	3.0 (±12.8)	1.9 (±12.3)	1.3 (±12.3)	0.4 (±13.2)	2.2 (±12.8)	
1st visit TG (mg/dL)							<0.001
Mean (SD)	135.1 (±71.1)	130.0 (±67.5)	124.3 (±62.9)	118.9 (±59.4)	115.8 (±59.4)	124.4 (±63.7)	
2nd visit TG (mg/dL)							<0.001
Mean (SD)	111.0 (±57.0)	120.3 (±60.1)	124.9 (±63.3)	127.6 (±65.4)	129.9 (±68.5)	123.9 (±63.4)	
%TG change							<0.001
Mean (SD)	−11.0 (±32.6)	−0.8 (±36.6)	5.4 (±33.7)	12.5 (±44.2)	17.7 (±42.7)	5.3 (±37.2)	

Table 2. *Cont.*

	Large Reduction (*N* = 1754)	Moderate Reduction (*N* = 2163)	Unchanged (*N* = 10,524)	Moderate Increase (*N* = 2664)	Large Increase (*N* = 1723)	Total (*N* = 18,828)	*p* Value
·t visit TG/HDL-C ratio							<0.001
Mean (SD)	3.2 (±2.2)	3.1 (±2.1)	2.9 (±1.9)	2.7 (±1.8)	2.6 (±1.8)	2.9 (±2.0)	
·d visit TG/HDL-C ratio							<0.001
Mean (SD)	2.5 (±1.7)	2.8 (±1.8)	2.9 (±1.9)	2.9 (±1.9)	2.9 (±2.0)	2.8 (±1.9)	
·_HDL_ratio_change							<0.001
Mean (SD)	−13.2 (±37.8)	−1.6 (±40.5)	5.3 (±37.9)	13.0 (±47.8)	19.7 (±47.9)	5.2 (±41.5)	

Abbreviations: BMI, body mass index; TG, triglycerides; HDL-C, high-density lipoprotein cholesterol; LDL, low-density lipoprotein.

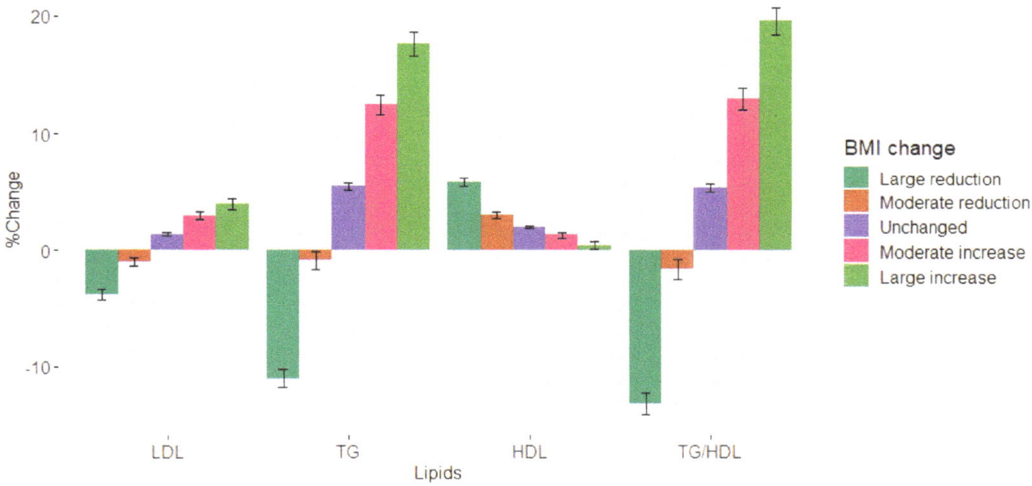

Figure 1. LDL-C, TG, HDL-C, and TG/HDL-C ratio change between visits across pre-specified BMI groups. Percent change in LDL-C, TG, HDL-C, and TG/HDL-C ratio between visits across pre-specified BMI groups. The analysis included 18,828 patients. *X*-axis from left to right represents LDL, TG, HDL, and TG/HDL-C ratio. *Y*-axis represents percent change in BMI. Abbreviations: LDL-C, low-density lipoprotein cholesterol; TG, triglycerides; HDL-C, high-density lipoprotein cholesterol; BMI, body mass index.

The proportion of patients with a >10% rise in the TG/HDL-C ratio progressively increased with the relative increases in BMI, with a 20.6%, 30.2%, 37.5%, 46.2%, and 50.2% increase for the "large reduction", "moderate reduction", "unchanged", "moderate increase", and "large increase" groups, respectively ($p < 0.01$) (Figure 2). Conversely, the proportion of patients with at least a 10% decrease in the TG/HDL-C ratio progressively declined with relative decreases in BMI: 60.5%, 46.7%, 37.7%, 30.5%, and 26.9% for "large reduction", "moderate reduction", "unchanged", "moderate increase", and "large increase", respectively ($p < 0.01$) (Figure 2).

In the multivariable logistic regression model, compared to the "unchanged" group, the odds ratio for TG/HDL-C ratio increases of at least 10% was 0.43, 0.73, 1.42, and 1.68 for the "large reduction", "moderate reduction", "moderate increase", and "large increase" groups, respectively ($p < 0.001$) (Figure 3). Concomitant DM was significantly associated with an elevated odds ratio for a >10% rise in the TG/HDL-C ratio ($p = 0.02$). Age, gender, initial BMI, IHD diagnosis, diagnosis of HTN, and obesity, which are clinically and epidemiologic relevant variables, did not show significant correlations with the TG/HDL-C ratio increase of at least 10% in multivariable logistic regression analysis (Figure 3).

Additional analyses excluding patients who were treated with statins, and subgroup analyses by gender, showed similar results regarding the initial TG/HDL-C ratio and baseline BMI.

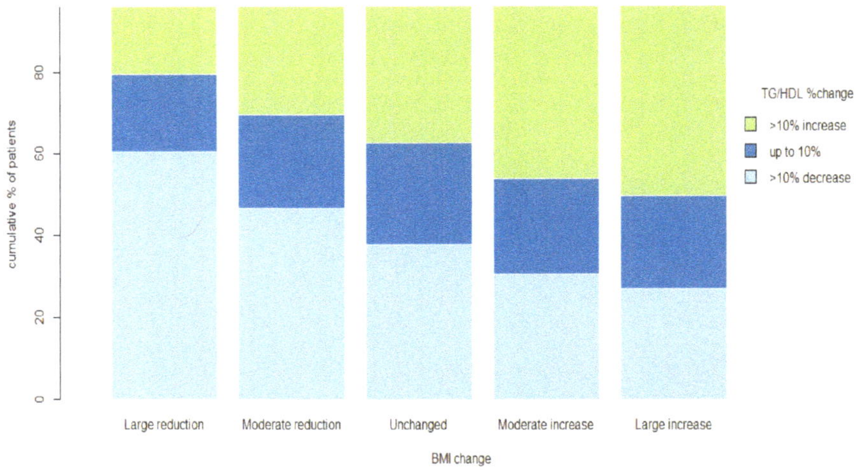

Figure 2. TG/HDL ratio %change according to the pre-specified BMI change. Percent change in TG/HDL-C ratio according to the pre-specified BMI change. Bars represent the pre-specified BMI change groups. Different colors represent the percent of patients in each pre-specified group with at least 10% increase in TG/HDL-C ratio from visit 1 to visit 2 (green), up to 10% change in TG/HDL-C ratio from visit 1 to visit 2 (blue) and at least 10% decrease in TG/HDL ratio from visit 1 to visit 2 (light blue). The analysis includes 18,828 patients. Abbreviations: BMI, body mass index; TG, triglycerides; HDL-C, high-density lipoprotein cholesterol.

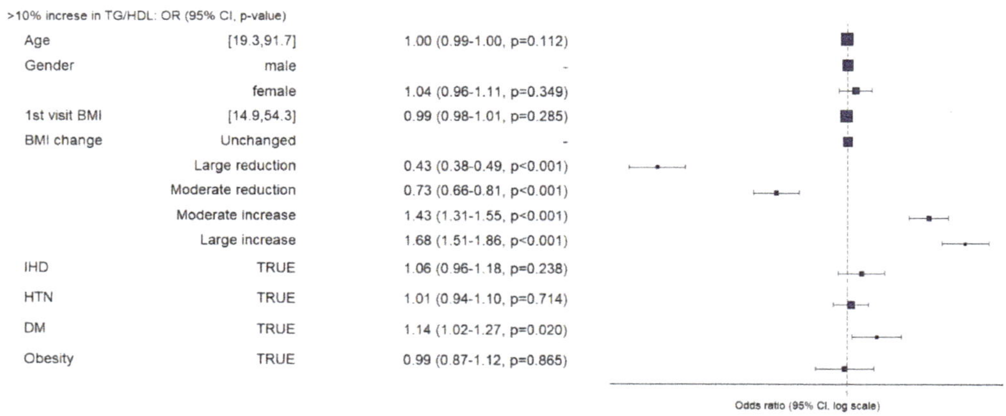

Figure 3. Relationship between baseline characteristics and increase of at least 10% in TG/HDL-C ratio. Logistic regression, presented as a forest plot, represents the relationship between baseline characteristics and an increase of at least 10% in the TG/HDL-C ratio on visit 2. The analysis includes 18,828 patients. Obesity is defined as BMI > 30 kg/m^2. Abbreviations: TG, triglycerides; HDL-C, high-density lipoprotein cholesterol; BMI, body mass index; IHD, ischemic heart disease; HTN, hypertension; DM, diabetes mellitus.

4. Discussion

In this study, we demonstrate that non-interventional weight changes are associated with significant alterations in the lipid profile. An increase in BMI, even when modest, was associated with a progressive rise in LDL-C and TG and a decrease in HDL-C. Conversely, a decrease in BMI was associated with a progressive decline in LDL-C and TG and an increase in HDL-C. The proportion of subjects with more than a 10% increase in TG/HDL-C progressively increased with a rise in BMI and conversely, patients with a decline in BMI showed a decline in their TG/HDL-C ratio.

Previous studies have shown that various interventional weight loss programs among overweight and obese individuals improve patients' lipid profiles [9,33,36,37]. A recent retrospective study shows that among a cohort of Japanese patients, non-interventional weight losses of 5% or more are associated with improved LDL-C, TG, and HDL-C levels [41]. Our results concur with these findings. However, our cohort is much larger, and we analyzed subtler BMI changes of 2.5% or more and assessed changes in the TG/HDL-C ratio as well.

An elevated TG/HDL-C ratio has been shown to predict metabolic syndrome occurrence [21], coronary artery disease [25,42,43], peripheral artery disease [44], and cerebrovascular disease [45]. The TG/HDL-C ratio was found to positively correlate with the degree of carotid plaque vulnerability and stenosis [26]. Higher TG/HDL ratios are also associated with the prevalence of CKD and its progression [27]. Arterial stiffness is a recognized predictor of CV mortality, and death and is also associated with the TG/HDL-C ratio [46]. TG/HDL-C was a better predictor than LDL-C for atherosclerosis development [47], and relative to LDL-C, total cholesterol, HDL-C, and triglycerides, TG/HDL-C showed the strongest association with the extent of coronary disease [48]. TG/HDL-C predicted all-cause mortality and major adverse cardiac events in patients presenting for coronary angiography, even after adjusting for known cardiovascular risk factors and CAD [28]. It has been shown that even when LDL-C levels are tightly controlled, a residual CV risk remains, which might be attributable to other lipid abnormalities, such as TG/HDL-C [25,47,49]. We believe that the mentioned association of higher TG/HDL-C with different cardiovascular diseases and the predictive value of higher ratios for worse prognoses highlights the potential of TG/HDL-C to serve as a CVD risk marker.

The drawback of the TG/HDL-C ratio is the absence of a universal unequivocal cutoff value, which limits its use as a predictive biomarker for CVD [25]. Some argue that the ideal cutoff for predicting CV outcomes with the TG/HDL-C ratio is above 2, while others recommend using ratios above 2.5 and even above 3 [25,28,50]. Notably, the TG/HDL-C ratio is an important prognosticator across different weight classes and not only for overweight or obese subjects. One study found that an increased TG/HDL-C ratio correlates with a significant increase in intracerebral hemorrhage and cerebral infarction, only in patients with normal BMI [24]. Another study showed that a higher TG/HDL-C ratio was a potential risk factor for prediabetes and insulin resistance in women, even in normal-weight women [50]. Interestingly, the mean BMI for our population was almost 28 kg/m^2, with the majority defined as either normal weight or overweight. We found that the association of non-interventional weight changes and alterations in lipid profile was independent of baseline BMI as well as gender.

In our cohort population, concomitant DM was significantly associated with an increased odds ratio of a $\geq$10% rise in the TG/HDL-C ratio. This finding is likely related to insulin resistance-mediated increased TG production by the liver and reduced clearance of TG-rich lipoproteins from the bloodstream [16] and concurs with the current literature, as the association between the TG/HDL-C ratio and insulin resistance has been widely explored. It has been shown that a high plasma TG/HDL-C ratio provides a simple means of identifying insulin-resistant obese patients who are likely to have increased risks for CVD [16,20,51,52]. In addition, the TG/HDL-C ratio significantly correlates with fasting insulin levels even among adults without DM [53], and the TG/HDL-C ratio is a valuable predictor of DM incidence [54]. Our findings highlight the importance of even minor weight changes, specifically among patients with DM, and suggest that individuals with DM who gain weight may be at a higher risk of worsening dyslipidemia and CVD development.

The TG/HDL-C ratio is potentially a modifiable risk factor as some studies suggest. It has been shown that specific dietary patterns obtained by a validated food frequency questionnaire are associated with changes in the TG/HDL-C ratio and ultimately with a reduced risk for DM [30]. In addition, in a randomized open-labeled trial, the consumption of fresh fish significantly reduced the TG/HDL-C ratio among patients with hyperlipidemia [32], and finally, a prospective cohort found that a greater adherence to the Western diet pattern increased the TG/HDL-C ratio and predicted a higher risk for abnormal lipids overall [31]. However, while the effect of different dietary patterns on lipid composition has been established, the influence of various diet compositions on weight loss is somewhat controversial. A large randomized trial showed that reduced-calorie diets result in clinically meaningful weight loss regardless of which macronutrients are consumed [33]. Other investigators have shown that the difference found in the effect of calorie-unrestricted low-carbohydrate/high-fat diets versus high-carbohydrate/low-fat diets on glycemic control and weight loss was not sustained three months after intervention [55]. Furthermore, in a recent study, a comparison of weight reduction using a very-low-carbohydrate diet versus a low-carbohydrate diet in obese patients yielded no significantly different outcomes, such as body weight and fat, lipid abnormalities, and liver function [34].

The aim of our study was to assess the association of non-interventional weight changes on the lipid profile and particularly, the TG/HDL-C ratio, regardless of any dietary habits or restrictions. Most patients do not participate in structured weight loss programs, yet we frequently observed modest weight changes, increases or decreases, between clinic visits. Therefore, we believed it to be prudent to evaluate the effects of these seemingly negligible weight changes on specific lipid parameters in this specific and very large proportion of clinic patients. Our findings, together with data from interventional weight programs, further highlight the importance of weight changes on the lipid profile and possibly on CV health.

One of our study's limitations is the lack of individual dietary data for our total cohort, which is attributed to the change in our EMR system from 2016. To partially overcome this limitation and to provide a general idea of our study population's dietary habits, we conducted an analysis of approximately 14,000 patients who were assessed in the same medical screening facility prior to 2016 and for whom dietary data exist. Our study has several other limitations. First, this is a retrospective study. Therefore, causality between BMI alterations and serum lipids could not be established. Second, data regarding the method for any weight changes obtained, including physical activity, are not available. In addition, our cohort had a clear male predominance (72%), which might reduce the generalization of our findings. However, in a subgroup analysis, we did not observe any gender-related significant differences in the association between weight changes and lipid profile.

5. Conclusions

In conclusion, we provide evidence that non-interventional weight changes, even when modest and subtle, are associated with changes in the lipid profile and in the TG/HDL-C ratio. Our findings concur with previous reports regarding the association between weight loss and alterations in lipid profile, specifically in the TG/HDL-C ratio.

Early detection of elevated TG/HDL-C ratios may serve as a strategy to prevent the development of atherosclerotic complications, especially in high-risk populations. Understanding that alterations in the TG/HDL-C ratio may be associated with modest, non-interventional weight changes may aid in better risk stratification and primary prevention of CV morbidity and mortality. Larger-scale prospective studies, with individual dietary data and long-term follow-up, are pivotal in evaluating and understanding the significance of modest non-interventional weight changes on CV morbidity and mortality.

Supplementary Materials: The following supporting information can be downloaded at https://www.mdpi.com/article/10.3390/nu16040486/s1, Figure S1: Pie chart representing the proportion of specific dietary restrictions and habits of 14,104 subjects, who were assessed in the same medical screening facility prior to 2016 and for whom dietary data exist.

Author Contributions: Conceptualization, S.W., E.M., A.K., T.H., A.L., E.G. and G.S.; Methodology, S.W., E.G. and G.S.; Data curation, S.W. and E.M.; Formal analysis, S.W.; Writing—original draft, S.W. and G.S.; Writing—review and editing, S.W., E.G. and G.S. All authors have read and agreed to the published version of the manuscript.

Funding: This research received no external funding.

Institutional Review Board Statement: This study was conducted in accordance with the Declaration of Helsinki and approved by the Institutional Ethics Committee of Chaim Sheba Medical Center (protocol code 4451-17-SMC, date of approval—3 December 2017).

Informed Consent Statement: Patient consent was waived because data were recorded anonymously.

Data Availability Statement: The data presented in this study are available on request from the corresponding author. The data are not publicly available due to privacy reasons.

Acknowledgments: We thank Tiran Golani for generating the graphical abstract for this manuscript.

Conflicts of Interest: The authors declare no conflicts of interest.

erences

Piché, M.E.; Tchernof, A.; Després, J.P. Obesity Phenotypes, Diabetes, and Cardiovascular Diseases. *Circ. Res.* **2020**, *126*, 1477–1500. [CrossRef] [PubMed]

Leggio, M.; Lombardi, M.; Caldarone, E.; Severi, P.; D'emidio, S.; Armeni, M.; Bravi, V.; Bendini, M.G.; Mazza, A. The relationship between obesity and hypertension: An updated comprehensive overview on vicious twins. *Hypertens. Res.* **2017**, *40*, 947–963. [CrossRef] [PubMed]

Wormser, D.; Kaptoge, S.; Di Angelantonio, E.; Wood, A.M.; Pennells, L.; Thompson, A.; Sarwar, N.; Kizer, J.R.; Lawlor, D.A.; Nordestgaard, B.G.; et al. Separate and combined associations of body-mass index and abdominal adiposity with cardiovascular disease: Collaborative analysis of 58 prospective studies. *Lancet* **2011**, *377*, 1085–1095. [CrossRef] [PubMed]

Hsu, C.Y.; McCulloch, C.E.; Iribarren, C.; Darbinian, J.; Go, A.S. Body mass index and risk for end-stage renal disease. *Ann. Intern. Med.* **2006**, *144*, 21–28. [CrossRef] [PubMed]

Al Rifai, M.; Silverman, M.G.; Nasir, K.; Budoff, M.J.; Blankstein, R.; Szklo, M.; Katz, R.; Blumenthal, R.S.; Blaha, M.J. The association of nonalcoholic fatty liver disease, obesity, and metabolic syndrome, with systemic inflammation and subclinical atherosclerosis: The Multi-Ethnic Study of Atherosclerosis (MESA). *Atherosclerosis* **2015**, *239*, 629–633. [CrossRef]

Koenen, M.; Hill, M.A.; Cohen, P.; Sowers, J.R. Obesity, Adipose Tissue and Vascular Dysfunction. *Circ. Res.* **2021**, *128*, 951–968. [CrossRef]

Navar-Boggan, A.M.; Peterson, E.D.; D'Agostino, R.B.; Neely, B.; Sniderman, A.D.; Pencina, M.J. Hyperlipidemia in early adulthood increases long-term risk of coronary heart disease. *Circulation* **2015**, *131*, 451–458. [CrossRef]

Kaneko, H.; Itoh, H.; Kiriyama, H.; Kamon, T.; Fujiu, K.; Morita, K.; Michihata, N.; Jo, T.; Takeda, N.; Morita, H.; et al. Lipid Profile and Subsequent Cardiovascular Disease among Young Adults Aged <50 Years. *Am. J. Cardiol.* **2021**, *142*, 59–65. [CrossRef]

Jiménez, J.-M.; Carbajo, M.-A.; López, M.; Cao, M.-J.; Rúiz-Tovar, J.; García, S.; Castro, M.-J. Changes in Lipid Profile, Body Weight Variables and Cardiovascular Risk in Obese Patients Undergoing One-Anastomosis Gastric Bypass. *Int. J. Environ. Res. Public Health* **2020**, *17*, 5858. [CrossRef]

Noakes, M.; Clifton, P.M. Weight loss and plasma lipids. *Curr. Opin. Lipidol.* **2000**, *11*, 65–70. [CrossRef]

Grundy, S.M. Metabolic syndrome update. *Trends Cardiovasc. Med.* **2016**, *26*, 364–373. [CrossRef]

Hasan, B.; Nayfeh, T.; Alzuabi, M.; Wang, Z.; Kuchkuntla, A.R.; Prokop, L.J.; Newman, C.B.; Murad, M.H.; Rajjo, T.I. Weight Loss and Serum Lipids in Overweight and Obese Adults: A Systematic Review and Meta-Analysis. *J. Clin. Endocrinol. Metab.* **2020**, *105*, 3695–3703. [CrossRef]

Welty, F.K. How Do Elevated Triglycerides and Low HDL-Cholesterol Affect Inflammation and Atherothrombosis? *Curr. Cardiol. Rep.* **2013**, *15*, 400. [CrossRef]

Kosmas, C.E.; Bousvarou, M.D.; Kostara, C.E.; Papakonstantinou, E.J.; Salamou, E.; Guzman, E. Insulin resistance and cardiovascular disease. *J. Int. Med. Res.* **2023**, *51*, 3000605231164548. [CrossRef]

Wong, N.D.; Sattar, N. Cardiovascular risk in diabetes mellitus: Epidemiology, assessment and prevention. *Nat. Rev. Cardiol.* **2023**, *20*, 685–695. [CrossRef]

Ormazabal, V.; Nair, S.; Elfeky, O.; Aguayo, C.; Salomon, C.; Zuñiga, F.A. Association between insulin resistance and the development of cardiovascular disease. *Cardiovasc. Diabetol.* **2018**, *17*, 122. [CrossRef]

17. Grundy, S.M. Hypertriglyceridemia, insulin resistance, and the metabolic syndrome. *Am. J. Cardiol.* **1999**, *83*, 25F–29F. [CrossRef] [PubMed]
18. Abbasi, F.; Kohli, P.; Reaven, G.M.; Knowles, J.W. Hypertriglyceridemia: A simple approach to identify insulin resistance and enhanced cardio-metabolic risk in patients with prediabetes. *Diabetes Res. Clin. Pract.* **2016**, *120*, 156–161. [CrossRef]
19. Kraegen, E.W.; Cooney, G.J.; Ye, J.; Thompson, A.L. Triglycerides, fatty acids and insulin resistance–hyperinsulinemia. *Exp. Clin. Endocrinol. Diabetes* **2001**, *109*, S516–S526. [CrossRef] [PubMed]
20. McLaughlin, T.; Abbasi, F.; Cheal, K.; Chu, J.; Lamendola, C.; Reaven, G. Use of metabolic markers to identify overweight individuals who are insulin resistant. *Ann. Intern. Med.* **2003**, *139*, 802–809. [CrossRef] [PubMed]
21. Abbasian, M.; Delvarianzadeh, M.; Ebrahimi, H.; Khosravi, F. Lipid ratio as a suitable tool to identify individuals with MetS risk: A case- control study. *Diabetes Metab. Syndr.* **2017**, *11* (Suppl. S1), S15–S19. [CrossRef]
22. Shao, Q.-Y.; Ma, X.-T.; Yang, Z.-Q.; Li, Q.-X.; Wang, Y.-F.; Liang, J.; Shen, H.; Liu, X.-L.; Zhou, Y.-J.; Shi, D.-M.; et al. Prognostic significance of multiple triglycerides-derived metabolic indices in patients with acute coronary syndrome. *J. Geriatr. Cardiol.* **2022**, *19*, 456–468. [CrossRef] [PubMed]
23. Wang, B.; Hua, J.; Ma, L. Triglyceride to High-Density Lipoprotein Ratio can predict coronary artery calcification. *Pakistan J. Med. Sci.* **2022**, *38*, 624–631. [CrossRef] [PubMed]
24. Sato, F.; Nakamura, Y.; Kayaba, K.; Ishikawa, S. TG/HDL-C ratio as a predictor of stroke in the population with healthy BMI: The Jichi Medical School Cohort Study. *Nutr. Metab. Cardiovasc. Dis.* **2022**, *32*, 1872–1879. [CrossRef] [PubMed]
25. Kosmas, C.E.; Rodriguez Polanco, S.; Bousvarou, M.D.; Papakonstantinou, E.J.; Peña Genao, E.; Guzman, E.; Kostara, C.E. The Triglyceride/High-Density Lipoprotein Cholesterol (TG/HDL-C) Ratio as a Risk Marker for Metabolic Syndrome and Cardiovascular Disease. *Diagnostics* **2023**, *13*, 929. [CrossRef] [PubMed]
26. Zhao, Z.; Wang, H.; Hou, Q.; Zhou, Y.; Zhang, Y. Non-traditional lipid parameters as potential predictors of carotid plaque vulnerability and stenosis in patients with acute ischemic stroke. *Neurol. Sci.* **2023**, *44*, 835–843. [CrossRef] [PubMed]
27. Nguyen, H.H.; Tran, H.H.; Nguyen, L.T.; Nguyen, T.; Nguyen, N.A.; Vi, M.T.; Nguyen, K.T. TG/HDL-C Ratio Is a Risk Factor Associated with CKD: Use in Assessing the Risk of Progression of CKD. *Pathophysiology* **2022**, *29*, 374–382. [CrossRef] [PubMed]
28. Sultani, R.; Tong, D.C.; Peverelle, M.; Lee, Y.S.; Baradi, A.; Wilson, A.M. Elevated Triglycerides to High-Density Lipoprotein Cholesterol (TG/HDL-C) Ratio Predicts Long-Term Mortality in High-Risk Patients. *Heart. Lung Circ.* **2020**, *29*, 414–4[illegible] [CrossRef] [PubMed]
29. Fechner, E.; Smeets, E.T.H.C.; Schrauwen, P.; Mensink, R.P. The Effects of Different Degrees of Carbohydrate Restriction and Carbohydrate Replacement on Cardiometabolic Risk Markers in Humans-A Systematic Review and Meta-Analysis. *Nutrients* **2020**, *12*, 991. [CrossRef]
30. Song, S.; Lee, J.E. Dietary Patterns Related to Triglyceride and High-Density Lipoprotein Cholesterol and the Incidence of Type Diabetes in Korean Men and Women. *Nutrients* **2018**, *11*, 8. [CrossRef]
31. Ushula, T.W.; Mamun, A.; Darssan, D.; Wang, W.Y.S.; Williams, G.M.; Whiting, S.J.; Najman, J.M. Dietary patterns and the risk of abnormal blood lipids among young adults: A prospective cohort study. *Nutr. Metab. Cardiovasc. Dis.* **2022**, *32*, 1165–11[illegible] [CrossRef]
32. Zibaeenezhad, M.J.; Ghavipisheh, M.; Attar, A.; Aslani, A. Comparison of the effect of omega-3 supplements and fresh fish lipid profile: A randomized, open-labeled trial. *Nutr. Diabetes* **2017**, *7*, 1. [CrossRef]
33. Sacks, F.M.; Bray, G.A.; Carey, V.J.; Smith, S.R.; Ryan, D.H.; Anton, S.D.; McManus, K.; Champagne, C.M.; Bishop, L.M.; Laran N.; et al. Comparison of weight-loss diets with different compositions of fat, protein, and carbohydrates. *N. Engl. J. Med.* **20[illegible]** *360*, 859–873. [CrossRef]
34. Kikuchi, T.; Kushiyama, A.; Yanai, M.; Kashiwado, C.; Seto, T.; Kasuga, M. Comparison of Weight Reduction, Change Parameters and Safety of a Very Low Carbohydrate Diet in Comparison to a Low Carbohydrate Diet in Obese Japanese Subje with Metabolic Disorders. *Nutrients* **2023**, *15*, 1342. [CrossRef]
35. Ma, C.; Avenell, A.; Bolland, M.; Hudson, J.; Stewart, F.; Robertson, C.; Sharma, P.; Fraser, C.; MacLennan, G. Effects of weight l interventions for adults who are obese on mortality, cardiovascular disease, and cancer: Systematic review and meta-analy *BMJ* **2017**, *359*, j4849. [CrossRef]
36. Santos, J.; Salgado, P.; Santos, C.; Mendes, P.; Saavedra, J.; Baldaque, P.; Monteiro, L.; Costa, E. Effect of bariatric surgery weight loss, inflammation, iron metabolism, and lipid profile. *Scand. J. Surg.* **2014**, *103*, 21–25. [CrossRef]
37. Wang, W.; Fann, C.S.J.; Yang, S.-H.; Chen, H.-H.; Chen, C.-Y. Weight loss and metabolic improvements in obese patients undergoing gastric banding and gastric banded plication: A comparison. *Nutrition* **2019**, *57*, 290–299. [CrossRef] [PubMed]
38. Unick, J.L.; Beavers, D.; Jakicic, J.M.; Kitabchi, A.E.; Knowler, W.C.; Wadden, T.A.; Wing, R.R.; Look AHEAD Research Gro Effectiveness of lifestyle interventions for individuals with severe obesity and type 2 diabetes: Results from the Look AHE trial. *Diabetes Care* **2011**, *34*, 2152–2157. [CrossRef] [PubMed]
39. Ayisi Addo, S.; Nti, C.; Vuvor, F.; Adjimani, J.; Steiner-Asiedu, M. Impact of Successful Weight Loss Maintenance on Seru Lipids and Glucose Concentrations of Previous Participants of a Weight Loss Programme in Accra, Ghana. *J. Nutr. Metab.* **20[illegible]** *2019*, 4729040. [CrossRef] [PubMed]
40. R Core Team. *R: A Language and Environment for Statistical Computing*; R Foundation for Statistical Computing: Vienna, A tria, 2022.

Kiriyama, H.; Kaneko, H.; Itoh, H.; Kamon, T.; Mizuno, Y.; Fujiu, K.; Morita, H.; Yamamichi, N.; Komuro, I. Association between changes in body weight and lipid profile in the general population: A community-based cohort study. *Eur. Heart J. Qual. Care Clin. Outcomes* **2021**, *7*, 109–110. [CrossRef]
Park, B.; Jung, D.H.; Lee, H.S.; Lee, Y.J. Triglyceride to HDL-Cholesterol Ratio and the Incident Risk of Ischemic Heart Disease Among Koreans Without Diabetes: A Longitudinal Study Using National Health Insurance Data. *Front. Cardiovasc. Med.* **2021**, *8*, 716698. [CrossRef] [PubMed]
Martínez-Marroquín, Y.; Meaney, A.; Samaniego-Méndez, V.; Nájera, N.; Ceballos, G.; Fernández-Barros, C.; Meaney, E. The TG/HDL-c Lipid Ratio as a Cardiovascular Risk Marker in a Mexican Urban Middle-Class Population: Do We Need a Risk Score Tailored for Mexicans? *J. Clin. Med.* **2023**, *12*, 6005. [CrossRef] [PubMed]
Mesut, E.; Cihan, A.; Orhan, G. Is it possible to predict the complexity of peripheral artery disease with atherogenic index? *Vascular* **2020**, *28*, 513–519. [CrossRef] [PubMed]
Gu, X.; Li, Y.; Chen, S.; Yang, X.; Liu, F.; Li, Y.; Li, J.; Cao, J.; Liu, X.; Chen, J.; et al. Association of Lipids with Ischemic and Hemorrhagic Stroke: A Prospective Cohort Study among 267,500 Chinese. *Stroke* **2019**, *50*, 3376–3384. [CrossRef] [PubMed]
Baba, M.; Maris, M.; Jianu, D.; Luca, C.T.; Stoian, D.; Mozos, I. The Impact of the Blood Lipids Levels on Arterial Stiffness. *J. Cardiovasc. Dev. Dis.* **2023**, *10*, 127. [CrossRef] [PubMed]
Edwards, M.K.; Blaha, M.J.; Loprinzi, P.D. Atherogenic Index of Plasma and Triglyceride/High-Density Lipoprotein Cholesterol Ratio Predict Mortality Risk Better than Individual Cholesterol Risk Factors, among an Older Adult Population. *Mayo Clin. Proc.* **2017**, *92*, 680–681. [CrossRef] [PubMed]
da Luz, P.L.; Favarato, D.; Faria-Neto, J.R.; Lemos, P.; Chagas, A.C.P. High ratio of triglycerides to HDL-cholesterol predicts extensive coronary disease. *Clinics* **2008**, *63*, 427–432. [CrossRef]
Dhindsa, D.S.; Sandesara, P.B.; Shapiro, M.D.; Wong, N.D. The Evolving Understanding and Approach to Residual Cardiovascular Risk Management. *Front. Cardiovasc. Med.* **2020**, *7*, 88. [CrossRef]
Borrayo, G.; Basurto, L.; González-Escudero, E.; Diaz, A.; Vázquez, A.; Sánchez, L.; Hernández-González, G.O.; Barrera, S.; Degollado, J.A.; Córdova, N.; et al. Tg/Hdl-C Ratio as Cardio-Metabolic Biomarker even in Normal Weight Women. *Acta Endocrinol.* **2018**, *14*, 261–267. [CrossRef]
McLaughlin, T.; Reaven, G.; Abbasi, F.; Lamendola, C.; Saad, M.; Waters, D.; Simon, J.; Krauss, R.M. Is there a simple way to identify insulin-resistant individuals at increased risk of cardiovascular disease? *Am. J. Cardiol.* **2005**, *96*, 399–404. [CrossRef]
Salazar, M.R.; Carbajal, H.A.; Espeche, W.G.; Leiva Sisnieguez, C.E.; Balbín, E.; Dulbecco, C.A.; Aizpurúa, M.; Marillet, A.G.; Reaven, G.M. Relation among the plasma triglyceride/high-density lipoprotein cholesterol concentration ratio, insulin resistance, and associated cardio-metabolic risk factors in men and women. *Am. J. Cardiol.* **2012**, *109*, 1749–1753. [CrossRef] [PubMed]
Li, C.; Ford, E.S.; Meng, Y.-X.; Mokdad, A.H.; Reaven, G.M. Does the association of the triglyceride to high-density lipoprotein cholesterol ratio with fasting serum insulin differ by race/ethnicity? *Cardiovasc. Diabetol.* **2008**, *7*, 4. [CrossRef] [PubMed]
Vega, G.L.; Barlow, C.E.; Grundy, S.M.; Leonard, D.; DeFina, L.F. Triglyceride-to-high-density-lipoprotein-cholesterol ratio is an index of heart disease mortality and of incidence of type 2 diabetes mellitus in men. *J. Investig. Med.* **2014**, *62*, 345–349. [CrossRef] [PubMed]
Hansen, C.D.; Gram-Kampmann, E.-M.; Hansen, J.K.; Hugger, M.B.; Madsen, B.S.; Jensen, J.M.; Olesen, S.; Torp, N.; Rasmussen, D.N.; Kjærgaard, M.; et al. Effect of Calorie-Unrestricted Low-Carbohydrate, High-Fat Diet Versus High-Carbohydrate, Low-Fat Diet on Type 2 Diabetes and Nonalcoholic Fatty Liver Disease: A Randomized Controlled Trial. *Ann. Intern. Med.* **2023**, *176*, 10–21. [CrossRef]

nutrients

Article

Effect of Intermittent Fasting on Cardiometabolic Health in the Chinese Population: A Meta-Analysis of Randomized Controlled Trials

Katy Cheung [1,†], Vicky Chan [2,†], Stephanie Chan [1], Martin Ming Him Wong [3], Gary Ka-Ki Chung [1], Wai-Yin Cheng [2,4], Kenneth Lo [2,4,5,*] and Fangfang Zeng [6,*]

1 JC School of Public Health and Primary Care, The Chinese University of Hong Kong, Hong Kong 999077, China; gchung@cuhk.edu.hk (G.K.-K.C.)
2 Department of Food Science and Nutrition, The Hong Kong Polytechnic University, Hong Kong 100872, China; vickycwk.chan@polyu.edu.hk (V.C.); wai-yin-nano.cheng@polyu.edu.hk (W.-Y.C.)
3 Institute of Epidemiology and Health Care, University College London, London WC1E 6BT, UK; ming.wong.23@ucl.ac.uk
4 Research Institute for Future Food, The Hong Kong Polytechnic University, Hong Kong 100872, China
5 Research Institute for Smart Ageing, The Hong Kong Polytechnic University, Hong Kong 100872, China
6 Department of Public Health and Preventive Medicine, School of Medicine, Jinan University, No. 601 Huangpu Road West, Guangzhou 510632, China
* Correspondence: kenneth.kh.lo@polyu.edu.hk (K.L.); zengff@jnu.edu.cn (F.Z.)
† These authors contributed equally to this work.

Abstract: The efficacy of intermittent fasting (IF), as an emerging weight management strategy, in improving cardiometabolic health has been evaluated in various populations, but that among Chinese individuals has not been systematically studied. A comprehensive search on multiple databases was performed to identify eligible randomized controlled trials (RCTs) up to October 2022. The primary outcome was post-intervention weight loss, and secondary outcomes included changes in cardiometabolic indicators. Effect estimates were meta-analyzed using a random-effects model. In total, nine RCTs with 899 Chinese participants were included. Time-restricted eating was the most adopted IF protocol in this study (six out of nine), followed by alternate-day fasting. The IF intervention significantly reduced body weight, body mass index, body fat mass, homeostatic model assessment of insulin resistance, low-density lipoprotein cholesterol, and triglycerides when compared with control groups. However, no statistically significant reductions in waist circumference, total cholesterol, high-density lipoprotein cholesterol, fasting glucose, systolic blood pressure, and diastolic blood pressure were found. To sum up, IF can be a weight management strategy and may improve the cardiometabolic health of Chinese adults, but more long-term trials using different IF strategies are required to generate robust evidence of its efficacy.

Keywords: cardiometabolic indicators; intermittent fasting; time-restricted eating; weight loss

1. Introduction

In the past decades, the rate of general and abdominal obesity has increased markedly among Chinese adults [1]. In 2019, more than 50% adults aged 18 or above were classified as overweight or obese according to body mass index (BMI) [2]. The number of Chinese people with overweight or obesity is estimated to grow to 790 million in 2030 [3]. As an established risk factor of cardiometabolic diseases, the obesity epidemic has increased the burden on the medical system in China [4]. By 2030, the medical cost attributed to overweight and obesity in China is predicted to be USD 61 billion [3]. Furthermore, at the same BMI values, Chinese individuals are at higher risk of cardiometabolic diseases than Black and White adults in the US [5]. Developing effective strategies for obesity prevention and management is important in the Chinese population.

Various forms of fasting have been developed, including intermittent fasting (IF), calorie restriction, long-term fasting, very low-calorie diet, and fasting-mimicking diet [6]. In recent years, IF has been an emerging dietary intervention for weight management. IF refers to diverse recurring eating patterns that require fasting for different time periods, ranging from hours to a few days [7], which includes alternate-day fasting (ADF), periodic fasting, and time-restricted eating (TRE). Previous studies demonstrated the potential benefits of IF with respect to obesity, insulin resistance, dyslipidaemia, hypertension, and inflammation [8,9].

Although IF is a potential weight management strategy, its efficacy may vary by dietary habits in the study population because of the adherence issue. A recent study reported that the average eating window of 1596 Chinese adults was 13.03 h, in which 45% of individuals commenced eating at 8:00–9:00 a.m., and 52% of participants ceased eating at 8:00 p.m. [10]. According to NHANES 2009–2014, the average eating window, first mealtime, and last mealtime of 15,341 adults aged 20 or above were 12.2 $\pm$ 0.06 h, 8:08 a.m., and 8:18 p.m., respectively [11]. With a potentially longer eating duration in the Chinese population than in the US, conducting IF by restricting the eating window may not have the same efficacy. In addition, whether IF is beneficial mainly because of calorie restriction is unclear. A one-year randomized controlled trial (RCT) with 139 Chinese participants found that early TRE (8:00 a.m. to 4:00 p.m.) combined with daily calorie restriction had similar effects as calorie restriction only on weight loss and body fat reduction in people with obesity [12], but more trials in the Chinese region are warranted to verify the finding.

In brief, the previous literature suggested a lack of systematic review of the efficacy of IF in improving cardiometabolic health of the Chinese population and whether the potential benefit of IF is independent of calorie restriction during the intervention. Gaining additional understanding on the efficacy of IF in the Chinese population may help health care professionals formulate evidence-based weight loss plans for individuals who are overweight and obese.

2. Materials and Methods

This meta-analysis was performed according to the Preferred Reporting Items for Systematic Reviews and Meta-Analyses 2020 statement [13]. The study protocol was registered in PROSPERO (CRD42022359891).

2.1. Search Strategy

Five databases, namely, Ovid MEDLINE, Embase (via Ovid), Ovid Emcare, WanFang, and the China Academic Journal Network Publishing Database (CNKI) were used to identify relevant RCTs that investigated the efficacy of IF on Chinese populations up to October 2022, using a combination of keywords related to IF (e.g., intermittent fasting or time-restricted feeding or periodic fasting) and RCT (e.g., RCT or clinical trial or controlled clinical trial or randomization or random assignment). Reference lists of the included studies were also retrieved for potential eligible studies. The details of the search terms that were used are summarized in Table S1.

2.2. Study Selection

Two independent reviewers (KC and KL) were involved in the two-stage process for the selection of studies. After duplicate studies were excluded, the titles and abstracts were first screened. The abstracts followed by full contents of studies that met the pre-specified eligibility criteria were assessed with reference to the inclusion and exclusion criteria.

2.3. Inclusion Criteria

1. RCTs evaluating the effects of IF on improving the cardiometabolic health of the ethnic Chinese population aged 18 years old or above, without restriction on the sex and health condition of the participants.

2. Intervention with duration more than 3 weeks to capture the treatment effects of long-term duration only, with reference to a previous meta-analysis of RCTs that examined the efficacy of nutritional intervention on weight loss and body composition [14].

2.4. Exclusion Criteria

1. Observational studies, review papers, comments, letters, news, notes, protocols, papers, or abstracts from conference proceedings.
2. Studies without an abstract or full text in English or Simplified/Traditional Chinese.
3. Studies without a control group.

2.5. Data Extraction

Data extraction was performed independently by two reviewers (KC and VC). The following study characteristics were extracted from each included study: (a) first author, (b) publication year, (c) location where the trial was conducted, (d) age and sex of participants, (e) sample size, (f) participants' weight and BMI at baseline, and (g) details of the trials (e.g., intervention duration, control group, IF methods adopted, outcomes, adverse events). Outcomes that appeared in at least three included studies were extracted to perform meta-analysis. For multiple post-intervention assessments, data from the assessments immediately after the intervention was extracted. If different units were used to report the same parameter in the studies, then the most frequently adopted unit was used for consistency. The reviewers reached a consensus on studies to be included before starting data analysis. Cases of inconsistencies were resolved via thorough discussions.

2.6. Quality and Risk-of-Bias Assessment

The guidelines from the Cochrane Handbook for Systematic Reviews of Interventions were followed for risk-of-bias assessment. The six domains of bias being assessed are selection bias, performance bias, detection bias, attrition bias, reporting bias, and other bias. The two reviewers (KC and KL) conducted the assessment independently and rated each item as low, unclear, or high risk. Funding of the included studies was assessed in terms of other bias. Studies that received industrial or commercial funding were rated as high risk [15].

2.7. Outcomes

IF interventions including ADF, 5:2 fasting, and daily TRE were evaluated. The IF interventions could be applied at different time intervals. The primary outcome was absolute weight loss after intervention. With reference to a previous meta-analysis of RCTs that examined cardiometabolic outcomes [16], cardiometabolic parameters, including BMI, waist circumference (WC), body fat mass (BFM), total cholesterol (TC), high-density lipoprotein-cholesterol (HDL-C), low-density lipoprotein cholesterol (LDL-C), triglycerides (TG), fasting plasma glucose (FPG)/fasting glucose (GLU), homeostatic model assessment of insulin resistance (HOMA-IR), systolic blood pressure (SBP), and diastolic blood pressure (DBP), were selected as secondary outcomes.

2.8. Statistical Analysis

Cochrane Collaboration Review Manager (version 5.4) was used for statistical analyses. Mean differences (MDs) were used to express the changes of outcomes between the pre- and post-intervention, with corresponding 95% confidence intervals (CIs). A p value of <0.05 was considered statistically significant. For studies with multiple IF interventions, the more commonly adopted intervention groups among other included studies were involved in the meta-analysis. For outcomes that were reported by at least three included studies, we stratified the analysis according to the control groups (ad libitum diet or calorie-restricted diet) to examine the relative advantage of the IF intervention over the calorie-restricted diet and also when IF is compared with the ad libitum diet. Random-effects model was adopted to combine outcomes from included studies and incorporate heterogeneity among studies [15]. The statistical heterogeneity of the included studies was estimated using

Cochran's Q test and I^2 statistics. Heterogeneity was described as moderate ($I^2 > 30\%$), substantial ($I^2 > 50\%$), and considerable ($I^2 > 75\%$). For studies identified as having high heterogeneity, input data were double-checked [15].

Sensitivity analysis was completed by excluding each included study one by one and recalculating the pooled estimate of the remaining studies to identify the studies that largely affected the summary effect or heterogeneity. For studies with multiple IF interventions, we recalculated the effect estimates by using the less commonly adopted intervention arms.

3. Results

3.1. Study Selection

The flow of study search, screening, and selection is described in Figure 1. A total of 746 articles were identified from the initial database search. After title and abstract screening, full text screening was conducted on 224 articles, and nine RCTs with 899 participants whose nationality were Chinese (excluding subjects in intervention groups irrelevant to the review) were included in the meta-analysis [12,17–24].

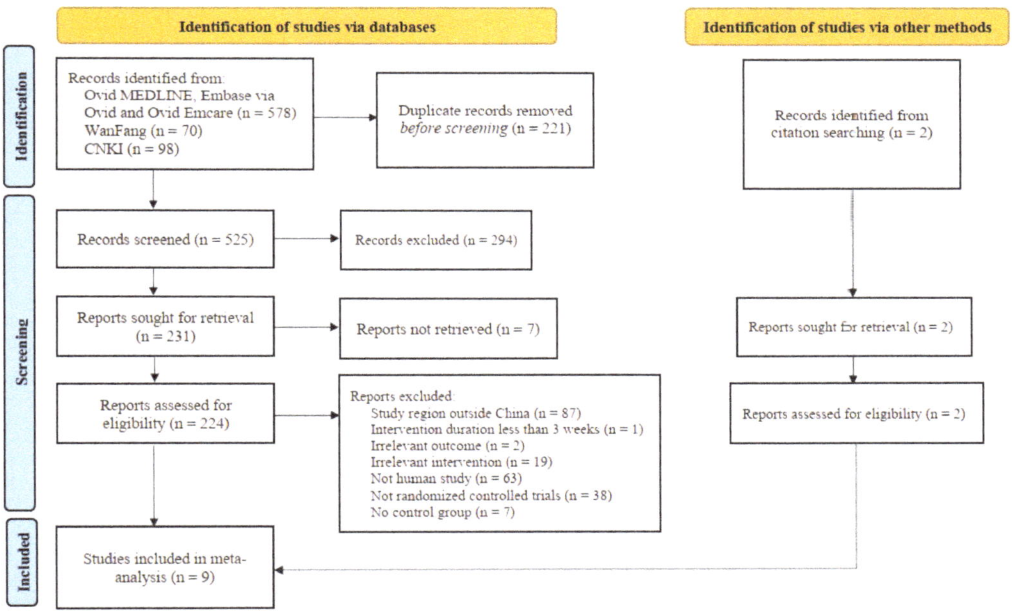

Figure 1. Flow diagram of study select.

3.2. Study Characteristics

The study characteristics of the nine RCTs included in the meta-analysis are summarized in Table 1. In general, three trials evaluated 16:8 TRE [12,21,23], one evaluated 14:10 TRE [19], two studies evaluated the 5:2 diet [20,22], one evaluated ADF [24], and two trials evaluated both 16:8 TRE and ADF [17,18]. Among them, three RCTs conducted interventions with multiple arms [17,18,23]. The follow-up period of trials ranged from 3 weeks to 12 months. Forest plots were not stratified by ad libitum and calorie-restricted groups, including both types of control, due to the limited number of studies (with fewer than three studies reporting the same outcome).

Table 1. Study characteristics of nine included studies.

Author, Year	Study Location	Follow-Up Period	Subject (n)	Comorbidities of Participants	IF Method	Comparator	Age ± SD	Gender (% of Male)	Baseline Weight ± SD (kg)	Weight Change (%)	Baseline BMI ± SD (kg/m^2)	Other Outcomes	Reported Adverse Events	Compliance to IF
Cai et al., 2019 [17]	Changsha, Hunan Province	12 weeks	264	Patients with non-alcoholic fatty liver dis	(i) 16:8 TRE (freely arranged) (n = 95) (ii) ADF (n = 90)	Consumed 80% of energy needs every day (n = 79)	Intervention: (i) TRE: 33.56 ± 6.23 (ii) ADF: 35.50 ± 4.42 Control group: 34.54 ± 6.96	33.0	Intervention: (i) TRE: 74.98 ± 8.02 (ii) ADF: 75.32 ± 8.53 Control: 72.94 ± 8.00	Intervention: (i) TRE: −4.4% (ii) ADF: −5.4% Control: −1.6%	Intervention: (i) TRE: 26.76 ± 1.59 (ii) ADF: 26.12 ± 2.21 Control: 26.34 ± 2.73	WC, BFM, TC, HDL-C, LDL-C, TG, GLU	No severe adverse events	Intervention: 97.5%
Chair et al., 2022 [18]	Changsha, Hunan Province	3 weeks	101	Overweight and obese individuals with prediabetes	(i) 16:8 TRE (freely arranged) (n = 33) (ii) ADF (n = 34)	Eating ad libitum (n = 34)	Intervention: (i) TRE: 36.06 ± 7.67 (ii) ADF: 34.68 ± 4.37 Control: 34.97 ± 6.23	36.7	Intervention: (i) TRE: 74.98 ± 8.02 (ii) ADF: 75.78 ± 8.46 Control: 72.15 ± 8.47	Intervention: (i) TRE: −6.1% (ii) ADF: −6.4% Control: −0.1%	Intervention: (i) TRE: 26.74 ± 1.58 (ii) ADF: 26.46 ± 2.36 Control: 26.47 ± 1.84	WC, TC, HDL-C, LDL-C, TG, GLU	No severe adverse events	Not available
Che et al., 2021 [19]	Tianjin	12 weeks	120	Overweight patients with type 2 diabetes	14:10 TRE (08:00–18:00) (n = 60)	Eating ad libitum (n = 60)	Intervention: 48.21 ± 9.32 Control: 48.78 ± 9.56	54.2	Intervention: 75.06 ± 4.42 Control: 74.68 ± 4.35	Intervention: −4.0% Control: −1.1%	Intervention: 26.42 ± 1.96 Control: 26.08 ± 2.14	TC, HDL-C, LDL-C, TG, FPG, HOMA-IR	No severe adverse events	Intervention: >6 days per week
Guo et al., 2021 [20]	Dongguan, Guangdong Province	8 weeks	39	Patients with metabolic syndrome	5:2 diet (n = 21)	Eating ad libitum (n = 18)	Intervention: 40.2 ± 5.7 Control: 42.7 ± 4.1	53.8	Intervention: 77.8 ± 13.6 Control: 74.1 ± 8.6	Intervention: −4.5% Control: −1.6%	Intervention: 28.0 ± 7.8 Control: 27.7 ± 2.3	WC, BFM, TC, HDL-C, LDL-C, TG, GLU, HOMA-IR, SBP, DBP	No severe adverse events	Intervention: 91.3% Control: 78.3%
Lin et al., 2022 [21]	Taiwan	8 weeks	63	Middle-aged peri-menopausal women with BMI > 24 kg/m^2 or WC > 80 cm	16:8 TRE (10:00–18:00 or 12:00–20:00) (n = 30)	Daily low-calorie diet of 1400 kcal (n = 33)	Intervention: 50.1 ± 7.5 Control: 54.2 ± 7.9	0	Intervention: 65.9 ± 9.7 Control: 65.8 ± 8.8	Intervention: −4.1% Control: −2.4%	Intervention: 25.9 ± 3.7 Control: 25.7 ± 3.8	WC, TC, HDL-C, LDL-C, TG, GLU, HOMA-IR, SBP, DBP	Not mentioned	Intervention: 84%
Liu, 2019 [22]	Nanchang, Jiangxi Province	20 weeks	54	Overweight and obese people	5:2 diet (n = 28)	Eating ad libitum with moderate exercise (n = 26)	Intervention: 43.04 ± 8.75 Control: 41.69 ± 8.56	31.5	Intervention: 72.96 ± 10.94 Control: 72.59 ± 8.26	Intervention: −7.4% Control: +0.6%	Intervention: 27.41 ± 2.52 Control: 27.94 ± 1.85	WC, TC, HDL-C, LDL-C, TG, FPG, SBP, DBP	Decreased concentration, thirsty, dizziness, low blood sugar level, abdominal bloating, constipation, unstable emotion	Not available
Liu et al., 2022 [12]	Guangzhou, Guangdong Province	12 months	139	Patients with obesity	16:8 TRE (08:00–16:00) (n = 69)	Daily calorie restriction by 75% (n = 70)	31.9 ± 9.1	51.1	88.2 ± 11.6	Intervention: −9.0% Control: −7.2%	Intervention: 31.8 ± 2.9 Control: 31.3 ± 2.6	WC, BFM, TC, HDL-C, LDL-C, TG, GLU, SBP, DBP, HOMA-IR	No deaths or serious adverse events, occurrences of mild adverse events were similar in the two groups	Intervention: 84.0% Control: 83.8%
Xie et al., 2022 [23]	Beijing	5 weeks	82	Healthy individuals without obesity	Early 16:8 TRE (06:00–15:00) (n = 28) Mid-day 16:8 TRE (11:00–20:00) (n = 26)	Eating ad libitum (n = 28)	Intervention: (i) eTRE: 28.68 ± 9.71 (ii) mTRE: 31.08 ± 8.44 Control: 33.57 ± 11.60	22.0	Intervention: (i) eTRE: 61.1 ± 8.8 (ii) mTRE: 61.0 ± 11.7 Control: 61.2 ± 9.9	Intervention: (i) eTRE: −2.6% (ii) mTRE: −0.3% Control: +0.5%	Intervention: (i) eTRE: 22.7 ± 3.1 (ii) mTRE: 21.4 ± 2.2 Control: 21.5 ± 2.9	BFM, FPG, HOMA-IR	No severe adverse events	Intervention: 96.8%
Zheng et al., 2021 [24]	Chengdu, Sichuan Province	8 weeks	37	Patients with spinal cord injury	ADF (n = 19)	Eating ad libitum (n = 18)	35.76 ± 6.92	91.9	Intervention: 61.06 ± 6.29 Control: 61.44 ± 5.29	Intervention: −3.3% Control: −0.3%	Intervention: 21.88 ± 1.59 Control: 22.34 ± 1.88	-	Nausea, dysphoria, pulmonary infection, hypoglycemia, hunger, irritability	Not available

Abbreviations: ADF, alternate-day fasting; BFM, body fat mass; BMI, body mass index; DBP, diastolic blood pressure; eTRE, early time-restricted eating; FPG, fasting plasma glucose; GLU, fasting glucose; HDL-C, high-density lipoprotein cholesterol; HOMA-IR, homeostatic model assessment of insulin resistance; IF, intermittent fasting; LDL-C, low-density lipoprotein cholesterol; mTRE, mid-day time-restricted eating; SBP, systolic blood pressure; SD, standard deviation; TC, total cholesterol; TG, triglycerides; TRE, time-restricted eating; and WC, waist circumference.

3.3. *Effect on Anthropometric Measurement*

Pooled analysis of all included studies with a total of 749 participants showed that adopting IF resulted in statistically significant reductions in body weight when comparing the IF intervention group with both control groups (ad libitum diet: MD = −2.61 kg, 95% CI = −3.37 to −1.85, I^2 = 76%) (calorie-restricted diet: MD = −1.40 kg, 95% CI = −1.60 to −1.20, I^2 = 0%). The overall MD was also statistically significant (MD = −2.20 kg, 95% CI = −2.75 to −1.66, I^2 = 87%) (Figure 2).

	Experimental			Control				Mean difference
Study or Subgroup	Mean	SD	Total	Mean	SD	Total	Weight	IV, Random, 95% CI
1.1.1 Ad libitum diet control group								
Chair et al. 2022	-4.55	3.1	33	-0.06	0.23	34	12.1%	-4.49 [-5.55 , -3.43]
Che et al. 2021	-2.98	0.43	60	-0.83	0.32	60	22.2%	-2.15 [-2.29 , -2.01]
Guo et al. 2021	-3.5	1.5	21	-1.2	1.5	18	13.4%	-2.30 [-3.24 , -1.36]
Liu 2019	-5.4	13.93	28	0.41	2.82	26	1.0%	-5.81 [-11.08 , -0.54]
Xie et al. 2022	-1.6	1.4	28	0.3	1.2	28	16.6%	-1.90 [-2.58 , -1.22]
Zheng et al. 2021	-2.01	4.36	19	-0.19	4.38	18	3.2%	-1.82 [-4.64 , 1.00]
Subtotal (95% CI)			**189**			**184**	**68.6%**	**-2.61 [-3.37 , -1.85]**
Heterogeneity: Tau² = 0.51; Chi² = 21.01, df = 5 (P = 0.0008); I² = 76%								
Test for overall effect: Z = 6.74 (P < 0.00001)								
1.1.2 Calorie restricted diet control group								
Cai et al. 2019	-3.25	0.67	95	-1.85	0.65	79	21.9%	-1.40 [-1.60 , -1.20]
Lin et al. 2022	-2.7	5.37	30	-1.6	3.36	33	4.7%	-1.10 [-3.34 , 1.14]
Liu et al. 2022	-8	6.66	69	-6.3	6.5	70	4.9%	-1.70 [-3.89 , 0.49]
Subtotal (95% CI)			**194**			**182**	**31.4%**	**-1.40 [-1.60 , -1.20]**
Heterogeneity: Tau² = 0.00; Chi² = 0.14, df = 2 (P = 0.93); I² = 0%								
Test for overall effect: Z = 14.06 (P < 0.00001)								
Total (95% CI)			**383**			**366**	**100.0%**	**-2.20 [-2.75 , -1.66]**
Heterogeneity: Tau² = 0.34; Chi² = 63.60, df = 8 (P < 0.00001); I² = 87%								
Test for overall effect: Z = 7.93 (P < 0.00001)								
Test for subgroup differences: Chi² = 9.16, df = 1 (P = 0.002), I² = 89.1%								

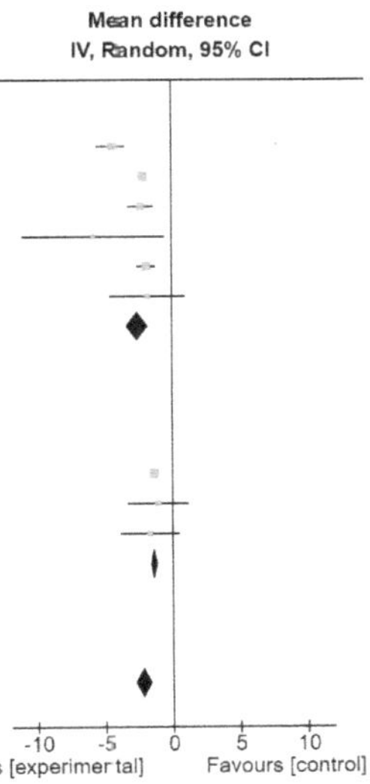

Figure 2. Forest plot for differences in body weight (in kg) between intermittent fasting and control groups [12,17–24]. Size of the green boxes represented study weight while the black diamond represented the pooled effect.

BMI analysis that involved 693 participants from eight studies also showed statistically significant reductions in comparison to both control groups (ad libitum diet: MD = −1.37 kg/m^2, 95% CI = −2.00 to −0.73, I^2 = 91%) (calorie-restricted diet: MD = −0.55 kg/m^2, 95% CI = −0.92 to −0.18, I^2 = 0%). The overall MD is also statistically significant (MD = −1.07 kg/m^2, 95% CI = −1.67 to −0.48, I^2 = 93%) (Figure S1).

Similarly, IF resulted in a statistically significant reduction in WC (MD = −4.04 cm, 95% CI = −7.09 to −0.99, I^2 = 65%) relative to the ad libitum diet control group. However, the result with the calorie-restricted diet control group was not statistically significant (MD = −0.42 cm, 95% CI = −1.46 to 0.62, I^2 = 0%). The overall result with 536 participants from six studies was not statistically significant (MD = −2.12 cm, 95% CI = −4.30 to 0.07, I^2 = 83%) (Figure S2).

3.4. *Effect on Body Fat Composition*

Amongst 408 participants from four studies, some showed that IF could lead to a statistically significant reduction in BFM (MD = −1.55 kg, 95% CI = −1.66 to −1.43, I^2 = 0%) (Figure S3). The consistency of the results was not affected despite the differences in body fat assessment methods.

3.5. *Effect on Blood Lipid Profile*

Eight studies involving 712 participants reported MDs in lipid profiles, including TC, HDL-C, LDL-C, and TG. No statistically significant differences in TC were found when compared with both control groups and the overall MD (ad libitum diet: MD = −1.43 mg/dL, 95% CI = −4.19 to 1.33, I^2 = 33%) (calorie-restricted diet: MD = 2.69 mg/dL, 95% CI = −2.85 to 8.23, I^2 = 0%) (overall: MD = −0.63 mg/dL, 95% CI = −3.20 to 1.94, I^2 = 30%) (Figure S4). A similar trend was found for HDL-C (ad libitum diet: MD = −0.92 mg/dL, 95% CI = −2.00 to 0.15, I^2 = 37%) (calorie-restricted diet: MD = 0.88 mg/dL, 95% CI = −0.70 to 2.45, I^2 = 0%) (overall: MD = −0.43 mg/dL, 95% CI = −1.29 to 0.44, I^2 = 31%) (Figure S5). Although the overall reduction was statistically significant for LDL-C, the result was insignificant when compared with that of the calorie-restricted control group (ad libitum diet: MD = −4.11 mg/dL, 95% CI = −7.66 to −0.57, I^2 = 66%) (calorie-restricted diet: MD = −0.01 mg/dL, 95% CI = −3.59 to 3.58, I^2 = 0%) (overall: MD = −2.86 mg/dL, 95% CI = −5.52 to −0.21, I^2 = 56%) (Figure S6). A statistically significant overall reduction in TG could be observed when compared with both control groups (ad libitum diet: MD = −2.22 mg/dL, 95% CI = −4.19 to −0.24, I^2 = 33%) (calorie-restricted diet: MD = −5.94 mg/dL, 95% CI = −6.28 to −5.59, I^2 = 0%) (overall: MD = −3.35 mg/dL, 95% CI = −6.13 to −0.58, I^2 = 97%) (Figure S7).

3.6. Effect on Blood Glucose

Data on FPG/GLU were reported in eight studies with 712 participants. A statistically significant reduction in FPG/GLU was observed when IF was compared with the ad libitum diet control group (MD = −8.42 mg/dL, 95% CI = −13.96 to −2.88, I^2 = 89%), but not for the calorie-restricted diet control group (MD = 1.65 mg/dL, 95% CI = −0.95 to 4.25, I^2 = 0%). The overall reduction was not statistically significant (MD = −4.61 mg/dL, 95% CI = −10.08 to 0.86, I^2 = 93%) (Figure S8). The study of Zheng et al. was not included in the pooled analysis because no exact figure of the MD, SD of MD, CI, and *p*-value was reported. A statistically significant reduction in HOMA-IR was observed (MD = −0.48, 95% CI = −0.80 to −0.17, I^2 = 51% (Figure S9), which included 417 participants from five studies.

3.7. Effect on Blood Pressure

Data on SBP and DBP were reported in five studies with 351 participants. IF did not lead to a statistically significant reduction in SBP (MD = −1.99 mmHg, 95% CI = −4.19 to 0.21, I^2 = 0%) (Figure S10) and DBP (MD = −1.84 mmHg, 95% CI = −4.64 to 0.96, I^2 = 56%) (Figure S11).

3.8. Risk-of-Bias Assessment

The risk-of-bias assessments for the included studies are summarized in Figure 3. Six studies described how a random sequence was generated, and three studies described how allocation concealment was achieved. For performance bias, seven and two studies were rated to have high and unclear level of bias, respectively. Seven studies were considered to have a high risk of blinding participants and personnel (performance bias) because masking the participants to their intervention was not possible. Two studies stated that none of the staff responsible for outcome measurements were informed of the assignment of participants and were rated with an unclear level of performance bias. The outcomes were detected entirely using machines, which is why the detection bias was low for all of the studies. For attrition bias, despite cases that were lost to follow-up, the attrition rate was relatively low for all of the studies. The reporting bias for all of the studies was uncertain given the lack of clarity on whether any measured, but not reported, outcomes based on the results only and without a trial protocol would be produced. None of the included studies indicated that their funding was from industrial or commercial sponsors, but three studies did not mention their sources of funding. Funnel plots to evaluate publication bias were not used in view of the small number of included studies (less than 10), where an appropriate level of the power of the tests to distinguish chance from real asymmetry could not be guaranteed [25].

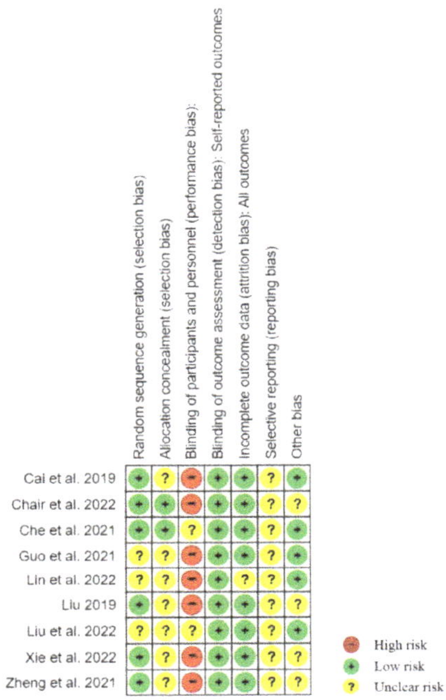

Figure 3. Risk-of-bias summary of the included studies [12,17–24].

3.9. Safety

Three studies reported the occurrence of mild adverse events (AE) such as dizziness, nausea, and constipation during the IF intervention [12,22,24]. One trial did not mention any AE [21]. No severe AEs were reported in the remaining five included studies [17–20,23]. Details of reported AEs are listed in Table S2.

3.10. Sensitivity Analysis

Sensitivity analysis was performed for each outcome. For most of the study outcomes, the statistical significance and heterogeneity remained similar regardless of the study being excluded. The following paragraphs summarize the substantial changes in heterogeneity and statistical significance after performing the leave-one-out approach. We also summarize the sensitivity analysis results of body weight and BMI, the primary outcomes, in Table S3. For body weight, after Cai et al. was excluded [17], I^2 decreased from 87% to 68%. Apart from this result, the results changed from significant to insignificant among the calorie-restricted diet subgroup, which could be due to the large sample size. More studies with the calorie-restricted diet as the control group should be performed to verify the significance of the findings. For BMI, after Che et al. were excluded [19], the I^2 reduced from 93% to 70% possibly because of the relatively larger sample size and weighting of each individual study.

Three included studies were three-armed [17,18,23], which is why data of another intervention group were selected for meta-analysis in the sensitivity analysis (Table S4). The second intervention group of Cai et al. and Chair et al. was ADF, which was less adopted among the other included studies. For Xie et al., the two intervention groups were early TRE (eTRE) and mid-day TRE (mTRE), and eTRE was included in the meta-analysis because it was suggested to be more effective than later TRE in improving insulin resistance, glycemic metabolism, and blood pressure, with reference to a previous network meta-analysis [26]. When the mTRE group was included instead of the eTRE group, or when the ADF group was included instead of the TRE group, neither the statistical significance nor the direction of intervention effects changed substantially (Table S4).

Given that TRE was the most adopted IF protocol in this work, further analysis was performed to compare TRE with the ad libitum diet or the calorie-restricted diet by removing non-TRE studies. For TC, when Guo et al. and Liu et al. were excluded [20,22], I^2 decreased from 30% to 8%, and the results changed from insignificant to significant (MD: −2.35 mg/dL [95% CI: −3.90, −0.81]). For LDL, when Guo et al. and Liu et al. were excluded [20,22], the results changed from significant to insignificant (MD: −1.36 mg/dL [95% CI: −4.04, 1.33]), while no substantial change in heterogeneity was observed. For HOMA-IR, when Guo et al. was removed [20], no substantial change in heterogeneity was observed, but the results changed from significant to insignificant (MD: −0.43 [95% CI: −0.87, 0.01]). For DBP, when Guo et al. and Liu et al. were excluded [20,22], the results changed from insignificant to significant (MD: −3.58 [95% CI: −7.09, −0.07]), while no substantial change in heterogeneity occurred.

4. Discussion

4.1. Summary of the Main Findings

The pooled analysis of nine RCTs that compared IF with ad libitum diet or calorie-restricted diet indicated that participants that engaged in IF showed significant reductions in body weight and BMI when compared with participants receiving the ad libitum diet and calorie-restricted diet. The IF intervention also reduced BFM, HOMA-IR, LDL-C, and TG significantly when compared with control groups. Meanwhile, no statistically significant overall reductions appeared in WC, TC, HDL-C, FPG/GLU, DBP, and SBP in the analyses. While the effect of IF on TG and LDL outcomes was statistically significant, the magnitude may be modest.

Similar to results of previous studies, IF did not lead to a significant change in blood glucose level but improved insulin sensitivity [27–30]. Insulin sensitivity indicates how the human body responds to insulin and regulates blood glucose level. Impaired insulin sensitivity will lead to insulin resistance, which is associated with metabolic syndromes (MetS) such as hypertension and dyslipidemia [31]. Energy depletion is achieved through IF, and this will lead to prolonged reduction of insulin secretion, which activates AMP-activated protein kinase and improves insulin sensitivity and glucose homeostasis by promoting glucose uptake and utilization [32]. Blood glucose level did not change significantly as a result of IF, possibly because of the mechanisms involved in maintaining blood glucose level and preventing hypoglycemia, namely, glycogenolysis and gluconeogenesis [33].

Moreover, IF improves the lipid profile by boosting fatty acid oxidation through nuclear expression of peroxisome proliferator-activated receptor alpha (PPARa) and peroxisome proliferator-activated receptor-gamma coactivator 1-alpha (PGC1a) and increasing apolipoprotein modulation in the liver [34]. Hepatic triglyceride accumulation was reduced because of increased fatty acid oxidation, thereby reducing very low-density lipoprotein (VLDL) production, followed by reduced serum levels of VLDL, low-density lipoprotein (LDL), and small and dense LDL (sdLDL) [34]. The apolipoprotein B level also decreased as it was one of the structural components of VLDL, LDL and sdLDL, while the apolipoprotein A level increased, which led to increasing the HDL level in the blood as it was the precursor of HDL [34]. This condition may explain why IF could reduce LDL-C and TG instead of the HDL-C level.

In the present meta-analysis, IF resulted in a significant reduction in body weight, which was consistent with that of previous studies [35–37]. BMI was calculated based on weight and height only, which is why the BMI value would decrease considerably when body weight decreased [38]. Moreover, waist circumference is an indicator of abdominal adiposity [37]. Previous evidence suggested that IF may have favorable effects on waist circumference reduction [9,18,39]. However, no significant results were observed in this meta-analysis, possibly because of the short duration of the IF intervention. The study duration of this meta-analysis ranged from 3 weeks to 12 months, and only one out of nine included studies that lasted for 12 months, which hindered its efficacy in long-term health outcomes. In the previous review, under prolonged fasting, the serum level of leptin decreased, whereas that of adiponectin did not change, which promoted fatty acid oxidation with an anti-inflammatory effect, and adiponectin was suggested to have an inverse correlation with visceral adiposity [40]. However, in exchange for short-term fasting, no change in the serum leptin level occurred [40]. Therefore, a short duration of the IF intervention may impact abdominal adiposity.

We also examined whether the statistically significant findings from meta-analysis may inform clinical practices. For body weight, at least 5% weight loss from baseline was considered clinically significant and could reduce the risk of developing type 2 diabetes and cardiovascular disease [41]. For the current analysis, the overall reduction in body weight after the IF intervention was statistically significant (MD = −2.20 kg, 95% CI = −2.75 to −1.66, I^2 = 87%), and the average weight loss after the IF intervention was 4.8%, which was close to the clinically significant value. Every 2 kg/m^2 incremental increase in BMI among the Chinese population was associated with an elevated relative risk of 15.4% for coronary heart disease, 6.1% for total stroke, and 18.8% for ischemic stroke [42]. Although the overall reduction in BMI after the IF intervention was statistically significant (MD = −1.07 kg/m^2, 95% CI = −1.67 to −0.48, I^2 = 93%), the finding might not be clinically significant. In addition, the pooled level of LDL-C reduction in the present meta-analysis was only −2.86 mg/dL, which was lower than the clinically significant value, i.e., each 38.7 mg/dL (1 mmol/L) lowering in LDL-C reduced the risk of cardiovascular mortality as demonstrated by another meta-analysis [43]. However, our observed results have not been consistent enough to propose recommendations for clinical practice, given limited studies and the heterogeneity in participants' characteristics such as their comorbidities. In this meta-analysis, most of the included studies were conducted among patients with diverse medical conditions (i.e., one study on non-alcoholic fatty liver disease [NAFLD], three on overweight or obese, two on prediabetes or diabetes, one on MetS, and one on spinal cord injury), and only one study was performed among healthy people. With reference to a previous meta-analysis, a statistically significant reduction in TC was observed among healthy people (WMD = −6.41 mg/dL, 95% CI = −9.64 to −3.18, I^2 = 76.8%), but not in people with a disease history including NAFLD, type 2 diabetes mellitus, and MetS (WMD = −13.23 mg/dL, 95% CI = −37.70 to 11.23, I^2 = 79.3%) [44]. Also, a higher TC reduction was observed among female participants (WMD = −18.71 mg/dL, 95% CI = −29.64 to −7.78, I^2 = 89.7%) than among male participants [44]. This finding implies that IF intervention effects could be affected by medical conditions and sex. Future studies controlling potential confounders are of vital importance to verify the health effects of IF among the Chinese population.

4.2. *Potential Mechanisms of Different IF Strategies*

While IF may exert health benefits via calorie restriction [39,45], additional potential mechanisms of how IF strategies benefit human health are still under discussion. For example, ADF was able to increase free fatty acid oxidation and deplete amino acids periodically, which accelerated adipose tissue lipolysis and hepatic amino acid uptake for gluconeogenesis. Thus, ADF was suggested to be beneficial in cardiovascular health and helpful for weight loss [46]. The 5:2 diet could reduce fasting serum insulin acutely during a two-day fast and moderately stimulate the release of adiponectin by adipose tissues, which improved insulin sensitivity and lowered the risks of developing cancer, heart disease, or diabetes [47]. TRE might improve oscillations in circadian clock gene expression and reset the molecular mechanisms of energy metabolism through a restricted eating window, which was beneficial for weight management [48,49]. Also, TRE was suggested to be able to alter the microbial community composition (i.e., increased the ratio of Firmicutes to Bacteroidetes) that resides in the intestinal tract and lower gut permeability, which lowered the risks of developing gut diseases [49]. One of the included studies in the present meta-analysis, in addition to the beneficial cardiometabolic effects, discussed the metabolic pathways of gut microbiota. Several gut microbial metabolites, namely, lipopolysaccharide (LPS), short-chain fatty acids (SCFAs), and trimethylamine *n*-oxide

(TMAO), play an important role in immunity and inflammation, which closely correlate with cardiovascular health [20]. After the IF intervention, plasma SCFAs were elevated from 4.97 ng/mL (95% CI: 4.09 to 5.86) to 6.14 ng/mL (95% CI: 4.90 to 7.37), while plasma LPS reduced from 156.1 ng/L (95% CI: 69.1 to 243.1) to 74.6 ng/L (95% CI: 36.5 to 112.7; $p = 0.011$), and no change in plasma TMAO was observed [20]. Authors have proposed that IF altered the gut microbiota and improved gut microbiota homeostasis, which was highly associated with improving cardiometabolic risk factors [20].

This meta-analysis indicates that IF is useful in weight loss. However, it is not beneficial to some cardiometabolic parameters, such as SBP and DBP. A previous meta-analysis with 694 participants showed similar findings, in which TRE could significantly reduce SBP (MD = −4.15 mmHg, 95% CI = −6.73 to −2.30; $p < 0.0001$) but not DBP [50]. In another one-year observational study with 1422 participants, regardless of sex, significant reductions of SBP (from 131.6 ± 0.7 mmHg to 120.7 ± 0.4 mmHg; $p < 0.001$) and DBP (from 83.7 ± 0.4 mmHg to 77.9 ± 0.3 mmHg; $p < 0.001$) were observed and were greater among people who fasted for longer [51]. From a physiological perspective, IF may trigger blood pressure reduction by increasing parasympathetic activity with brain-derived neurotrophic factor production, promoting renal Na excretion, and improving sensitivity of natriuretic peptides and insulin receptors [51]. Only four RCTs were included for the analysis because of the limited studies. Therefore, further studies should be conducted to verify the effects of IF on blood pressure among the Chinese population.

4.3. Additional Benefits of IF Compared with the Calorie-Restricted Diet

Another controversial issue is the additional weight loss effects of IF when compared with the calorie-restricted diet. Unlike people who are on a calorie-restricted diet, people adopting IF are not necessarily required to limit their calorie intake [52]. However, IF emphasizes the importance of staying in sync with natural circadian rhythms instead of restricting total calorie intake [52]. A previous meta-analysis with 205 participants with obesity reported that IF was more beneficial than the calorie-restricted diet for weight loss (SMD = −0.21 kg, 95% CI = −0.40 to −0.02; $p = 0.028$) but no difference was observed in BMI reduction (SMD = 0.02 kg/m^2, 95% CI = −0.16 to 0.20; $p = 0.848$) [39]. Another review suggested that IF and the calorie-restricted diet were equally effective in body weight loss (IF: 4–8% vs. calorie-restricted diet: 5–8%) and fat mass reduction (IF: 11–16% vs. calorie-restricted diet: 10–20%), but IF outperformed the calorie-restricted diet in lean mass retention [53]. Moreover, an earlier meta-analysis suggested that IF was comparable to the calorie-restricted diet (MD = −0.26 kg, 95% CI = −0.31 to 0.84; $p = 0.37$) and could be a reliable weight loss alternative [54]. The current meta-analysis pooled the effects from multiple studies conducted in China and showed statistically significant overall reductions in body weight, BMI, and TG when compared with the calorie-restricted diet and the ad libitum diet. While more large-scale studies with a longer study duration should be conducted, the current findings demonstrate the potential clinical significance of IF in cardiometabolic health, which warrants in-depth investigation.

4.4. Adherence to IF Strategies in China

Weight loss is important in reducing the risk of various cardiometabolic diseases [55]. Hence, good adherence to a weight loss strategy is crucial.

In China, the eating habits of the Chinese population are a potential barrier that lowers people's acceptance and adherence to IF. The average eating window of Chinese adults is 13.03 ± 2.02 h per day [10]. People with fixed-time jobs or living in urban areas have busy schedules and commonly have irregular meals [10]. Moreover, midnight snacks are a common food culture in southern China and Hong Kong [56]. Chinese individuals who are accustomed to having many dinner gatherings and have a habit of enjoying midnight snacks may find it difficult to adopt IF. Hence, the significance of evening gatherings with family or friends should be taken into consideration to improve IF adherence in the Chinese population [57].

In this meta-analysis, six studies reported IF adherence rates ranging from 84% to 97.5%, which suggested that IF is feasible in the short term. However, good adherence to IF in the long term could not be concluded due to small sample sizes (39 to 174) and varied study durations (5 weeks to 12 months). Also, in one study, participants were not blinded, so they might have already been interested in TRE, which resulted in high adherence rates [23].

4.5. Adverse Events of IF in the Chinese Population

Although IF is gaining popularity, studies reporting the safety of IF strategies are insufficient. Common adverse events include vertigo, nausea, insomnia, headaches, and exhaustion [58]. In the current meta-analysis, no serious adverse events were disclosed. However, people with chronic diseases such as diabetes, heart failure, asthma, and cancers are suggested to be more likely to experience adverse events [58].

4.6. Limitations of the Study

This meta-analysis has some limitations that should be noted for cautious interpretation. First, most included RCTs had a small number of recruited subjects and a short follow-up period, with only one study lasting for 12 months [12]. Second, different IF methods were pooled for the meta-analysis because of the limited data for comparison with two control groups (ad libitum diet and calorie-restricted diet). The comparison between IF and the calorie-restricted diet has not been comprehensively assessed. Third, considerable heterogeneity was observed in multiple meta-analysis results, which may limit the interpretation accuracy. The between-study differences, such as adherence to fasting regimes, metabolic status, diet, and exercise level of the subjects, which were rarely reported in the included studies, might also contribute to the high heterogeneity [59]. The number of eligible studies in this work was very limited, and the results had considerable heterogeneity. Thus, the findings of recent studies may not be consistent enough to inform clinical recommendations. Age, sex, intervention duration, and morbidity status were considered potential sources of heterogeneity in previous meta-analysis, and meta-regression analyses were performed to explore the heterogeneity [54,60,61]. However, different studies obtained inconsistent results. For example, Pascual et al. concluded that intervention duration did not have a confounding effect [54], while Jahrami et al. revealed that fasting duration was a confounding factor, but age and sex were not [61]. Faris et al. suggested that diet, fasting duration, body weight and health status before fasting, and exercise level were considerable interfering factors [60]. More future studies on the effect of IF among the Chinese population with different characteristics and morbidities should be conducted to explore the heterogeneity and investigate how these factors are associated with the effect of IF interventions [15].

5. Conclusions

Among Chinese adults, adopting IF for at least three weeks can result in some degree of weight loss and improvement in cardiometabolic health. IF may have potential roles in weight management, but more well-designed studies are necessary to provide robust evidence of its effects on weight management by considering the effects of sex and meal timing and to account for the dietary habits of the Chinese population. Moreover, the possible adverse incidents and long-term effects of IF interventions need to be studied by conducting more long-term and large-scale clinical trials.

Supplementary Materials: The following supporting information can be downloaded at https://www.mdpi.com/article/10.3390/nu16030357/s1, Figure S1: Forest plot for differences in body mass index (in kg/m^2) between intermittent fasting and control groups; Figure S2: Forest plot for differences in waist circumference (in cm) between intermittent fasting and control groups; Figure S3: Forest plot for differences in body fat mass (in kg) between intermittent fasting and control groups; Figure S4: Forest plot for differences in total cholesterol (in mg/dL) between intermittent fasting and control groups; Figure S5: Forest plot for differences in high-density lipoprotein cholesterol (in mg/dL) between intermittent fasting and control groups; Figure S6: Forest plot for differences in low-density lipoprotein cholesterol (in mg/dL) between intermittent fasting and control groups; Figure S7: Forest plot for differences in triglycerides (in mg/dL) between intermittent fasting and control groups; Figure S8: Forest plot for differences in fasting glucose or fasting plasma glucose (in mg/dL) between intermittent fasting and control groups; Figure S9: Forest plot for differences in homeostatic model assessment of insulin resistance between intermittent fasting and control groups; Figure S10: Forest plot for differences in systolic blood pressure (in mmHg) between intermittent fasting and control groups; Figure S11: Forest plot for differences in diastolic blood pressure (in mmHg) between intermittent fasting and control groups; Table S1: Search terms used in the literature review; Table S2: Reported adverse events of the included studies; Table S3: Sensitivity analysis summary of the included studies in body weight and BMI; Table S4: Pooled MDs when another intervention group in multi-arm studies was included.

Author Contributions: Conceptualization, K.L.; formal analysis, K.C. and V.C.; funding acquisition, K.L.; methodology, K.L.; supervision, K.L. and F.Z.; visualization, V.C.; writing—original draft, K.C. and V.C.; Writing—review and editing, K.C., V.C., S.C., M.M.H.W., G.K.-K.C., W.-Y.C., K.L. and F.Z. All authors have read and agreed to the published version of the manuscript.

Funding: K.L. received funding from the Projects of RISA CD69 and Start-up Fund for New Recruits BE91.

Institutional Review Board Statement: Not applicable.

Informed Consent Statement: Not applicable.

Data Availability Statement: The data presented in this study are available on request from the corresponding authors.

Conflicts of Interest: The authors declare no conflict of interest.

References

1. Ma, S.; Xi, B.; Yang, L.; Sun, J.; Zhao, M.; Bovet, P. Trends in the prevalence of overweight, obesity, and abdominal obesity a Chinese adults between 1993 and 2015. *Int. J. Obes.* **2021**, *45*, 427–437. [CrossRef] [PubMed]
2. Chen, K.; Shen, Z.; Gu, W.; Lyu, Z.; Qi, X.; Mu, Y.; Ning, Y. Prevalence of obesity and associated complications in C A cross-sectional, real-world study in 15.8 million adults. *Diabetes Obes. Metab.* **2023**, *25*, 3390–3399. [CrossRef]
3. Hu, G. More vigorous efforts are needed to fight obesity, a serious public health problem in China. *Obesity* **2021**, *29*, 1580 [CrossRef] [PubMed]
4. Report on Cardiovascular Health and Diseases in China 2021: An Updated Summary. *Biomed. Environ. Sci.* **2022**, *35*, 57 [CrossRef]
5. Pan, W.H.; Flegal, K.M.; Chang, H.Y.; Yeh, W.T.; Yeh, C.J.; Lee, W.C. Body mass index and obesity-related metabolic disord Taiwanese and US whites and blacks: Implications for definitions of overweight and obesity for Asians. *Am. J. Clin. Nutr.* *79*, 31–39. [CrossRef]
6. Wilhelmi de Toledo, F.; Grundler, F.; Sirtori, C.R.; Ruscica, M. Unravelling the health effects of fasting: A long road from ol treatment to healthy life span increase and improved cognition. *Ann. Med.* **2020**, *52*, 147–161. [CrossRef]
7. Anton, S.D.; Moehl, K.; Donahoo, W.T.; Marosi, K.; Lee, S.A.; Mainous, A.G.; Leeuwenburgh, C.; Mattson, M.P. Flippir Metabolic Switch: Understanding and Applying the Health Benefits of Fasting: Flipping the Metabolic Switch. *Obesity* **20** 254–268. [CrossRef]
8. De Cabo, R.; Mattson, M.P. Effects of Intermittent Fasting on Health, Aging, and Disease. *N. Engl. J. Med.* **2019**, *381*, 2541– [CrossRef]
9. Yang, F.; Liu, C.; Liu, X.; Pan, X.; Li, X.; Tian, L.; Sun, J.; Yang, S.; Zhao, R.; An, N.; et al. Effect of Epidemic Intermittent Fa on Cardiometabolic Risk Factors: A Systematic Review and Meta-Analysis of Randomized Controlled Trials. *Front. Nutr.* *8*, 669325. [CrossRef]
10. Tang, R.; Wang, J.; Zhang, W.; Fu, W.; Zhuo, L.; Yang, J.; Wang, Q.; Kun, Y. Eating window and eating habits of adults in C A cross-sectional study. *Heliyon* **2023**, *9*, e17233. [CrossRef]
11. Kant, A.K. Eating patterns of US adults: Meals, snacks, and time of eating. *Physiol. Behav.* **2018**, *193*, 270–278. [CrossRef]
12. Liu, D.; Huang, Y.; Huang, C.; Yang, S.; Wei, X.; Zhang, P.; Guo, D.; Lin, J.; Xu, B.; Li, C.; et al. Calorie Restriction with or wi Time-Restricted Eating in Weight Loss. *N. Engl. J. Med.* **2022**, *386*, 1495–1504. [CrossRef] [PubMed]
13. Page, M.J.; McKenzie, J.E.; Bossuyt, P.M.; Boutron, I.; Hoffmann, T.C.; Mulrow, C.D.; Shamseer, L.; Tetzlaff, J.M.; Akl, Brennan, S.E.; et al. The PRISMA 2020 statement: An updated guideline for reporting systematic reviews. *BMJ* **2021**, *372*, [CrossRef]

lenezhad, N.; Mohammadi, M.; Ramezani-Jolfaie, N.; Mozaffari-Khosravi, H.; Salehi-Abargouei, A. Effects of l-carnitine upplementation on weight loss and body composition: A systematic review and meta-analysis of 37 randomized controlled inical trials with dose-response analysis. *Clin. Nutr. ESPEN* **2020**, *37*, 9–23. [CrossRef] [PubMed]

iggins, J.P.T.; Thomas, J.; Chandler, J.; Cumpston, M.; Li, T.; Page, M.J.; Welch, V.A. (Eds.) *Cochrane Handbook for Systematic eviews of Interventions Version 6.3*; Cochrane: Oxford, UK, 2022. Available online: https://training.cochrane.org/handbook ccessed on 17 July 2023).

'ong, J.; Chan, K.Y.; Lo, K. Sodium-glucose co-transporter 2 inhibitors on weight change and cardiometabolic profiles in dividuals with overweight or obesity and without diabetes: A meta-analysis. *Obes. Rev.* **2021**, *22*, e13336. [CrossRef]

ai, H.; Qin, Y.L.; Shi, Z.Y.; Chen, J.H.; Zeng, M.J.; Zhou, W.; Chen, R.Q.; Chen, Z.Y. Effects of alternate-day fasting on body eight and dyslipidaemia in patients with non-alcoholic fatty liver disease: A randomised controlled trial. *BMC Gastroenterol.* **)19**, *19*, 219. [CrossRef]

hair, S.Y.; Cai, H.; Cao, X.; Qin, Y.; Cheng, H.Y.; Ng, M.T. Intermittent Fasting in Weight Loss and Cardiometabolic Risk eduction: A Randomized Controlled Trial. *J. Nurs. Res.* **2022**, *30*, e185. [CrossRef] [PubMed]

'he, T.; Yan, C.; Tian, D.; Zhang, X.; Liu, X.; Wu, Z. Time-restricted feeding improves blood glucose and insulin sensitivity in verweight patients with type 2 diabetes: A randomised controlled trial. *Nutr. Metab.* **2021**, *18*, 88. [CrossRef]

Guo, Y.; Luo, S.; Ye, Y.; Yin, S.; Fan, J.; Xia, M. Intermittent Fasting Improves Cardiometabolic Risk Factors and Alters Gut Microbiota in Metabolic Syndrome Patients. *J. Clin. Endocrinol. Metab.* **2021**, *106*, 64–79. [CrossRef]

in, Y.J.; Wang, Y.T.; Chan, L.C.; Chu, N.F. Effect of time-restricted feeding on body composition and cardio-metabolic risk in niddle-aged women in Taiwan. *Nutrition* **2022**, *93*, 111504. [CrossRef]

.iu, D. The Effects of Intermittent Fasting with Appropriate amount of Exercise on Overweight and Obese People: A randomized Controlled Trial. Master's Thesis, Nanchang University, Nanchang, China, 2019.

.ie, Z.; Sun, Y.; Ye, Y.; Hu, D.; Zhang, H.; He, Z.; Zhao, H.; Yang, H.; Mao, Y. Randomized controlled trial for time-restricted ating in healthy volunteers without obesity. *Nat. Commun.* **2022**, *13*, 1003. [CrossRef] [PubMed]

Zheng, J.; Liu, J.; Jiang, Y.; Pang, R.; Yang, X.; Liu, H.; Lin, N.; Li, Y.; Xiong, D.; Chen, X.; et al. Safety of Every-Other-Day Fasting in the Treatment of Spinal Cord Injury: A Randomized Controlled Trial. *Am. J. Phys. Med. Rehabil.* **2021**, *100*, 1184–1189. [CrossRef] PubMed]

Yin, C.; Li, Z.; Xiang, Y.; Peng, H.; Yang, P.; Yuan, S.; Zhang, X.; Wu, Y.; Huang, M.; Li, J. Effect of Intermittent Fasting on Non-Alcoholic Fatty Liver Disease: Systematic Review and Meta-Analysis. *Front. Nutr.* **2021**, *8*, 709683. [CrossRef]

.iu, J.; Yi, P.; Liu, F. The Effect of Early Time-Restricted Eating vs Later Time-Restricted Eating on Weight Loss and Metabolic Health. *J. Clin. Endocrinol. Metab.* **2023**, *108*, 1824–1834. [CrossRef] [PubMed]

Antoni, R.; Johnston, K.L.; Collins, A.L.; Robertson, M.D. Intermittent v. continuous energy restriction: Differential effects on postprandial glucose and lipid metabolism following matched weight loss in overweight/obese participants. *Br. J. Nutr.* **2018**, *119*, 507–516. [CrossRef]

Cienfuegos, S.; Gabel, K.; Kalam, F.; Ezpeleta, M.; Wiseman, E.; Pavlou, V.; Lin, S.; Oliveira, M.L.; Varady, K.A. Effects of 4- and 6-h Time-Restricted Feeding on Weight and Cardiometabolic Health: A Randomized Controlled Trial in Adults with Obesity. *Cell. Metab.* **2020**, *32*, 366–378.e363. [CrossRef] [PubMed]

Gabel, K.; Kroeger, C.M.; Trepanowski, J.F.; Hoddy, K.K.; Cienfuegos, S.; Kalam, F.; Varady, K.A. Differential Effects of Alternate-Day Fasting Versus Daily Calorie Restriction on Insulin Resistance. *Obesity* **2019**, *27*, 1443–1450. [CrossRef]

Sutton, E.F.; Beyl, R.; Early, K.S.; Cefalu, W.T.; Ravussin, E.; Peterson, C.M. Early Time-Restricted Feeding Improves Insulin Sensitivity, Blood Pressure, and Oxidative Stress Even without Weight Loss in Men with Prediabetes. *Cell Metab.* **2018**, *27*, 1212–1221.e1213. [CrossRef]

Ferrannini, E. Is insulin resistance the cause of the metabolic syndrome? *Ann. Med.* **2006**, *38*, 42–51. [CrossRef]

Albosta, M.; Bakke, J. Intermittent fasting: Is there a role in the treatment of diabetes? A review of the literature and guide for primary care physicians. *Clin. Diabetes Endocrinol.* **2021**, *7*, 3. [CrossRef]

Rui, L. Energy metabolism in the liver. *Compr. Physiol.* **2014**, *4*, 177–197. [CrossRef]

Santos, H.O.; Macedo, R.C.O. Impact of intermittent fasting on the lipid profile: Assessment associated with diet and weight loss. *Clin. Nutr. ESPEN* **2018**, *24*, 14–21. [CrossRef] [PubMed]

Harris, L.; Hamilton, S.; Azevedo, L.B.; Olajide, J.; De Brún, C.; Waller, G.; Whittaker, V.; Sharp, T.; Lean, M.; Hankey, C.; et al. Intermittent fasting interventions for treatment of overweight and obesity in adults: A systematic review and meta-analysis. *JBI Database System. Rev. Implement. Rep.* **2018**, *16*, 507–547. [CrossRef] [PubMed]

Morales-Suarez-Varela, M.; Collado Sánchez, E.; Peraita-Costa, I.; Llopis-Morales, A.; Soriano, J.M. Intermittent Fasting and the Possible Benefits in Obesity, Diabetes, and Multiple Sclerosis: A Systematic Review of Randomized Clinical Trials. *Nutrients* **2021**, *13*, 3179. [CrossRef]

Park, J.; Seo, Y.G.; Paek, Y.J.; Song, H.J.; Park, K.H.; Noh, H.M. Effect of alternate-day fasting on obesity and cardiometabolic risk: A systematic review and meta-analysis. *Metabolism* **2020**, *111*, 154336. [CrossRef]

Khanna, D.; Peltzer, C.; Kahar, P.; Parmar, M.S. Body Mass Index (BMI): A Screening Tool Analysis. *Cureus* **2022**, *14*, e22119. [CrossRef]

Zhang, Q.; Zhang, C.; Wang, H.; Ma, Z.; Liu, D.; Guan, X.; Liu, Y.; Fu, Y.; Cui, M.; Dong, J. Intermittent Fasting versus Continuous Calorie Restriction: Which Is Better for Weight Loss? *Nutrients* **2022**, *14*, 1781. [CrossRef]

40. Varkaneh Kord, H.; Tinsley, G.M.; Santos, H.O.; Zand, H.; Nazary, A.; Fatahi, S.; Mokhtari, Z.; Salehi-Sahlabadi, A.; Ta Rahmani, J.; et al. The influence of fasting and energy-restricted diets on leptin and adiponectin levels in humans: A syst review and meta-analysis. *Clin. Nutr.* **2021**, *40*, 1811–1821. [CrossRef]
41. Williamson, D.A.; Bray, G.A.; Ryan, D.H. Is 5% weight loss a satisfactory criterion to define clinically significant weig *Obesity* **2015**, *23*, 2319–2320. [CrossRef]
42. Zhou, B.F. Effect of body mass index on all-cause mortality and incidence of cardiovascular diseases-report for meta-ana prospective studies open optimal cut-off points of body mass index in Chinese adults. *Biomed. Environ. Sci.* **2002**, *15*, 245-
43. Khan, S.U.; Michos, E.D. Cardiovascular mortality after intensive LDL-Cholesterol lowering: Does baseline LDL-Chol really matter? *Am. J. Prev. Cardiol.* **2020**, *1*, 100013. [CrossRef]
44. Meng, H.; Zhu, L.; Kord-Varkaneh, H.; Santos, H.O.; Tinsley, G.M.; Fu, P. Effects of intermittent fasting and energy-restricte on lipid profile: A systematic review and meta-analysis. *Nutrition* **2020**, *77*, 110801. [CrossRef]
45. Aksungar, F.B.; Sarıkaya, M.; Coskun, A.; Serteser, M.; Unsal, I. Comparison of Intermittent Fasting Versus Caloric Restric Obese Subjects: A Two Year Follow-Up. *J. Nutr. Health Aging* **2017**, *21*, 681–685. [CrossRef]
46. Stekovic, S.; Hofer, S.J.; Tripolt, N.; Aon, M.A.; Royer, P.; Pein, L.; Stadler, J.T.; Pendl, T.; Prietl, B.; Url, J.; et al. Alternate Day F Improves Physiological and Molecular Markers of Aging in Healthy, Non-obese Humans. *Cell Metab.* **2019**, *30*, 462–47 [CrossRef]
47. Harvie, M.N.; Pegington, M.; Mattson, M.P.; Frystyk, J.; Dillon, B.; Evans, G.; Cuzick, J.; Jebb, S.A.; Martin, B.; Cutler, R.G The effects of intermittent or continuous energy restriction on weight loss and metabolic disease risk markers: A randomize in young overweight women. *Int. J. Obes.* **2011**, *35*, 714–727. [CrossRef]
48. Patterson, R.E.; Sears, D.D. Metabolic Effects of Intermittent Fasting. *Annu. Rev. Nutr.* **2017**, *37*, 371–393. [CrossRef] [Pub
49. Cheng, W.Y.; Desmet, L.; Depoortere, I. Time-restricted eating for chronodisruption-related chronic diseases. *Acta Physiol 239*, e14027. [CrossRef] [PubMed]
50. Wang, W.; Wei, R.; Pan, Q.; Guo, L. Beneficial effect of time-restricted eating on blood pressure: A systematic meta-analys meta-regression analysis. *Nutr. Metab.* **2022**, *19*, 77. [CrossRef] [PubMed]
51. Wilhelmi de Toledo, F.; Grundler, F.; Bergouignan, A.; Drinda, S.; Michalsen, A. Safety, health improvement and well- during a 4 to 21-day fasting period in an observational study including 1422 subjects. *PLoS ONE* **2019**, *14*, e0209353. [Cro [PubMed]
52. Dong, T.A.; Sandesara, P.B.; Dhindsa, D.S.; Mehta, A.; Arneson, L.C.; Dollar, A.L.; Taub, P.R.; Sperling, L.S. Intermittent Fa A Heart Healthy Dietary Pattern? *Am. J. Med.* **2020**, *133*, 901–907. [CrossRef]
53. Varady, K.A. Intermittent versus daily calorie restriction: Which diet regimen is more effective for weight loss? *Obes. Rev. 12*, e593–e601. [CrossRef] [PubMed]
54. Elortegui Pascual, P.; Rolands, M.R.; Eldridge, A.L.; Kassis, A.; Mainardi, F.; Lê, K.A.; Karagounis, L.G.; Gut, P.; Varady, K meta-analysis comparing the effectiveness of alternate day fasting, the 5:2 diet, and time-restricted eating for weight loss. *C* **2023**, *31* (Suppl. S1), 9–21. [CrossRef] [PubMed]
55. Sattar, N.; Gill, J.M.R.; Alazawi, W. Improving prevention strategies for cardiometabolic disease. *Nat. Med.* **2020**, *26*, 32 [CrossRef]
56. Zhou, Y.; Wang, J.; Duan, Y.; Luo, X.; Wan, Z.; Luo, Y.; Li, Y.; Wang, Y.; Xie, J. Dietary diversity and determinants of young a in central China: A cross-sectional study from 2015 to 2020. *Front. Nutr.* **2022**, *9*, 931107. [CrossRef]
57. Parr, E.B.; Devlin, B.L.; Hawley, J.A. Perspective: Time-Restricted Eating-Integrating the What with the When. *Adv. Nutr. 13*, 699–711. [CrossRef]
58. Grajower, M.M.; Horne, B.D. Clinical Management of Intermittent Fasting in Patients with Diabetes Mellitus. *Nutrients 11*, 873. [CrossRef]
59. Chew, H.S.J.; Ang, W.H.D.; Tan, Z.Y.A.; Ang, W.W.; Chan, K.S.; Lau, Y. Umbrella review of time-restricted eating on weight fasting blood glucose, and lipid profile. *Nutr. Rev.* **2022**, *81*, 1180–1199. [CrossRef]
60. Faris, M.A.; Jahrami, H.; BaHammam, A.; Kalaji, Z.; Madkour, M.; Hassanein, M. A systematic review, meta-analysis, meta-regression of the impact of diurnal intermittent fasting during Ramadan on glucometabolic markers in healthy sub *Diabetes Res. Clin. Pract.* **2020**, *165*, 108226. [CrossRef] [PubMed]
61. Jahrami, H.A.; Alsibai, J.; Clark, C.C.T.; Faris, M.A.E. A systematic review, meta-analysis, and meta-regression of the impa diurnal intermittent fasting during Ramadan on body weight in healthy subjects aged 16 years and above. *Eur. J. Nutr.* *59*, 2291–2316. [CrossRef] [PubMed]

MDPI AG
Grosspeteranlage 5
4052 Basel
Switzerland
Tel.: +41 61 683 77 34

Nutrients Editorial Office
E-mail: nutrients@mdpi.com
www.mdpi.com/journal/nutrients

www.ingramcontent.com/pod-product-compliance
Lightning Source LLC
Chambersburg PA
CBHW041952260926
51850CB00019B/2622
* 9 7 8 3 7 2 5 8 7 1 5 4 4 *